The Unofficial Guide to Radiology

100 Practice Chest X-rays

SECOND EDITION

EDITION
2

The Unofficial Guide to Radiology

100 Practice Chest X-rays

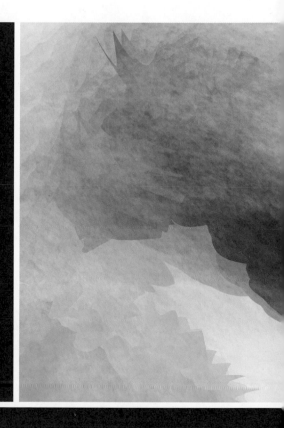

Edited by

Ali B.A.K. Al-Hadithi MB BChir, MA (Cantab),
MRCP (UK), AFHEA, PGCert (Med Ed)
Academic Clinical Fellow (Cardiology and Internal Medicine)
University of Cambridge
Cambridge, United Kingdom

Cambridge University Hospitals NHS Foundation Trust
Cambridge, United Kingdom

Series Editor
Zeshan Qureshi BM, BSc (Hons), MSc, MRCPCH,
FAcadMEd, MRCPS (Glasg)
Paediatric Registrar
London Deanery
United Kingdom

ELSEVIER

First edition 2017. Published by Zeshan Qureshi.

Notices

Practitioners and researchers must always rely on their own experience and knowledge in evaluating and using any information, methods, compounds or experiments described herein. Because of rapid advances in the medical sciences, in particular, independent verification of diagnoses and drug dosages should be made. To the fullest extent of the law, no responsibility is assumed by Elsevier, authors, editors or contributors for any injury and/or damage to persons or property as a matter of products liability, negligence or otherwise, or from any use or operation of any methods, products, instructions, or ideas contained in the material herein.

ISBN: 978-0-443-10917-1

Content Strategist: Trinity Hutton
Content Project Manager: Tapajyoti Chaudhuri
Design: Hitchen Miles
Marketing Manager: Deborah Watkins

Printed in India

Last digit is the print number: 9 8 7 6 5 4 3 2 1

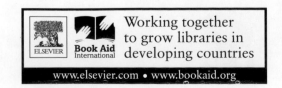

Ali would like to dedicate this book to his family Bara, Suhair, Ahmed and Miriam for their continuous support.

Contents

Series Editor Foreword

The Unofficial Guide to Medicine is not just about helping students study, it is also about allowing those that learn to take back control of their own education. Since its inception, it has been driven by the voices of students, and through this, democratized the process of medical education, blurring the line between learners and teachers.

Medical education is an evolving process, and the latest iteration of our titles has been rewritten to bring them up to date with modern curriculums, after extensive deliberation and consultation. We have kept the series up to date, incorporating new guidelines and perspectives from a wide range of students, junior doctors and senior clinicians. There is greater consistency across the titles, more illustrations, and through these and other changes, I hope the books will now be even better study aids.

These books though are a process of continual improvement. By reading this book, I hope that you not only get through your exams but also consider contributing to a future edition. You may be a student now, but you are also the future of medical education.

I wish you all the best with your future career and any upcoming exams.

Zeshan Qureshi
November 2022

Introduction

Almost every patient has some form of medical imaging performed during his or her investigations and management. The commonest type of imaging modality remains the X-ray. Chest X-rays are a frequently performed and particularly important test that all doctors should be able to interpret.

Despite its universal importance, X-ray interpretation is often an overlooked subject in the medical school curriculum, making it difficult and daunting for many medical students and junior doctors. *The Unofficial Guide to Radiology: 100 Practice Chest X-rays* aims to help address this.

The key to interpreting X-rays is having a systematic method for assessment, and then getting lots of practice looking at and presenting X-rays. The best-selling core radiology text *The Unofficial Guide to Radiology* was specifically designed for medical students, radiographers, physician's associates and junior doctors. It outlines a comprehensive system for assessing X-rays, in addition to clinical and radiology-based MCQs to contextualize the radiographs to real clinical scenarios. Its approach led to recognition from the British Medical Association, the British Institute of Radiology and the Royal College of Radiologists. This follow-up textbook builds upon these foundations, providing readers with the opportunity to practise and consolidate their chest X-ray assessment and presenting skills.

There are lots of radiology textbooks available, but many have important limitations. Most have small, often poor-quality images which are not ideal for displaying the radiological findings. The findings are usually only described in a figure below the image, and it may be difficult to know exactly what part of the image corresponds to which finding! Many textbooks deal with X-rays in isolation rather than in a useful clinical context.

We have designed this book to allow readers to practice interpreting X-rays in as useful and clinically relevant way as possible. There are:

- 100 large, high-quality chest X-rays to assess.
- Cases presented in the context of a clinical scenario and covering a wide range of common and important findings (in line with the Royal College of Radiologists' Undergraduate Radiology Curriculum).
- Detailed on-image colour annotations to highlight key findings.
- Comprehensive systematic X-ray reports.
- Relevant further investigations and management are discussed for each case.
- Our second edition offers an additional 3 questions per case, listed at the end of the book.

The cases are divided by difficulty into standard, intermediate and advanced based on the imaging findings and clinical implications. Each begins with a clinical scenario and a chest X-ray for you to interpret. You can then turn over the page and find a fully annotated version of the same X-ray with a comprehensive report. Each systematically structured report is colour-coded to match the corresponding labelled image.

Each report is based on an ABCDE approach to chest X-ray interpretation, as recommended in *The Unofficial Guide to Radiology*:

Technical features: Patient ID, projection, penetration, inspiration, rotation.
Airway: Tracheal position.
Breathing: Lung parenchyma, pleural spaces, pulmonary vasculature.
Circulation and mediastinum: Heart size/shape/borders, aorta, mediastinum, hila.
Diaphragm and delicates: Diaphragm position/shape, pneumoperitoneum, skeleton, soft tissues.
Extras: Anything else, e.g. ECG clips, line, tubes, surgical staples.
Review areas: Lung apices/hila/behind heart/costophrenic angles/below the diaphragm.
Summary: Putting together the salient findings of the X-ray with a differential diagnosis.
Investigations and management: The next steps in management after taking on board X-ray findings.

With this textbook, we hope you will become more confident and competent interpreting chest X-rays, both in examination situations and in clinical practice.

Case

13

A 2-year-old female presents with her parents to ED after swallowing a coin. There is no significant past medical history. On examination, she has oxygen saturations of 100% in air and is afebrile. Lung fields are resonant throughout, with good bilateral air entry. A chest X-ray is requested to assess the position of the foreign body.

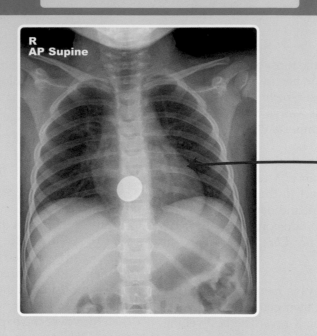

R
AP Supine

REPORT – SWALLOWED FOREIGN BODY

TECHNICAL INFORMATION

Patient ID: Anonymous
Projection: AP supine
Penetration: Adequate – vertebral bodies just visible behind heart
Inspiration: Limited – five anterior ribs visible
Rotation: The patient is not rotated

● **AIRWAY**
The trachea is central.

● **BREATHING**
The lungs are clear.
The lungs are not hyperinflated.
The pleural spaces are clear.
Normal pulmonary vascularity.

● **CIRCULATION AND MEDIASTINUM**
The heart does not appear enlarged, although its size cannot be accurately assessed on an AP X-ray.

The heart borders are clear.

The aorta appears normal.

The mediastinum is central, not widened, with normal thymic contours.

There is a circular radio-opaque foreign body projected over the lower mediastinum.

There is no evidence of pneumomediastinum.

Normal size, shape and position of both hila.

● **DIAPHRAGM AND DELICATES**

Normal appearance and position of the hemidiaphragms.

No pneumoperitoneum visible although the supine projection makes this difficult to assess.

The imaged skeleton is intact with no fractures or destructive bony lesions visible.

The visible soft tissues are unremarkable.

● **EXTRAS AND REVIEW AREAS**

No vascular lines, tubes or surgical clips.
Lung apices: Normal.
Hila: Normal.
Behind heart: Radio-opaque foreign body projected centrally over the lower mediastinum.
Costophrenic angles: Normal.
Below the diaphragm: Normal.

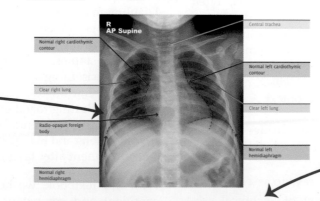

R
AP Supine

Central trachea

Normal right cardiothymic contour

Normal left cardiothymic contour

Clear right lung

Clear left lung

Radio-opaque foreign body

Normal left hemidiaphragm

Normal right hemidiaphragm

SUMMARY, INVESTIGATIONS AND MANAGEMENT

This X-ray demonstrates a radio-opaque foreign body projected centrally over the lower mediastinum. Assuming it is not outwith the patient (i.e. on their skin or clothing), it is in keeping with a swallowed foreign body in the lower oesophagus.

Ingested coins in the lower oesophagus do not necessarily need to be removed – their progress through the GI tract can be assessed with serial X-rays. However, endoscopic removal should be considered if the coin appears stuck or is not progressing.

Acknowledgements

Thank you to the following contributors for their contribution to the first edition:

Mark Rodrigues
Mohammed Rashid Akhtar
Na'eem Ahmed
Nihad Khan

Abbreviations

AC joint	acromioclavicular joint	**HR**	heart rate
ACE	angiotensin-converting enzyme	**HRCT**	high-resolution computed tomography
AP	anterior–posterior	**ITU**	intensive treatment unit
ARDS	acute respiratory distress syndrome	**IV**	intravenous
ATLS	advanced trauma life support	**JVP**	jugular venous pulse
BPM	beats per minute	**LFTs**	liver function tests
CABG	coronary artery bypass graft	**LLL**	left lower lobe
COPD	chronic obstructive pulmonary disease	**MDT**	multidisciplinary team
CRP	c-reactive protein	**MI**	myocardial infarction
CT	computed tomography	**NG tube**	nasogastric tube
CTPA	computed tomography pulmonary angiography	**PA**	posterior–anterior
		PE	pulmonary embolism
CURB-65	confusion	**PICC**	peripherally inserted central catheter
	urea >7 mmol/L	**PSA**	prostate-specific antigen
	respiratory rate ≥30	**RR**	respiratory rate
	sbp <90 mmHg or dbp ≤60 mmHg	**RSB**	retained surgical foreign bodies
	age ≥65	**SLE**	systemic lupus erythematosus
ED	emergency department	**SVC**	superior vena cava
ECG	electrocardiogram	**TB**	tuberculosis
ECHO	echocardiogram	**TFT**	thyroid function test
ESR	erythrocyte sedimentation rate	**U&Es**	urea and electrolytes
ET tube	endotracheal tube	**VATS**	video-assisted thoracic surgery
FBC	full blood count		
GORD	gastrooesophageal reflux disease		

Contributors

SERIES EDITOR

Zeshan Qureshi
BM, BSc (Hons), MSc, MRCPCH, FAcadMEd,
MRCPS (Glasg)
Paediatric Registrar, London Deanery,
United Kingdom

EDITOR

Ali B.A.K. Al-Hadithi
MB BChir, MA (Cantab), MRCP (UK), AFHEA,
PGCert (Med Ed)
Academic Clinical Fellow (Cardiology and Internal
Medicine), University of Cambridge, Cambridge,
United Kingdom

Cambridge University Hospitals NHS Foundation
Trust, Cambridge, United Kingdom

AUTHORS

Nishaanth Dalavaye
BSc (Hons)
School of Medicine, Cardiff University, Cardiff,
United Kingdom

Liza Y.W. Chong
BMedSc (Hons)
Medical student, University of Edinburgh,
United Kingdom

Lauren Franklin
Medical student, Keele University, United Kingdom

Rebecca Jenkins
Medical student, Hull York Medical School,
United Kingdom

A 70-year-old male who lives in a residential home presents to ED with increasing confusion. He has a productive cough and a fever. He has a past medical history of hypertension, angina and mild cognitive impairment. He has a 25 pack-year smoking history. On examination, he has oxygen saturations of 89% in air and is febrile with a temperature of 38.8°C. There is dullness to percussion and coarse crackles in the right upper zone. A chest X-ray is requested to assess for possible pneumonia or collapse.

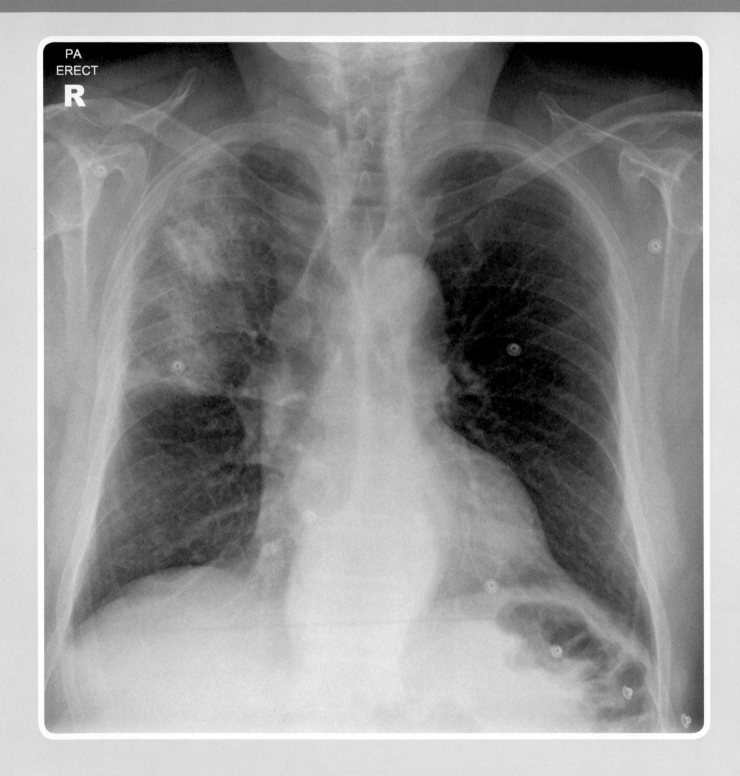

PA
ERECT
R

TECHNICAL INFORMATION

Patient ID: Anonymous
Projection: PA
Penetration: Adequate – vertebral bodies just visible behind heart
Inspiration: Adequate – eight anterior ribs visible
Rotation: Not rotated

● AIRWAY

The upper trachea is central. The lower trachea is displaced to the right by the aortic arch.

● BREATHING

There is heterogeneous air space opacification in the right upper zone. This has a relatively well-defined inferior margin, which is likely to represent the horizontal fissure. There is a focal area of increased opacification in the right upper zone, which may represent focal consolidation or an underlying mass. The remainder of the lungs are clear. The lungs are not hyperinflated.

The pleural spaces are clear.

Normal pulmonary vascularity.

● CIRCULATION AND MEDIASTINUM

The heart is not enlarged.

The heart borders are clear.

There is unfolding of the thoracic aorta, which displaces the lower trachea to the right.

The mediastinum is central, not widened, with clear borders. There is a well-defined density projected over the lower mediastinum, which is in keeping with a hiatus hernia.

Normal size, shape and position of both hila.

● DIAPHRAGM AND DELICATES

Normal appearance and position of hemidiaphragms.

No pneumoperitoneum.

The imaged skeleton is intact with no fractures or destructive bony lesions visible.

The visible soft tissues are unremarkable.

● EXTRAS AND REVIEW AREAS

ECG electrodes in situ.

No vascular lines, tubes or surgical clips.
Lung apices: Heterogeneous right apical consolidation. Normal left apex.
Hila: Normal.
Behind heart: There is a retrocardiac density, which represents a hiatus hernia.
Costophrenic angles: Normal.
Below the diaphragm: Normal.

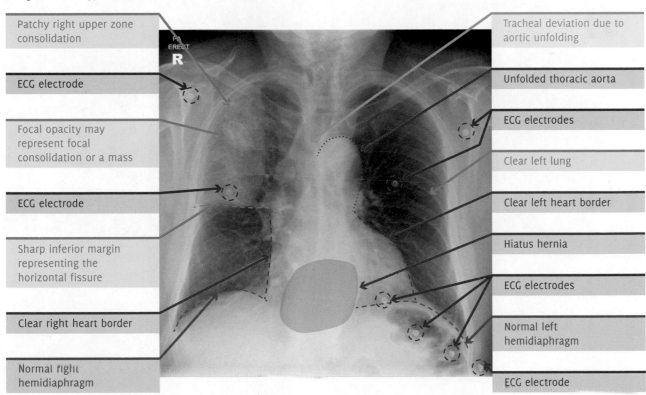

Patchy right upper zone consolidation

ECG electrode

Focal opacity may represent focal consolidation or a mass

ECG electrode

Sharp inferior margin representing the horizontal fissure

Clear right heart border

Normal right hemidiaphragm

Tracheal deviation due to aortic unfolding

Unfolded thoracic aorta

ECG electrodes

Clear left lung

Clear left heart border

Hiatus hernia

ECG electrodes

Normal left hemidiaphragm

ECG electrode

SUMMARY, INVESTIGATIONS AND MANAGEMENT

This X-ray demonstrates heterogeneous right upper zone consolidation in keeping with pneumonia. The consolidation has a relatively abrupt inferior margin in keeping with the horizontal fissure, indicating this is right upper lobe pneumonia. A focal opacity in this region may represent focal consolidation or a mass. Incidentally, there is also a hiatus hernia.

Initial blood tests may include FBC, U&Es, blood cultures and CRP. A sputum culture may also be taken.

The patient should be treated with appropriate antibiotics for community-acquired pneumonia, and a follow-up chest X-ray performed in 4 to 6 weeks to ensure resolution. The antibiotics may be oral or intravenous depending on the severity of pneumonia (CURB-65).

If the focal opacity in the right upper zone does not resolve, then a CT of the chest and abdomen with IV contrast would be appropriate to assess for a lung tumour. It would also be useful to review previous imaging and case notes to see if there was an abnormality at this site before.

A 71-year-old female presents to ED with chest pain and breathlessness. She had a left total hip replacement 2 weeks ago. She is a nonsmoker. On examination, she has oxygen saturations of 91% in air and is afebrile. Lung fields are resonant throughout, with good air entry bilaterally. A chest X-ray is requested to assess for possible pneumonia, collapse, effusion or pulmonary embolism.

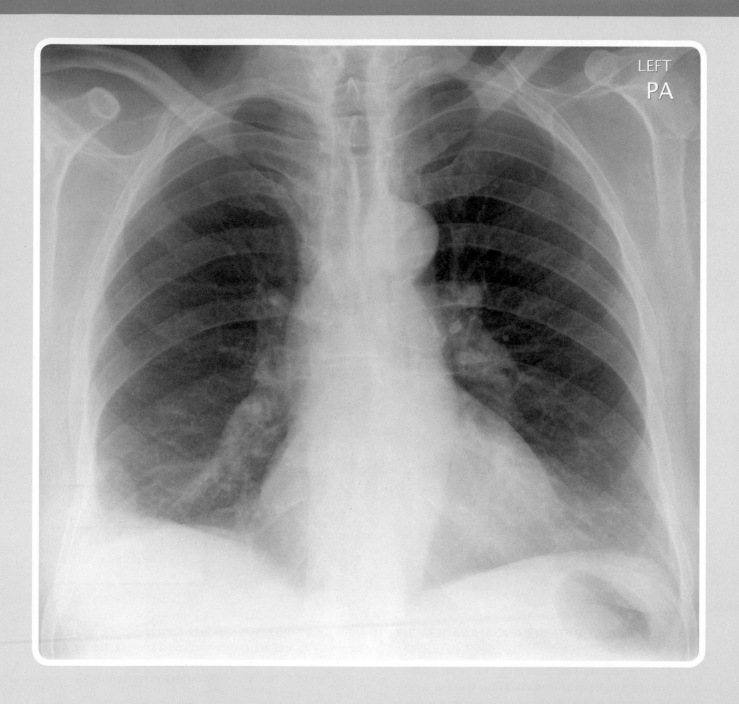

LEFT

PA

TECHNICAL INFORMATION

Patient ID: Anonymous
Projection: PA
Penetration: Adequate – vertebral bodies just visible behind heart
Inspiration: Adequate – six anterior ribs visible
Rotation: Not rotated

● AIRWAY

The trachea is central.

● BREATHING

There is blunting of the right costophrenic angle in keeping with a small pleural effusion. A small area of heterogeneous opacification is visible in the adjacent lung.

The lungs are otherwise clear. They are not hyperinflated.

The left-sided pleural space is clear. Normal pulmonary vascularity.

● CIRCULATION AND MEDIASTINUM

The heart is not enlarged.

The heart borders are clear.

There is mild unfolding of the thoracic aorta.

The mediastinum is central, not widened, with clear borders.

Normal size, shape and position of both hila.

● DIAPHRAGM AND DELICATES

The lateral aspect of the right hemidiaphragm is obscured. Normal position and appearance of the left hemidiaphragm.

No pneumoperitoneum.

The imaged skeleton is intact with no fractures or destructive bony lesions visible.

The visible soft tissues are unremarkable.

● EXTRAS AND REVIEW AREAS

No vascular lines, tubes or surgical clips.
Lung apices: Normal.
Hila: Normal.
Behind heart: Normal.
Costophrenic angles: Blunting of right costophrenic angle. Normal left costophrenic angle.
Below the diaphragm: Normal.

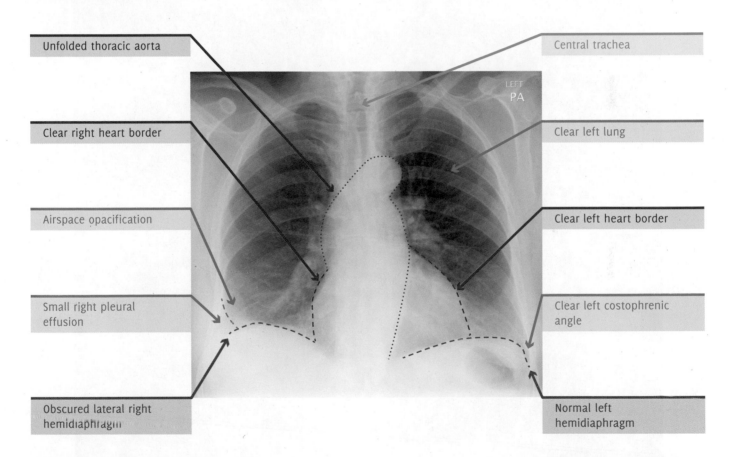

Unfolded thoracic aorta	Central trachea
Clear right heart border	Clear left lung
Airspace opacification	Clear left heart border
Small right pleural effusion	Clear left costophrenic angle
Obscured lateral right hemidiaphragm	Normal left hemidiaphragm

SUMMARY, INVESTIGATIONS AND MANAGEMENT

This X-ray demonstrates a small right pleural effusion with minor associated consolidation. This may reflect pneumonia with a parapneumonic effusion. The other main differential, especially given recent surgery, is a pulmonary embolism with infarction (consolidation) and an effusion.

Supplementary oxygen should be given.

Initial blood tests may include an arterial blood gas, FBC, U&Es, LFTs, blood cultures, coagulation and a CRP. Sputum cultures would also be helpful. D-dimer is unlikely to be helpful given the recent surgery. A CT pulmonary angiogram should be considered.

Treatment with either antibiotics or low-molecular-weight heparin will be guided by the results of the investigations.

A 60-year-old female presents to her GP with fatigue, weight loss and wheeze. There is no significant past medical history. She is a nonsmoker. On examination, she has oxygen saturations of 99% in air and is afebrile. There is wheeze in the right upper zone. A chest X-ray is requested to assess for malignancy or COPD.

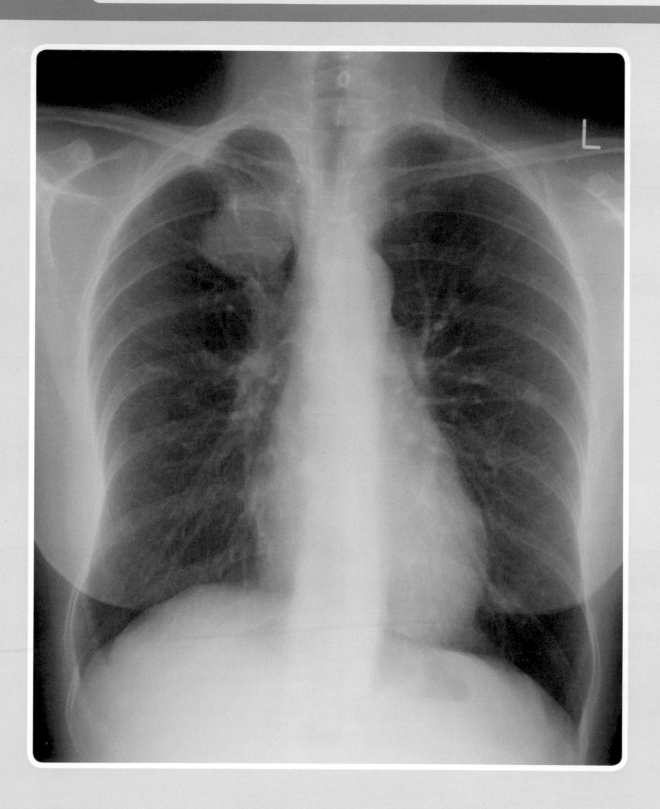

TECHNICAL INFORMATION

Patient ID: Anonymous
Projection: PA
Penetration: Adequate – vertebral bodies just visible behind heart
Inspiration: Adequate – seven anterior ribs visible
Rotation: The patient is slightly rotated to the right

● AIRWAY

The trachea is central after factoring in patient rotation.

● BREATHING

There is a right upper zone mass projected over the anterior aspects of the right first and second ribs. There are multiple small pulmonary nodules visible within the left hemithorax.

The lungs are not hyperinflated.

There is pleural thickening at the right lung apex.

Normal pulmonary vascularity.

● CIRCULATION AND MEDIASTINUM

The heart is not enlarged.

The heart borders are clear.

The aorta appears normal.

The mediastinum is central and not widened. The right upper zone mass appears contiguous with the superior mediastinum.

The right hilum is abnormally dense. It also appears higher than the left. Normal size, shape and position of the left hilum.

● DIAPHRAGM AND DELICATES

Normal appearance and position of the hemidiaphragms.

No pneumoperitoneum.

The imaged skeleton is intact with no fractures or destructive bony lesions visible.

The visible soft tissues are unremarkable.

● EXTRAS AND REVIEW AREAS

No vascular lines, tubes or surgical clips.
Lung apices: Right apical pleural thickening.
Hila: Dense right hilum, normal left hilum.
Behind heart: Normal.
Costophrenic angles: Normal.
Below the diaphragm: Normal.

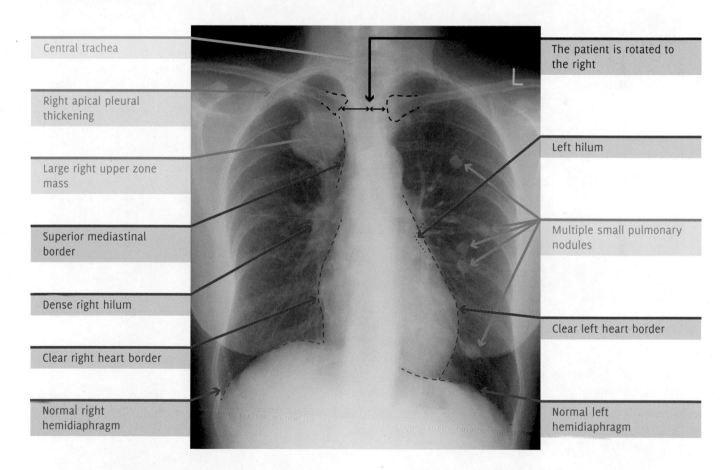

Central trachea

Right apical pleural thickening

Large right upper zone mass

Superior mediastinal border

Dense right hilum

Clear right heart border

Normal right hemidiaphragm

The patient is rotated to the right

Left hilum

Multiple small pulmonary nodules

Clear left heart border

Normal left hemidiaphragm

SUMMARY, INVESTIGATIONS AND MANAGEMENT

This X-ray demonstrates a large, rounded right upper lobe lung lesion associated with multiple smaller nodules. This is highly suspicious of a right upper lobe primary lung cancer with lung metastases. The dense right hilum is suspicious for hilar nodal disease. The significance of the right apical pleural thickening is not clear.

Initial blood tests may include FBC, U&Es, CRP, LFTs and bone profile.

A staging CT chest and abdomen with IV contrast should be performed.

The patient should be referred to respiratory/oncology services for further management, which may include biopsy and MDT discussion. Treatment, which may include surgery, radiotherapy, chemotherapy or palliative treatment, will depend on the outcome of the MDT discussion, investigations and the patient's wishes.

A 55-year-old male presents to ED with a 2-week history of a productive cough and shortness of breath. There is a history of gastro-oesophageal reflux. He is a nonsmoker. On examination, he has oxygen saturations of 100% in air and is afebrile. Lungs are resonant throughout, with good bilateral air entry. A chest X-ray is requested to assess for possible pneumonia, effusion or collapse.

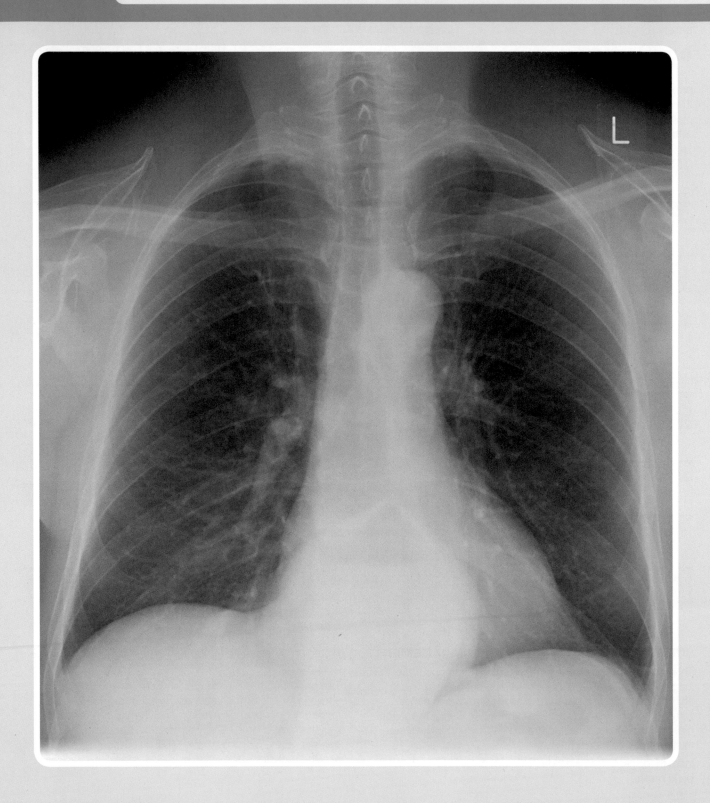

TECHNICAL INFORMATION

Patient ID: Anonymous

Projection: PA

Penetration: Adequate – vertebral bodies just visible behind heart

Inspiration: Adequate – six anterior ribs visible

Rotation: The patient is slightly rotated to the left

● AIRWAY

The trachea is central after factoring in patient rotation.

● BREATHING

The lungs are clear.

They are not hyperinflated.

The pleural spaces are clear.

Normal pulmonary vascularity.

● CIRCULATION AND MEDIASTINUM

There is a mass projected centrally over the lower mediastinum/heart. An air-fluid level is visible.

The heart is not enlarged.

The heart borders are clear.

The aorta appears normal.

The mediastinum is central, not widened, with clear borders.

Normal size, shape and position of both hila.

● DIAPHRAGM AND DELICATES

Normal appearance and position of the hemidiaphragms.

No pneumoperitoneum.

The imaged skeleton is intact with no fractures or destructive bony lesions visible.

The visible soft tissues are unremarkable.

● EXTRAS AND REVIEW AREAS

No vascular lines, tubes or surgical clips.

Lung apices: Normal.

Hila: Normal.

Behind heart: Retrocardiac opacity with an air-fluid level.

Costophrenic angles: Normal.

Below the diaphragm: Normal.

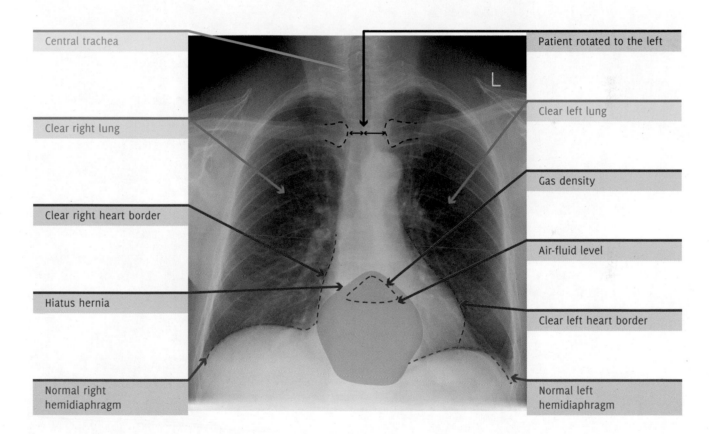

SUMMARY, INVESTIGATIONS AND MANAGEMENT

This X-ray demonstrates a retrocardiac opacity with an air-fluid level consistent with a moderately sized hiatus hernia. The lungs are clear.

Initial blood tests may include FBC, U&Es and CRP to look for possible infection.

Treatment may be required if the gastrooesophageal reflux disease is symptomatic; otherwise no treatment for the hiatus hernia is necessary.

A non binary 54-year-old presents to ED with acute shortness of breath. They have a background of ischaemic heart disease and have a 20 pack-year smoking history. On examination, they are apyrexial, with oxygen saturations of 90% in air. HR is 100 bpm with a RR of 22. There is dullness and inspiratory crackles in both lower zones. The JVP is raised 4 cm. A chest X-ray is performed to look for pulmonary oedema.

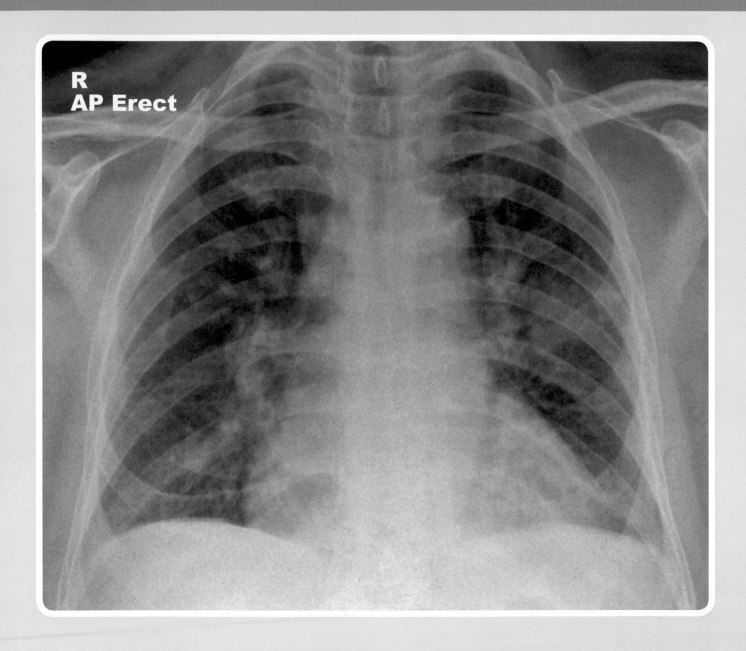

R
AP Erect

TECHNICAL INFORMATION

Patient ID: Anonymous
Projection: AP erect
Penetration: Adequate – vertebral bodies just visible behind heart
Inspiration: Adequate – six anterior ribs visible
Rotation: The patient is mildly rotated to the right

● AIRWAY

The trachea is central.

● BREATHING

There is interstitial opacification throughout both lungs. Prominent pulmonary vessels within the upper lobes are in keeping with upper lobe venous diversion.

The lungs are not hyperinflated.

The pleural spaces are clear.

● CIRCULATION AND MEDIASTINUM

The heart appears enlarged although its size cannot be accurately assessed on an AP X-ray.

The heart borders are clear.

There is unfolding of the thoracic aorta.

The mediastinum is central, not widened, with clear borders.

The hila are enlarged, which is likely vascular in origin, but they are in a normal position, with no increased density.

● DIAPHRAGM AND DELICATES

There is blunting of the costophrenic angles in keeping with small pleural effusions. The hemidiaphragms are otherwise normal.

No pneumoperitoneum.

The imaged skeleton is intact with no fractures or destructive bony lesions visible.

The visible soft tissues are unremarkable.

● EXTRAS AND REVIEW AREAS

No vascular lines, tubes or surgical clips.
Lung apices: Upper lobe venous blood diversion.
Hila: Enlarged.
Behind heart: Normal.
Costophrenic angles: Blunting consistent with small effusions.
Below the diaphragm: Normal.

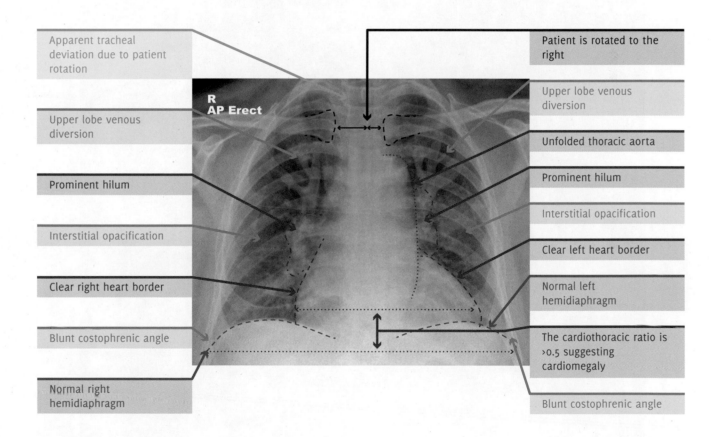

Apparent tracheal deviation due to patient rotation

Upper lobe venous diversion

Prominent hilum

Interstitial opacification

Clear right heart border

Blunt costophrenic angle

Normal right hemidiaphragm

R
AP Erect

Patient is rotated to the right

Upper lobe venous diversion

Unfolded thoracic aorta

Prominent hilum

Interstitial opacification

Clear left heart border

Normal left hemidiaphragm

The cardiothoracic ratio is >0.5 suggesting cardiomegaly

Blunt costophrenic angle

SUMMARY, INVESTIGATIONS AND MANAGEMENT

This X-ray demonstrates features of heart failure (cardiomegaly, interstitial opacification, upper lobe venous diversion and small pleural effusions).

U&Es should be performed to assess renal function, along with FBC to look for any associated anaemia. An ECG would be helpful to look for any new electrical changes. An echocardiogram (ECHO) would allow assessment of the left ventricular function. The patient should be managed for acute pulmonary oedema/heart failure. A repeat chest X-ray can be used to help monitor response to treatment.

A 50-year-old female presents to the ED with shortness of breath. She also reports weight loss of 10 kg in the last month. She has an 80 pack-year smoking history. On examination, she is cachexic, has oxygen saturations of 100% in air and is afebrile. The lungs are resonant throughout, with good air entry bilaterally. There is tar staining of the fingernails. A chest X-ray is requested to assess for possible malignancy.

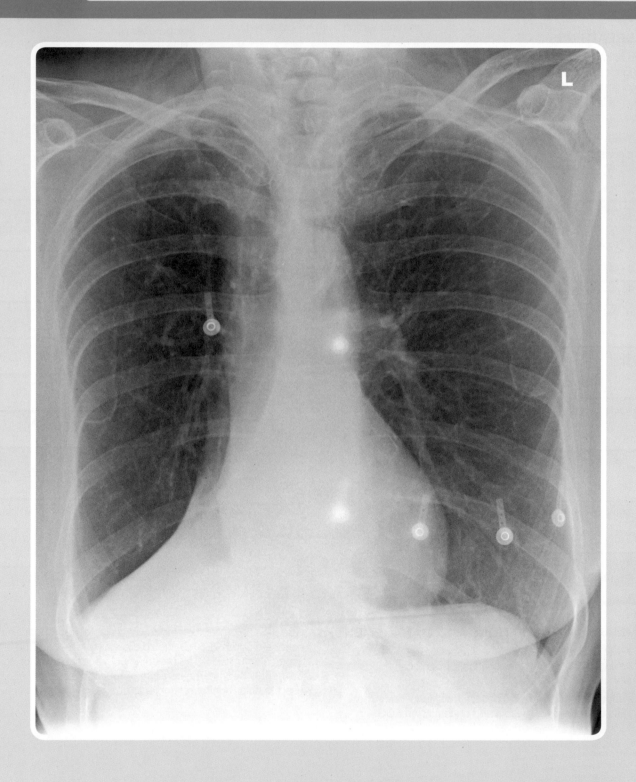

TECHNICAL INFORMATION

Patient ID: Anonymous
Projection: PA
Penetration: Underpenetrated – vertebral bodies not visible behind heart
Inspiration: Adequate – seven anterior ribs visible
Rotation: Not rotated

● AIRWAY

The trachea is deviated to the right.

● BREATHING

There is a homogeneous triangular-shaped opacity in the medial aspect of the right lower zone that involves the right retrocardiac area, in keeping with the sail sign. The right hemithorax appears smaller than the left indicating volume loss. The left lung appears hyperexpanded with some coarsening of the bronchovascular markings.

The lungs are otherwise clear.

The pleural spaces are clear, apart from mild bilateral apical pleural thickening.

Normal pulmonary vascularity.

● CIRCULATION AND MEDIASTINUM

The heart is not enlarged.

The heart borders are clear.

The aorta appears normal.

The mediastinum is displaced to the right.

The right hilum is difficult to identify and probably depressed. Normal size, shape and position of the left hilum.

● DIAPHRAGM AND DELICATES

The right hemidiaphragm is indistinct, indicating right lower lobe pathology.

Normal position and appearance of the left hemidiaphragm.

No pneumoperitoneum.

The imaged skeleton is intact with no fractures or destructive bony lesions visible.

The visible soft tissues are unremarkable.

● EXTRAS AND REVIEW AREAS

ECG clips in situ.

No vascular lines, tubes or surgical clips.
Lung apices: Mild apical pleural thickening.
Hila: Right hilum is difficult to identify and probably depressed. Normal left hilum.
Behind heart: Increased right retrocardiac opacification.
Costophrenic angles: Normal.
Below the diaphragm: Normal.

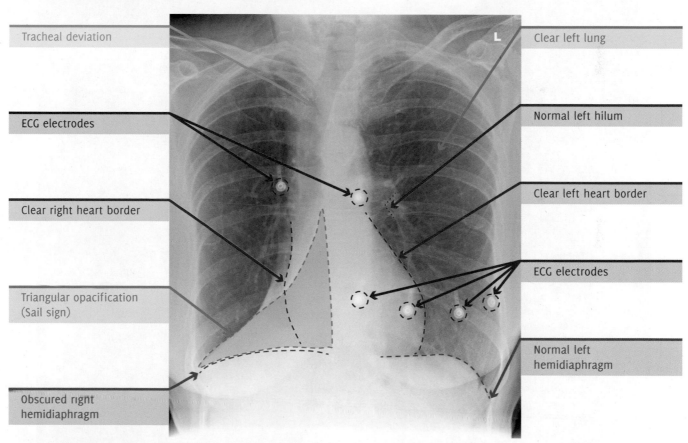

Labels around image:
- Tracheal deviation
- ECG electrodes
- Clear right heart border
- Triangular opacification (Sail sign)
- Obscured right hemidiaphragm
- L
- Clear left lung
- Normal left hilum
- Clear left heart border
- ECG electrodes
- Normal left hemidiaphragm

SUMMARY, INVESTIGATIONS AND MANAGEMENT

This X-ray shows a right lower lobe collapse (increased triangular opacity medially in the right lower zone which obscured the right hemidiaphragm – sail sign). There is resultant right-sided volume loss with probable depression of the right hilum. No definite mass can be seen, but given the history, malignancy is the most concerning differential. Other differentials for collapse include mucus plugging and an inhaled foreign body.

Initial blood tests may include FBC, U&Es, LFTs, bone profile, CRP, ESR and TFTs. A CT chest with IV contrast should be

performed to assess for an underlying tumour. A CT of the abdomen will usually also be acquired at the same time to enable lung cancer staging.

The patient should be referred to respiratory/oncology services for further management, which may include biopsy and MDT discussion. Treatment, which may include surgery, radiotherapy, chemotherapy or palliative treatment, will depend on the outcome of the MDT and the patient's wishes.

A 43-year-old female presents to ED with worsening shortness of breath and inspiratory chest pain. She has had a cough for the last few weeks as well as general flu-like symptoms. She has a 30 pack-year smoking history. On examination, oxygen saturations are 91% in air and she is afebrile. There is reduced air entry in the right upper zone, with associated dullness to percussion. A chest X-ray is requested to assess for possible malignancy, collapse or consolidation.

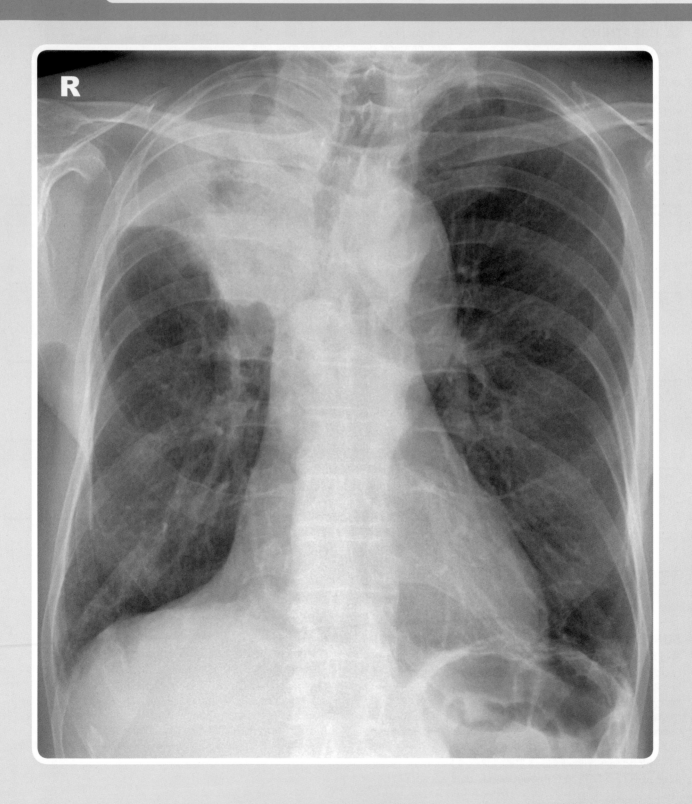

TECHNICAL INFORMATION

Patient ID: Anonymous
Projection: PA
Penetration: Adequate – vertebral bodies just visible behind heart
Inspiration: Adequate – six anterior ribs visible
Rotation: Not rotated

● AIRWAY

The trachea is deviated to the right and appears attenuated distally.

● BREATHING

There is an area of increased density in the right upper zone. It has a concave inferior margin, consistent with elevation of the horizontal fissure. The inferomedial margin has a convex contour, suggestive of a central mass. A small, rounded opacity is present at the left costophrenic angle.

The lungs are otherwise clear.

The lungs are not hyperinflated.

The pleural spaces are clear.

Normal pulmonary vascularity.

● CIRCULATION AND MEDIASTINUM

The heart is not enlarged.

The heart borders are clear.

There is mild unfolding of the thoracic aorta.

The mediastinum is central.

The right hilum is elevated and bulky. The right main bronchus appears compressed. The right side of the upper mediastinum is indistinct. Normal size, shape and position of the left hilum.

● DIAPHRAGM AND DELICATES

Normal position and appearance of the hemidiaphragms.

No pneumoperitoneum.

The imaged skeleton is intact with no fractures or destructive bony lesions visible.

The visible soft tissues are unremarkable.

● EXTRAS AND REVIEW AREAS

No vascular lines, tubes or surgical clips.
Lung apices: Opacification of the right apex. Normal left apex.
Hila: Elevated, bulky right hilum. Normal left hilum.
Behind heart: Normal.
Costophrenic angles: Rounded opacity at the left costophrenic angle.
Below the diaphragm: Normal.

Opacification of the partially collapsed right upper lobe

Elevated horizontal fissure

Convex medial/concave lateral contour consistent with a central mass (Golden S sign)

Compressed right main bronchus

Abnormal right hilar/subcarinal density

Clear right heart border

Normal right hemidiaphragm

Tracheal deviation and attenuation

Unfolded thoracic aorta

Normal left main bronchus

Clear left heart border

Subtle nodule/mass

Normal left hemidiaphragm

SUMMARY, INVESTIGATIONS AND MANAGEMENT

This X-ray demonstrates a right upper lobe collapse (increased opacity in the right upper zone, concave inferior margin representing the displaced horizontal fissure). There is resultant volume loss demonstrated by tracheal deviation and elevation of the right hilum. The inferior margin of the collapse has a convex contour medially, in keeping with a proximal tumour (Golden S sign).

The distal trachea and right main bronchus appear attenuated by a mass. The small rounded opacity at the left costophrenic angle may represent a pulmonary nodule/metastasis.

The most likely differential for a hilar lung mass is a primary lung malignancy. Pulmonary metastases are less likely.

Supplementary oxygen should be given.

Initial blood tests may include FBC, U&Es, LFTs, bone profile, CRP and ESR. A CT chest with IV contrast should be performed to assess for underlying tumour. A CT of the abdomen will usually also be acquired at the same time to enable lung cancer staging.

The patient should be referred to respiratory/oncology services for further management, which may include biopsy and MDT discussion. Treatment, which may include surgery, radiotherapy, chemotherapy or palliative treatment, will depend on the outcome of the MDT and the patient's wishes.

A 33-year-old female presents to ED with a productive cough and feeling generally unwell. There is no significant past medical history. She is a nonsmoker. On examination, she has oxygen saturations of 96% in air and is afebrile. There is dullness to percussion and reduced air entry at the left lung base. A chest X-ray is requested to assess for possible pneumonia, effusion or collapse.

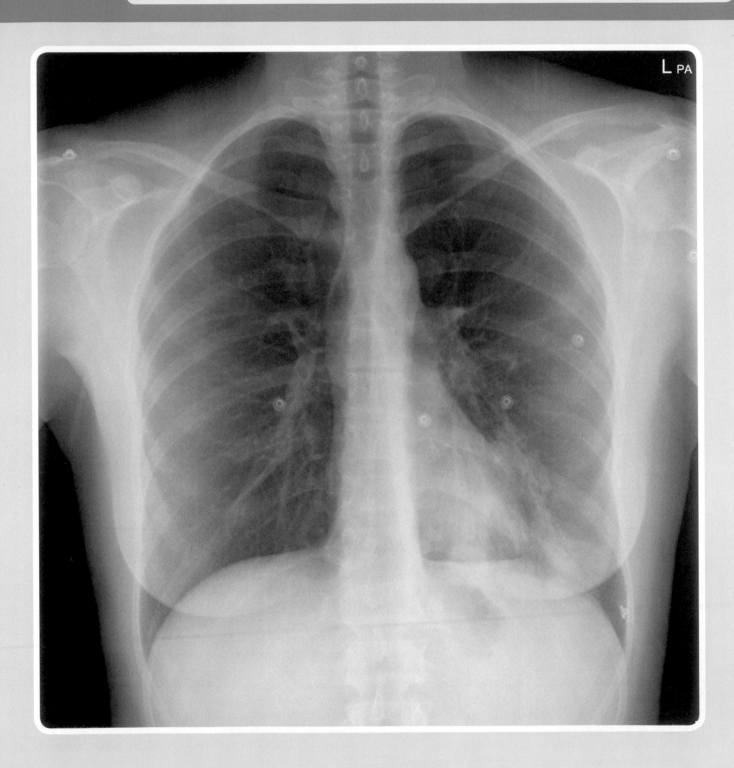

TECHNICAL INFORMATION

Patient ID: Anonymous
Projection: PA
Penetration: Adequate – vertebral bodies just visible behind heart
Inspiration: Adequate – six anterior ribs visible
Rotation: The patient is slightly rotated to the right

● AIRWAY

The trachea is central after factoring in patient rotation.

● BREATHING

There is heterogeneous airspace opacification in the left lower zone, in keeping with consolidation. The rest of the lungs are clear. The lungs are not hyperinflated.

The pleural spaces are clear.

Normal pulmonary vascularity.

● CIRCULATION AND MEDIASTINUM

The heart is not enlarged.

The heart borders are clear.

The aorta appears normal.

The mediastinum is central, not widened, with clear borders.

Normal size, shape and position of the hila.

● DIAPHRAGM AND DELICATES

Normal position and appearance of the right hemidiaphragm. The left hemidiaphragm is partially obscured by overlying consolidation.

No pneumoperitoneum.

The imaged skeleton is intact with no fractures or destructive bony lesions visible.

The visible soft tissues are unremarkable.

● EXTRAS AND REVIEW AREAS

ECG electrodes in situ.

No vascular lines, tubes or surgical clips.
Lung apices: Normal.
Hila: Normal.
Behind heart: Heterogeneous left retrocardiac consolidation.
Costophrenic angles: Normal.
Below the diaphragm: Normal.

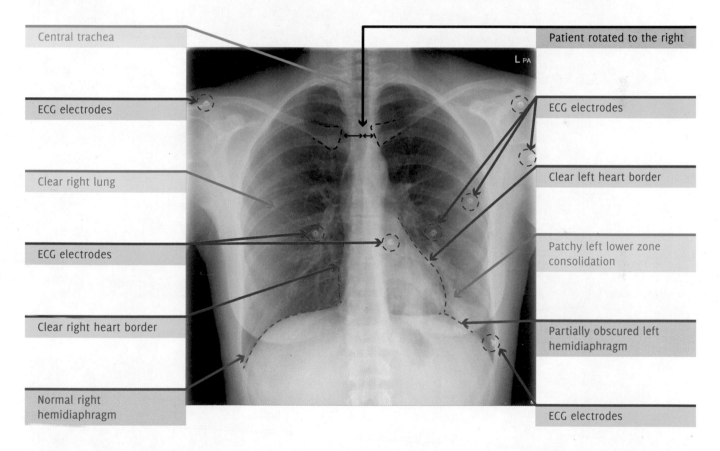

Central trachea

Patient rotated to the right

ECG electrodes

ECG electrodes

Clear right lung

Clear left heart border

ECG electrodes

Patchy left lower zone consolidation

Clear right heart border

Partially obscured left hemidiaphragm

Normal right hemidiaphragm

ECG electrodes

SUMMARY, INVESTIGATIONS AND MANAGEMENT

This X-ray demonstrates left lower zone consolidation, which partially obscures the left hemidiaphragm. The left heart border is preserved. The findings are consistent with left lower lobe pneumonia.

Initial blood tests may include FBC, U&Es, LFTs, bone profile, CRP and blood cultures. Sputum culture can also be checked.

Appropriate antibiotics should be given to treat a community-acquired pneumonia, which may be oral or intravenous depending on the severity of pneumonia (CURB-65). A follow-up chest X-ray in 4 to 6 weeks should be taken to ensure resolution.

A 31-year-old male is brought to the ED with acute onset breathlessness and wheeze. He is a known asthmatic, on regular inhaled corticosteroid therapy and a β2 agonist when required. He is a nonsmoker. On examination, he is apyrexial, with oxygen saturations of 82% in air. There is widespread wheeze. There is decreased air entry on the left side and the lungs are resonant throughout. An urgent chest X-ray is requested to assess for a possible pneumothorax.

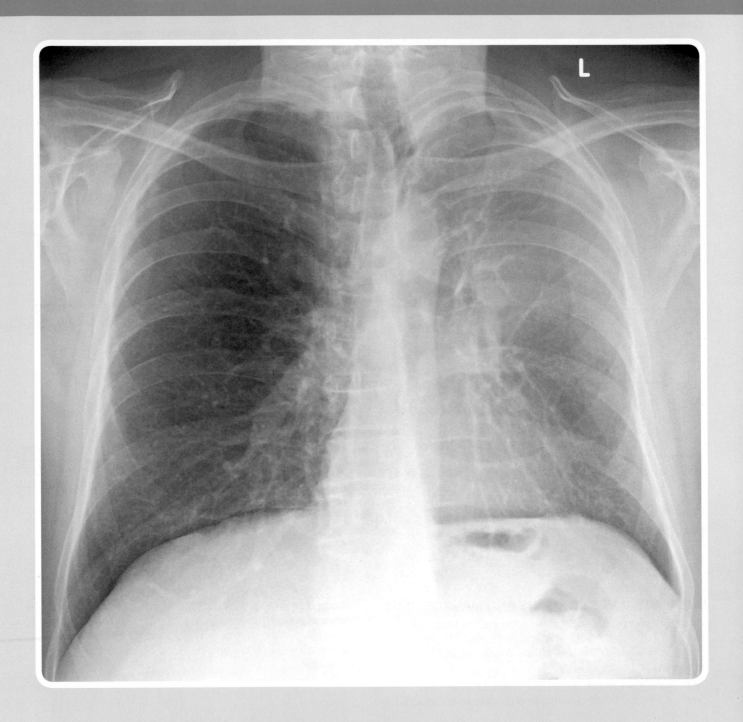

TECHNICAL INFORMATION

Patient ID: Anonymous
Projection: PA
Penetration: Adequate – vertebral bodies just visible behind heart
Inspiration: Adequate – eight anterior ribs visible
Rotation: The patient is slightly rotated to the left

● AIRWAY

The trachea is deviated to the left, even when allowing for the patient rotation.

● BREATHING

There is diffuse, veil-like opacification of the left hemithorax.

The right lung is clear apart from mild right apical scarring.

The lungs are not hyperinflated.

The pleural spaces are clear.

Normal pulmonary vascularity.

● CIRCULATION AND MEDIASTINUM

The heart is not enlarged.

The left heart border is indistinct. The right heart border is displaced to the left, being projected over the spine. It appears clear.

The aorta appears normal.

The mediastinum is displaced to the left.

Normal size, shape and position of both hila.

● DIAPHRAGM AND DELICATES

Normal appearance and position of the hemidiaphragms.

No pneumoperitoneum.

The imaged skeleton is intact with no fractures or destructive bony lesions visible.

The visible soft tissues are unremarkable.

● EXTRAS AND REVIEW AREAS

No vascular lines, tubes or surgical clips.
Lung apices: Left apical opacification. Right apical scarring.
Hila: Normal.
Behind heart: Normal.
Costophrenic angles: Normal.
Below the diaphragm: Normal.

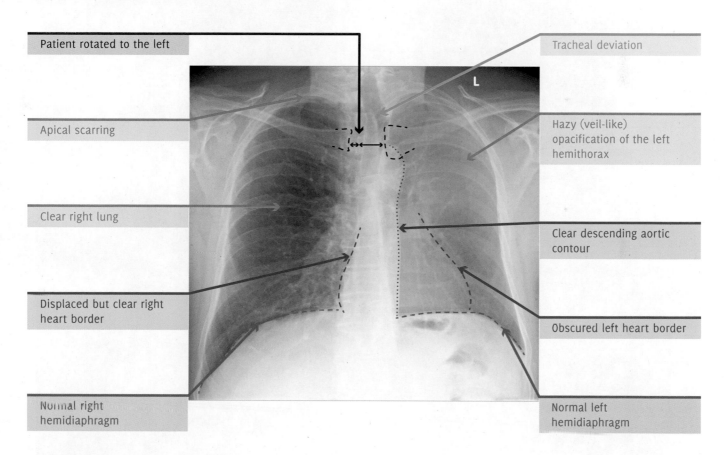

Patient rotated to the left

Tracheal deviation

Apical scarring

Hazy (veil-like) opacification of the left hemithorax

Clear right lung

Clear descending aortic contour

Displaced but clear right heart border

Obscured left heart border

Normal right hemidiaphragm

Normal left hemidiaphragm

SUMMARY, INVESTIGATIONS AND MANAGEMENT

This X-ray shows a left upper lobe collapse ('veil-like' opacification of the left hemithorax) with resultant volume loss demonstrated by mediastinal shift to the left.

Given the patient's age and the asthma history, the most likely diagnosis is collapse secondary to mucus plugging. An inhaled foreign body is another possibility. Malignancy is unlikely in this context.

The acute asthma exacerbation should be managed using an ABCDE approach, with oxygen, nebulized bronchodilators and corticosteroids initially. Bloods may not be necessary if there is a rapid improvement with initial treatment. Chest physiotherapy may help relieve mucus plugging and a follow-up chest X-ray should be performed to ensure resolution of the collapse.

Respiratory referral should be considered.

A 40-year-old male presents to ED with shortness of breath and a 6-week history of cough. He has a history of testicular cancer, which was treated with surgery. He is a nonsmoker. On examination, he has oxygen saturations of 100% in air and is afebrile. Lungs are resonant throughout with good bilateral air entry. A chest X-ray is requested to assess for possible malignancy.

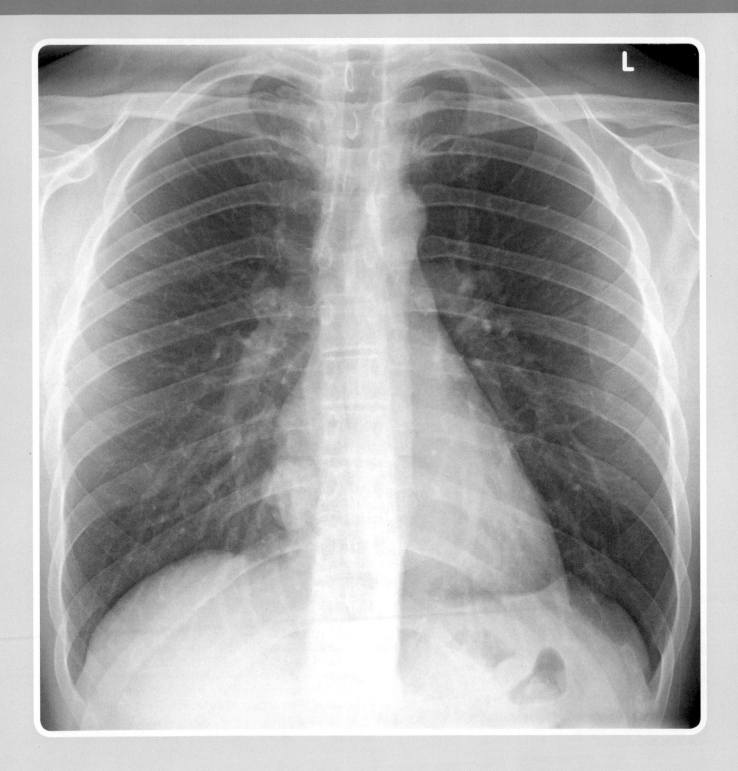

TECHNICAL INFORMATION

Patient ID: Anonymous
Projection: PA
Penetration: Adequate – vertebral bodies just visible behind heart
Inspiration: Adequate – eight anterior ribs visible
Rotation: Not rotated

AIRWAY

The trachea is central.

BREATHING

There is a small, lobulated mass medially in the right lower zone. It is partially projected over the right heart border. The lungs are otherwise clear.

The lungs are not hyperinflated.

The pleural spaces are clear.

Normal pulmonary vascularity.

CIRCULATION AND MEDIASTINUM

The heart is not enlarged.

The heart borders are clear. A mass is projected over the right heart border, although the border remains visible.

The aorta appears normal.

The mediastinum is central, not widened, with clear borders.

Normal size, shape and position of both hila.

DIAPHRAGM AND DELICATES

Normal appearance and position of the hemidiaphragms.

No pneumoperitoneum.

The imaged skeleton is intact with no fractures or destructive bony lesions visible.

The visible soft tissues are unremarkable.

EXTRAS AND REVIEW AREAS

No vascular lines, tubes or surgical clips.
Lung apices: Normal.
Hila: Normal.
Behind heart: Mass projected over the right heart border.
Costophrenic angles: Normal.
Below the diaphragm: Normal.

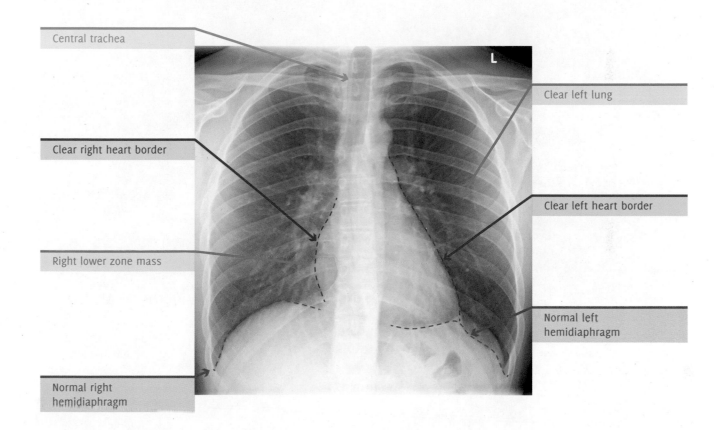

Central trachea

Clear left lung

Clear right heart border

Clear left heart border

Right lower zone mass

Normal left hemidiaphragm

Normal right hemidiaphragm

SUMMARY, INVESTIGATIONS AND MANAGEMENT

This X-ray demonstrates a small rounded mass medially in the right lower zone. The mass is projected over the right cardiac border, which remains visible, indicating the mass is not in the middle lobe or anterior mediastinum. Given the history of previous malignancy, this is suspicious for a metastasis.

Initial blood tests may include FBC, U&Es, LFTs and bone profile.

A staging CT chest, abdomen and pelvis with IV contrast should be performed to identify any underlying malignancy.

The patient should be referred to oncology services for further management, which may include biopsy and MDT discussion.

Treatment, which may include surgery, radiotherapy, chemotherapy or palliative treatment, will depend on the outcome of the MDT discussion, investigations and the patient's wishes.

A 40-year-old male presents to ED with shortness of breath. He has been off work for a week with a productive cough and feeling feverish. On examination, he has oxygen saturations of 98% in air and is febrile at 39°C. There is decreased air entry, dullness to percussion and crackles in the left lower zone. A chest X-ray is requested to assess for possible pneumonia, effusion or collapse.

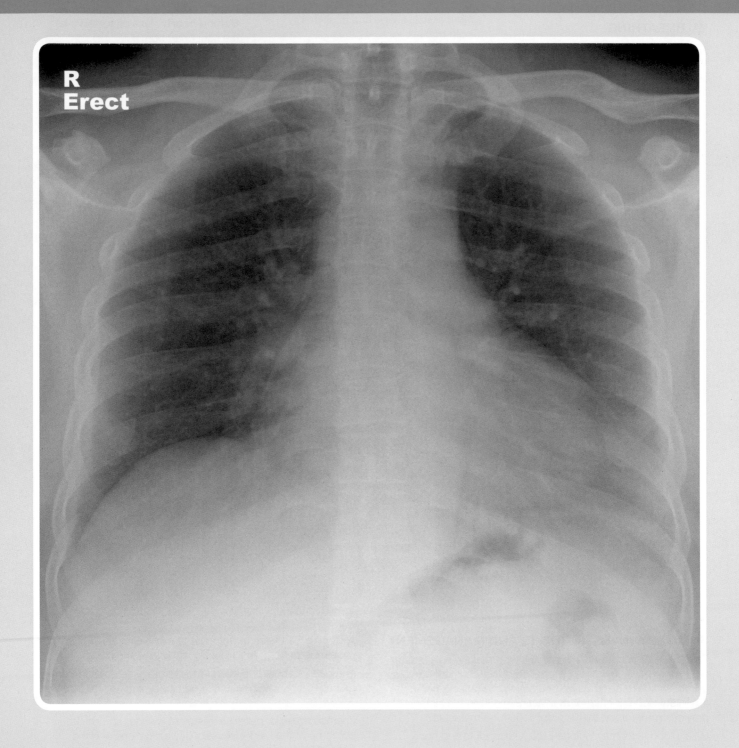

TECHNICAL INFORMATION

Patient ID: Anonymous
Projection: AP
Penetration: Adequate – vertebral bodies just visible behind heart
Inspiration: Adequate – seven anterior ribs visible
Rotation: Not rotated

● AIRWAY

The trachea is central.

● BREATHING

There is heterogeneous opacification peripherally in the left lower zone consistent with consolidation. The rest of the lungs are clear. The lungs are not hyperinflated.

The left costophrenic angle is difficult to define, which may be due to pneumonia or a small effusion. The right-sided pleural spaces are clear.

Normal pulmonary vascularity.

● CIRCULATION AND MEDIASTINUM

The heart does not appear enlarged, although its size cannot be accurately assessed on an AP X-ray.

The cardiac borders are clear.

The aorta appears normal.

The mediastinum is central, not widened, with clear borders.

Normal size, shape and position of both hila.

● DIAPHRAGM AND DELICATES

The left hemidiaphragm is obscured. Normal position and appearance of the right hemidiaphragm.

No pneumoperitoneum.

The imaged skeleton is intact with no fractures or destructive bony lesions visible.

The visible soft tissues are unremarkable.

● EXTRAS AND REVIEW AREAS

No vascular lines, tubes or surgical clips.
Lung apices: Normal.
Hila: Normal.
Behind heart: Normal.
Costophrenic angles: Left costophrenic angle blunting.
Below the diaphragm: Normal.

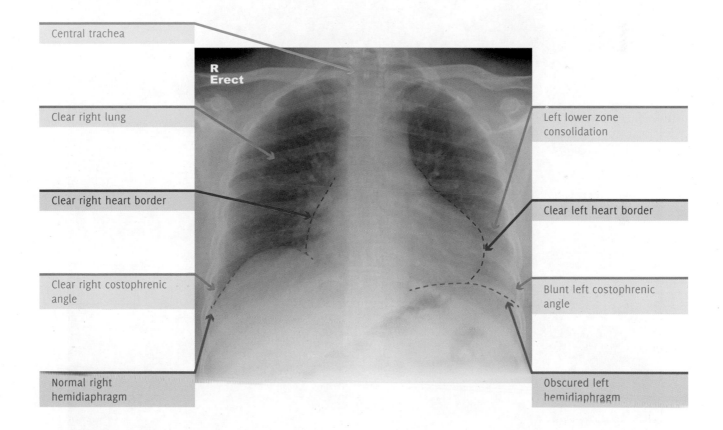

Central trachea

R Erect

Clear right lung

Clear right heart border

Clear right costophrenic angle

Normal right hemidiaphragm

Left lower zone consolidation

Clear left heart border

Blunt left costophrenic angle

Obscured left hemidiaphragm

SUMMARY, INVESTIGATIONS AND MANAGEMENT

This X-ray demonstrates consolidation in the left lower zone. The consolidation obscures the left hemidiaphragm but not the left heart border consistent with left lower lobe pneumonia. There may be a small left pleural effusion.

Initial blood tests may include FBC, U&Es, blood cultures and CRP. A sputum culture may also be taken.

The patient should be treated with appropriate antibiotics for community-acquired pneumonia and a follow-up chest X-ray performed to ensure resolution. The antibiotics may be oral or intravenous depending on the severity of pneumonia (CURB-65). Ultrasound could be used to further assess the volume of the pleural effusion, particularly if a diagnostic pleural aspiration is being considered.

A 35-year-old male presents to ED with coryzal symptoms, fever and a productive cough with green sputum. There is no significant past medical history. He has a 15 pack-year smoking history. On examination, he has oxygen saturations of 94% in air and is febrile with a temperature of 38.9°C. There is dullness to percussion and crackles in the left mid zone. A chest X-ray is requested to assess for possible pneumonia.

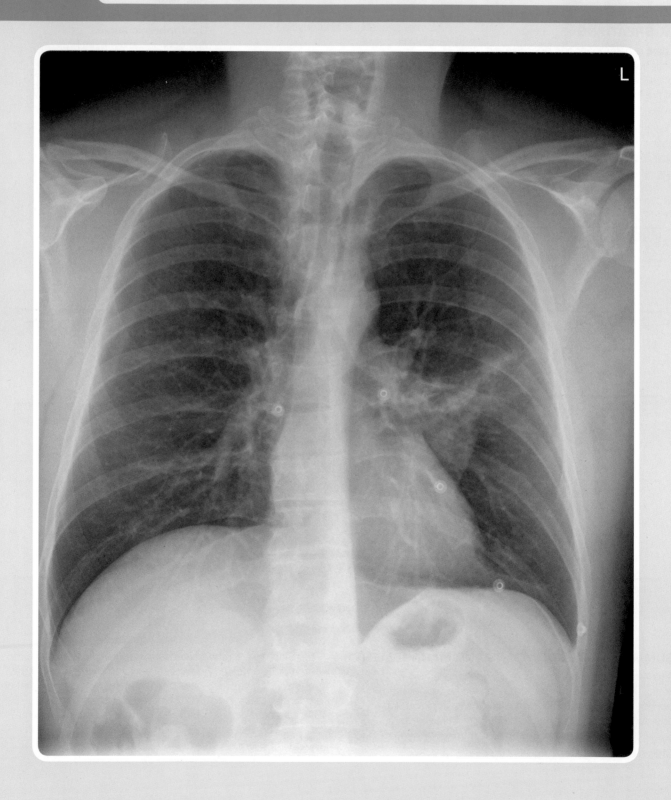

L

TECHNICAL INFORMATION

Patient ID: Anonymous
Projection: PA
Penetration: Adequate – vertebral bodies just visible behind heart
Inspiration: Adequate – seven anterior ribs visible
Rotation: The patient is rotated to the right

● AIRWAY

The trachea is central after factoring in patient rotation.

● BREATHING

There is heterogeneous airspace opacification in the medial aspect of the left mid zone consistent with consolidation. This obscures the superior aspect of the left heart border. The lungs are otherwise clear. The lungs are not hyperinflated.

The pleural spaces are clear.
Normal pulmonary vascularity.

● CIRCULATION AND MEDIASTINUM

The heart is not enlarged.

The superior aspect of the left heart border is obscured by consolidation. The right heart border is difficult to identify due to patient rotation.

The aorta appears normal.

The mediastinum is central, not widened, with clear borders.

The left hilum is obscured by consolidation. Normal size, shape and position of the right hilum.

● DIAPHRAGM AND DELICATES

Normal position and appearance of the hemidiaphragms.

No pneumoperitoneum.

The imaged skeleton is intact with no fracture or destructive bony lesion visible.

The visible soft tissues are unremarkable.

● EXTRAS AND REVIEW AREAS

There are ECG electrodes in situ.

No vascular lines, tubes or surgical clips.
Lung apices: Normal.
Hila: The left hilum is obscured by consolidation. Normal right hilum.
Behind heart: Normal.
Costophrenic angles: Normal.
Below the diaphragm: Normal.

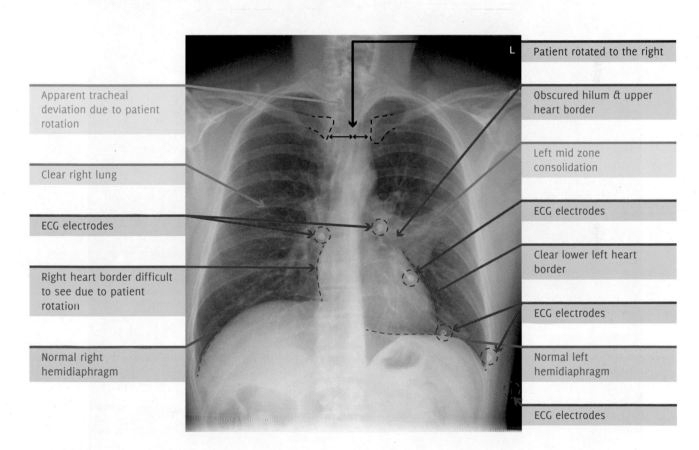

Apparent tracheal deviation due to patient rotation

Clear right lung

ECG electrodes

Right heart border difficult to see due to patient rotation

Normal right hemidiaphragm

Patient rotated to the right

Obscured hilum & upper heart border

Left mid zone consolidation

ECG electrodes

Clear lower left heart border

ECG electrodes

Normal left hemidiaphragm

ECG electrodes

SUMMARY, INVESTIGATIONS AND MANAGEMENT

This X-ray demonstrates left mid zone consolidation which partially obscures the left heart border. The findings are in keeping with pneumonia affecting the lingual segment of the left upper lobe.

Initial blood tests may include FBC, U&Es, CRP and blood cultures. A sputum culture may also be obtained.

The patient should be treated with appropriate antibiotics for community-acquired pneumonia and a follow-up chest X-ray performed to ensure resolution. The antibiotics may be oral or intravenous depending on the severity of pneumonia (CURB-65).

A 2-year-old female presents with her parents to ED after swallowing a coin. There is no significant past medical history. On examination, she has oxygen saturations of 100% in air and is afebrile. Lung fields are resonant throughout, with good bilateral air entry. A chest X-ray is requested to assess the position of the foreign body.

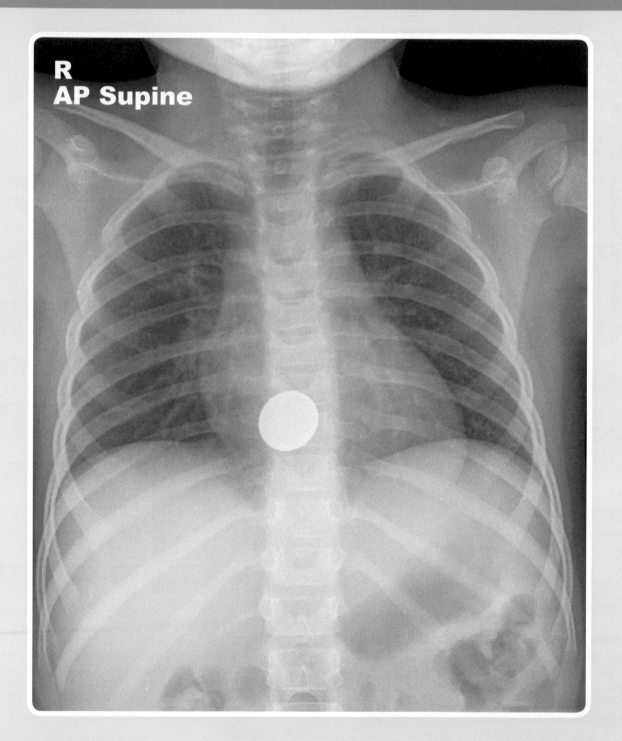

TECHNICAL INFORMATION

Patient ID: Anonymous
Projection: AP supine
Penetration: Adequate – vertebral bodies just visible behind heart
Inspiration: Limited – five anterior ribs visible
Rotation: The patient is not rotated

● AIRWAY

The trachea is central.

● BREATHING

The lungs are clear.

The lungs are not hyperinflated.

The pleural spaces are clear.

Normal pulmonary vascularity.

● CIRCULATION AND MEDIASTINUM

The heart does not appear enlarged, although its size cannot be accurately assessed on an AP X-ray.

The heart borders are clear.

The aorta appears normal.

The mediastinum is central, not widened, with normal thymic contours.

There is a circular radio-opaque foreign body projected over the lower mediastinum.

There is no evidence of pneumomediastinum.

Normal size, shape and position of both hila.

● DIAPHRAGM AND DELICATES

Normal appearance and position of the hemidiaphragms.

No pneumoperitoneum visible although the supine projection makes this difficult to assess.

The imaged skeleton is intact with no fractures or destructive bony lesions visible.

The visible soft tissues are unremarkable.

● EXTRAS AND REVIEW AREAS

No vascular lines, tubes or surgical clips.
Lung apices: Normal.
Hila: Normal.
Behind heart: Radio-opaque foreign body projected centrally over the lower mediastinum.
Costophrenic angles: Normal.
Below the diaphragm: Normal.

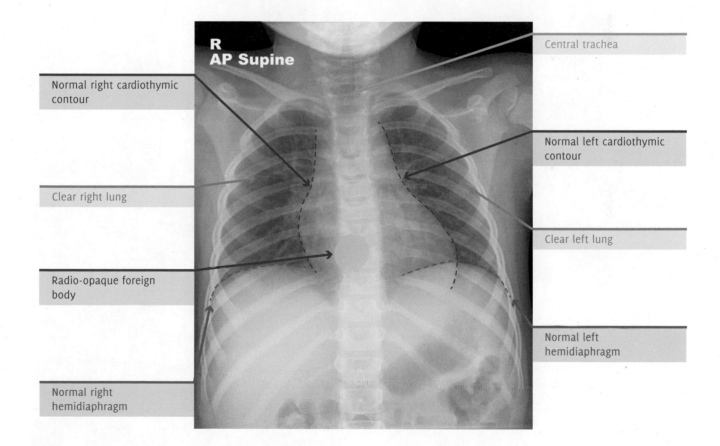

R
AP Supine

Central trachea

Normal right cardiothymic contour

Normal left cardiothymic contour

Clear right lung

Clear left lung

Radio-opaque foreign body

Normal left hemidiaphragm

Normal right hemidiaphragm

SUMMARY, INVESTIGATIONS AND MANAGEMENT

This X-ray demonstrates a radio-opaque foreign body projected centrally over the lower mediastinum. Assuming it is not outwith the patient (i.e. on their skin or clothing), it is in keeping with a swallowed foreign body in the lower oesophagus.

Ingested coins in the lower oesophagus do not necessarily need to be removed – their progress through the GI tract can be assessed with serial X-rays. However, endoscopic removal should be considered if the coin appears stuck or is not progressing.

A 25-year-old male presents to ED with worsening abdominal pain. He has a background of ulcerative colitis and has been having diarrhoea and rectal bleeding over the last week. He is a nonsmoker. On examination, he has oxygen saturations of 86% in air, RR 23, HR 128 bpm, and is febrile with a temperature of 38°C. Lungs are resonant throughout with good bilateral air entry. The abdomen is extremely tender, with absent bowel sounds and percussion tenderness. An erect chest X-ray is requested to assess for possible perforation.

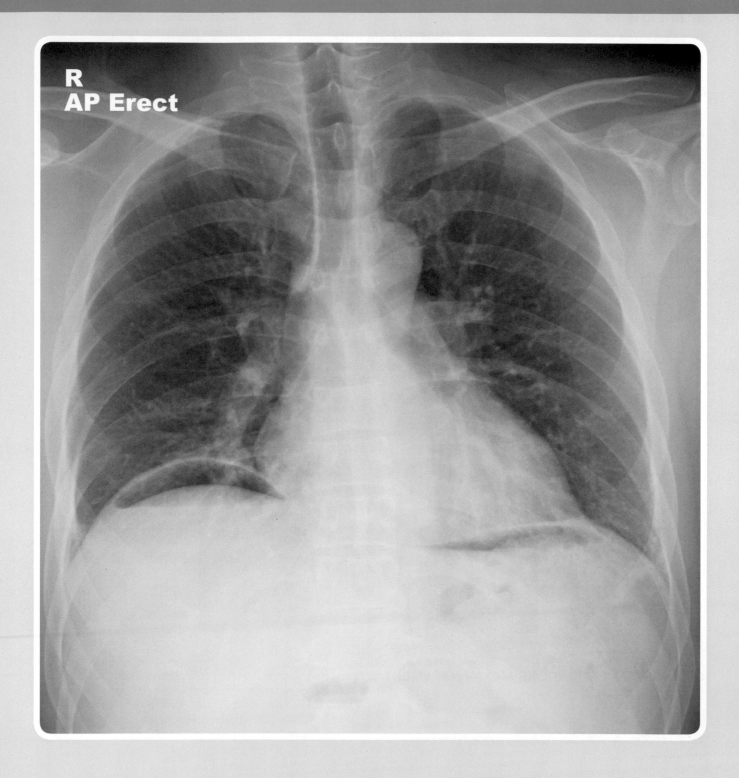

TECHNICAL INFORMATION

Patient ID: Anonymous
Projection: AP erect
Penetration: Adequate – vertebral bodies just visible behind heart
Inspiration: Adequate – six anterior ribs visible
Rotation: The patient is slightly rotated to the right

● AIRWAY

The trachea is central after factoring in patient rotation.

● BREATHING

The lungs are clear. They are not hyperinflated.

The pleural spaces are clear.

Normal pulmonary vascularity.

● CIRCULATION AND MEDIASTINUM

The heart does not appear enlarged, although its size cannot be accurately assessed on an AP X-ray.

The heart borders are clear.

The aorta appears normal.

The mediastinum is central, not widened, with clear borders.

Normal size, shape and position of both hila.

● DIAPHRAGM AND DELICATES

Normal position and appearance of both hemidiaphragms.

There are crescentic lucencies beneath both the left and right hemidiaphragms, in keeping with a pneumoperitoneum.

The imaged skeleton is intact with no fractures or destructive bony lesions visible.

The visible soft tissues are unremarkable.

● EXTRAS AND REVIEW AREAS

No vascular lines, tubes or surgical clips.
Lung apices: Normal.
Hila: Normal.
Behind heart: Normal.
Costophrenic angles: Normal.
Below the diaphragm: Pneumoperitoneum.

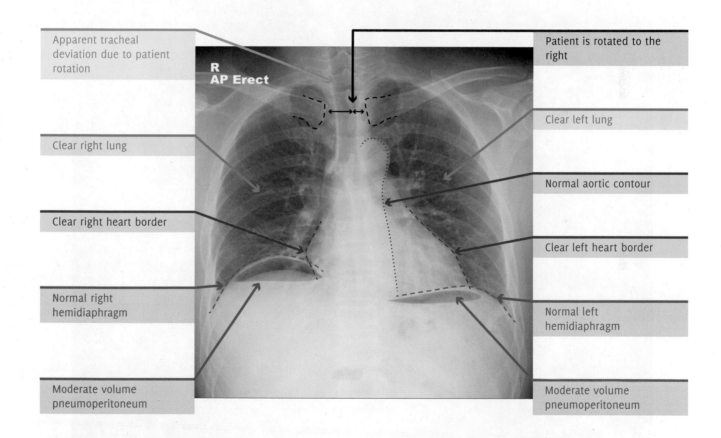

Apparent tracheal deviation due to patient rotation

R
AP Erect

Patient is rotated to the right

Clear right lung

Clear left lung

Normal aortic contour

Clear right heart border

Clear left heart border

Normal right hemidiaphragm

Normal left hemidiaphragm

Moderate volume pneumoperitoneum

Moderate volume pneumoperitoneum

SUMMARY, INVESTIGATIONS AND MANAGEMENT

This X-ray demonstrates pneumoperitoneum. Given the clinical information, it may be related to perforation of a toxic megacolon.

The patient should be urgently resuscitated using an ABCDE approach. Oxygen should be administered, wide-bore cannulae should be inserted, and a fluid bolus should be given, as well as appropriate antibiotics for abdominal sepsis. Initial blood tests may include FBC, U&Es, LFTs, CRP, coagulation, group/save and blood cultures.

Urgent surgical review is required. Depending on the clinical picture, the patient may be taken straight to theatre, have an urgent CT abdomen/pelvis with IV contrast (to identify the site and cause of the perforation) or require further stabilization before any action.

A 30-year-old female presents to ED 2 weeks postpartum feeling unwell, with a productive cough. On examination, she has oxygen saturations of 90% in air and is afebrile. There is dullness to percussion, crackles and reduced air entry at both lung bases. A chest X-ray is requested to assess for possible pneumonia, effusion or collapse.

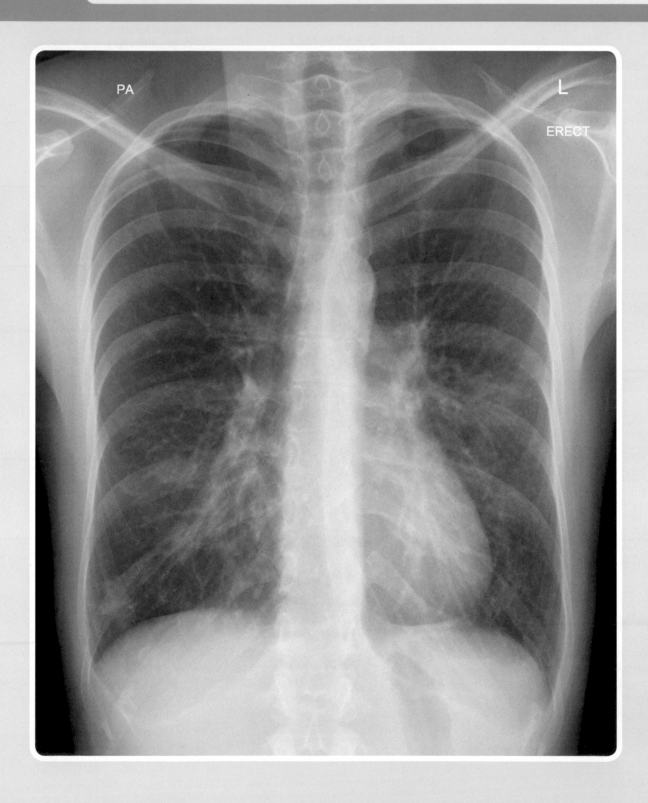

PA

L

ERECT

TECHNICAL INFORMATION

Patient ID: Anonymous
Projection: PA
Penetration: Adequate – vertebral bodies just visible behind heart
Inspiration: Adequate – seven anterior ribs visible
Rotation: The patient is slightly rotated to the right

● AIRWAY

The trachea is central.

● BREATHING

There is heterogeneous airspace opacification of the right lower zone and left mid zone consistent with consolidation. The rest of the lungs are clear. The lungs are not hyperinflated.

The pleural spaces are clear.
Normal pulmonary vascularity.

● CIRCULATION AND MEDIASTINUM

The heart is not enlarged.

The left heart border is clear. The right heart border is obscured by consolidation.

The mediastinum is central, not widened, with clear borders.

Normal size, shape and position of both hila.

● DIAPHRAGM AND DELICATES

Normal position and appearance of the hemidiaphragms.

No pneumoperitoneum.

The imaged skeleton is intact with no fractures or destructive bony lesions visible.

The visible soft tissues are unremarkable.

● EXTRAS AND REVIEW AREAS

No vascular lines, tubes or surgical clips.
Lung apices: Normal.
Hila: Normal.
Behind heart: Normal.
Costophrenic angles: Normal.
Below the diaphragm: Normal.

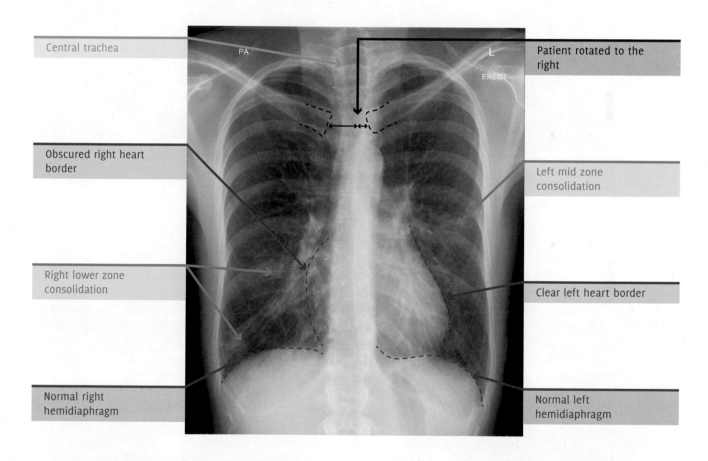

Central trachea

PA

L

ERECT

Patient rotated to the right

Obscured right heart border

Left mid zone consolidation

Right lower zone consolidation

Clear left heart border

Normal right hemidiaphragm

Normal left hemidiaphragm

SUMMARY, INVESTIGATIONS AND MANAGEMENT

The X-ray demonstrates consolidation involving the right lower and left mid zones, in keeping with pneumonia. The right heart border is obscured, indicating middle lobe pneumonia. The left heart border and hemidiaphragm are preserved, making it difficult to determine which lobe the left-sided pneumonia is affecting.

Supplementary oxygen should be given. Initial blood tests may include FBC, U&Es, blood cultures and CRP. A sputum culture may also be taken.

The patient should be treated with appropriate antibiotics for community-acquired pneumonia and have a follow-up chest X-ray performed in 4 to 6 weeks to ensure resolution. The antibiotics may be oral or intravenous depending on the severity of pneumonia (CURB-65). The choice of antibiotics may need to be modified if the patient is breastfeeding.

A 30-year-old female presents to ED with sudden onset right-sided pleuritic chest pain and breathlessness. She has no significant past medical history. She is a nonsmoker. On examination, she has oxygen saturations of 91% in air and is afebrile. HR is 92 bpm, and BP is 120/80 mmHg. There is increased resonance in the right hemithorax and reduced air entry. A chest X-ray is requested to assess for a possible pneumothorax.

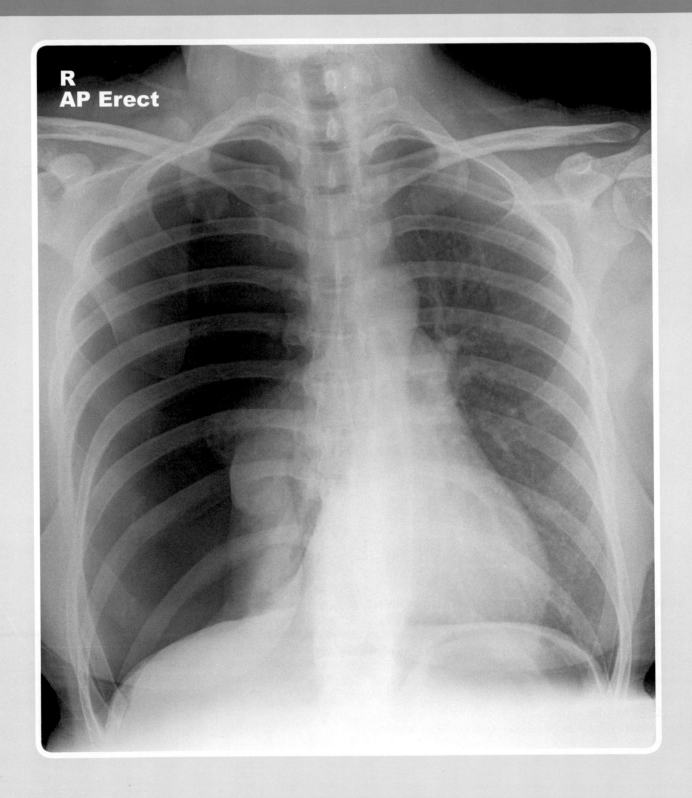

TECHNICAL INFORMATION

Patient ID: Anonymous
Projection: AP erect
Penetration: Adequate – vertebral bodies just visible behind heart
Inspiration: Adequate – six anterior ribs visible
Rotation: The patient is slightly rotated to the right

● AIRWAY

The trachea is central after factoring in patient rotation.

● BREATHING

A lung edge is visible in the right hemithorax, beyond which no lung markings are seen, consistent with a large pneumothorax. There is almost complete collapse of the underlying right lung.

The left lung is clear. It is not hyperexpanded.

The left pleural spaces are clear, and there is normal pulmonary vascularity.

● CIRCULATION AND MEDIASTINUM

The heart does not appear enlarged, although its size cannot be accurately assessed on an AP X-ray.

The right heart border is difficult to identify (probably due to patient rotation and the adjacent collapsed right lung). The left heart border is clear.

The mediastinum is central allowing for patient rotation. It is not widened, with clear borders.

The right hilum is difficult to identify due to the adjacent collapsed lung. Normal size, shape and position of the left hilum.

● DIAPHRAGM AND DELICATES

Normal appearance and position of hemidiaphragms.

No pneumoperitoneum.

The imaged skeleton is intact with no fractures or destructive bony lesions visible.

The visible soft tissues are unremarkable. Of note, there is no surgical emphysema.

● EXTRAS AND REVIEW AREAS

No vascular lines, tubes or surgical clips.
Lung apices: Right pneumothorax. Normal left apex.
Hila: Right hilum is difficult to identify. Normal left hilum.
Behind heart: Normal.
Costophrenic angles: Normal.
Below the diaphragm: Normal.

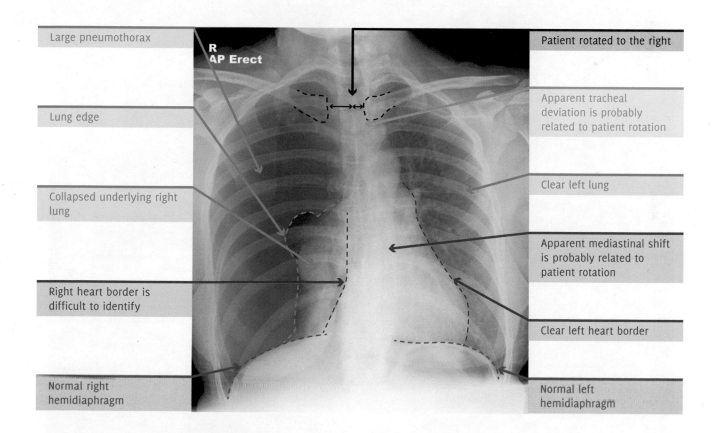

- Large pneumothorax
- Lung edge
- Collapsed underlying right lung
- Right heart border is difficult to identify
- Normal right hemidiaphragm
- R AP Erect
- Patient rotated to the right
- Apparent tracheal deviation is probably related to patient rotation
- Clear left lung
- Apparent mediastinal shift is probably related to patient rotation
- Clear left heart border
- Normal left hemidiaphragm

SUMMARY, INVESTIGATIONS AND MANAGEMENT

This X-ray demonstrates a large right-sided pneumothorax with almost complete collapse of the underlying lung. The apparent mediastinal shift to the left is likely due to rotation; however, the patient should be assessed for clinical evidence of a tension pneumothorax.

The patient should be given supplementary oxygen.

The pneumothorax will require active intervention due to its large size. Needle aspiration of the pneumothorax should be performed in the first instance. An intercostal chest drain may still be required depending on the success of the aspiration.

The patient should be referred to respiratory and follow-up chest X-rays performed until the pneumothorax has resolved.

A 32-year-old female on the surgical ward develops shortness of breath and a fever 36 hours post-appendicectomy. There is no other significant past medical history. She is a nonsmoker. On examination, she has oxygen saturations of 91% in air, RR of 25, HR of 120, and is febrile with a temperature of 39.5°C. There is reduced air entry and crackles in the right lung base. A chest X-ray is requested to assess for possible pneumonia or effusion.

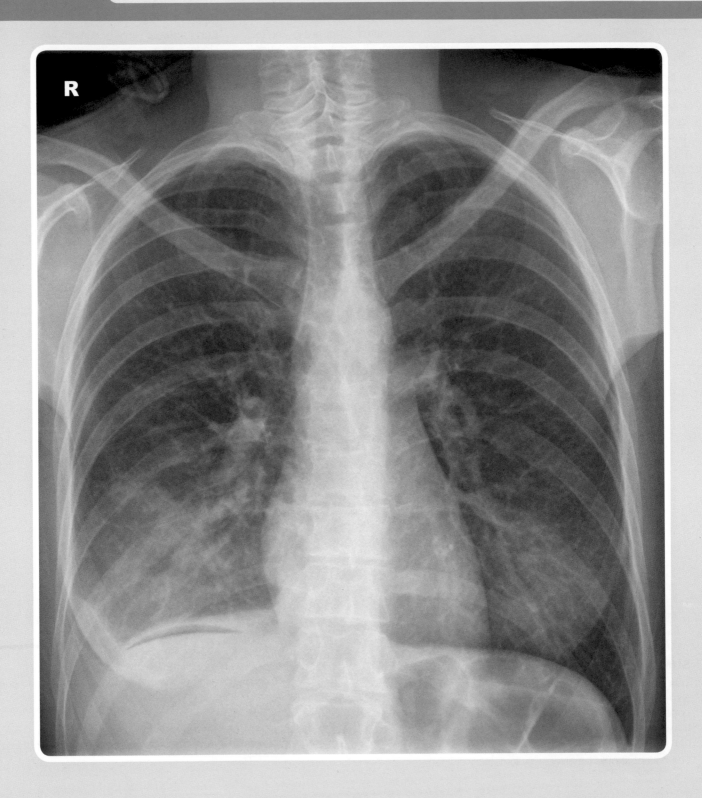

TECHNICAL INFORMATION

Patient ID: Anonymous
Projection: PA
Penetration: Adequate – vertebral bodies just visible behind heart
Inspiration: Adequate – seven anterior ribs visible
Rotation: The patient is slightly rotated to the right

● AIRWAY

The trachea is central after factoring in patient rotation.

● BREATHING

There is right lower zone air space opacification in keeping with consolidation. The remainder of the lungs are clear. The lungs are not hyperinflated.

There is blunting of the right costophrenic angle, consistent with a small pleural effusion. The left pleural space is clear.

Normal pulmonary vascularity.

● CIRCULATION AND MEDIASTINUM

The heart is not enlarged.

The heart borders are clear.

The aorta appears normal.

The mediastinum is central, not widened, with clear borders.

Normal size, shape and position of both hila.

● DIAPHRAGM AND DELICATES

The lateral aspect of the right hemidiaphragm is obscured by the pleural effusion. The remainder of the diaphragm is clear.

There is a lucent crescent below the right hemidiaphragm consistent with a small volume of pneumoperitoneum.

The imaged skeleton is intact with no fractures or destructive bony lesions visible.

The visible soft tissues are unremarkable.

● EXTRAS AND REVIEW AREAS

No vascular lines, tubes or surgical clips.
Lung apices: Normal.
Hila: Normal.
Behind heart: Increased right retrocardiac opacification consistent with consolidation.
Costophrenic angles: Blunting of the right costophrenic angle. Normal left costophrenic angle.
Below the diaphragm: Small-volume pneumoperitoneum beneath the right hemidiaphragm.

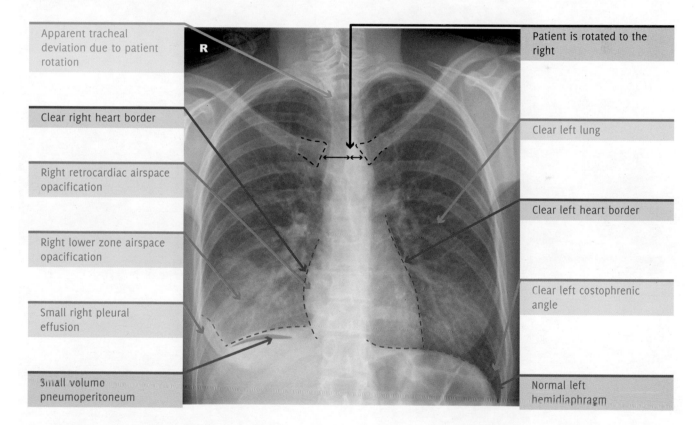

Apparent tracheal deviation due to patient rotation

Clear right heart border

Right retrocardiac airspace opacification

Right lower zone airspace opacification

Small right pleural effusion

Small volume pneumoperitoneum

Patient is rotated to the right

Clear left lung

Clear left heart border

Clear left costophrenic angle

Normal left hemidiaphragm

SUMMARY, INVESTIGATIONS AND MANAGEMENT

The X-ray demonstrates right lower zone consolidation, associated with a pleural effusion. This is consistent with pneumonia and a parapneumonic effusion. There is also a small-volume pneumoperitoneum, which is in keeping with the recent surgery.

The patient should be started on supplementary oxygen. Initial blood tests may include FBC, U&Es, blood cultures and CRP. A sputum culture may also be taken.

She will require IV fluids and appropriate antibiotics for hospital-acquired pneumonia, and a follow-up X-ray to ensure resolution of the consolidation should be performed. An ultrasound could be considered to assess the size of the parapneumonic effusion and permit ultrasound-guided aspiration/drainage if required.

A 38-year-old female has had a PICC inserted for chemotherapy. She has a past medical history of breast cancer. She is a nonsmoker. On examination, she has oxygen saturations of 100% in air and is afebrile. Lungs are resonant throughout, with good bilateral air entry. A routine postprocedure chest X-ray is requested to assess PICC position.

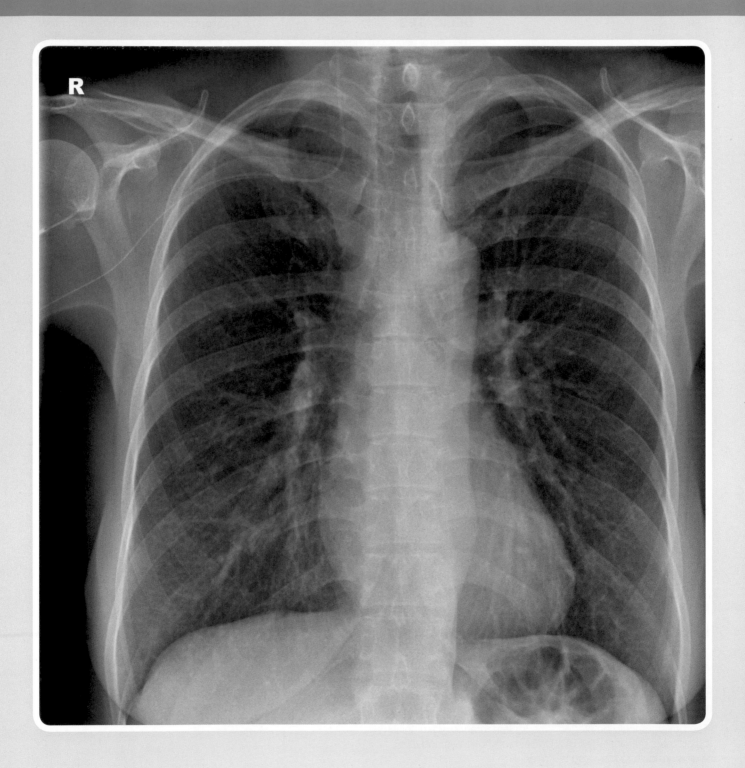

TECHNICAL INFORMATION

Patient ID: Anonymous
Projection: PA
Penetration: Adequate – vertebral bodies just visible behind heart
Inspiration: Adequate – seven anterior ribs visible
Rotation: The patient is slightly rotated to the right

● AIRWAY

The trachea is central after factoring in patient rotation.

● BREATHING

The lungs are clear.

The lungs are not hyperinflated.

The pleural spaces are clear. No pneumothorax.

Normal pulmonary vascularity.

● CIRCULATION AND MEDIASTINUM

The heart is not enlarged.

The heart borders are clear.

The aorta appears normal.

The mediastinum is central, not widened, with clear borders.

Normal size, shape and position of both hila.

● DIAPHRAGM AND DELICATES

Normal position and appearance of the hemidiaphragms.

No pneumoperitoneum.

The imaged skeleton is intact with no fractures or destructive bony lesions visible.

The visible soft tissues are unremarkable.

● EXTRAS AND REVIEW AREAS

The right PICC is projected over the right axillary and subclavian veins. It then courses cranially to enter the right internal jugular vein, rather than going into the superior vena cava.
Lung apices: Normal.
Hila: Normal.
Behind heart: Normal.
Costophrenic angles: Normal.
Below the diaphragm: Normal.

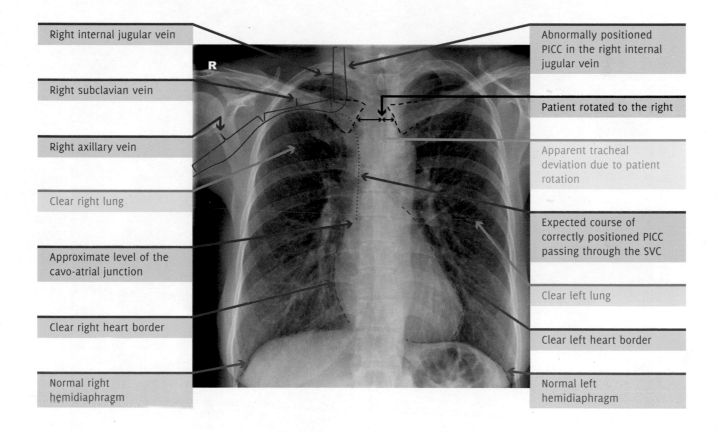

Right internal jugular vein

Right subclavian vein

Right axillary vein

Clear right lung

Approximate level of the cavo-atrial junction

Clear right heart border

Normal right hemidiaphragm

Abnormally positioned PICC in the right internal jugular vein

Patient rotated to the right

Apparent tracheal deviation due to patient rotation

Expected course of correctly positioned PICC passing through the SVC

Clear left lung

Clear left heart border

Normal left hemidiaphragm

SUMMARY, INVESTIGATIONS AND MANAGEMENT

This X-ray demonstrates the right PICC is malpositioned, with its tip in the right internal jugular vein.

The right PICC needs to be resited, and its position checked with a repeat X-ray prior to use.

A 40-year-old female presents to ED with a 1-week history of cough and fever. There is no significant past medical history and she is a nonsmoker. On examination, she has oxygen saturations of 85% in air and is febrile with a temperature of 38.2°C. There is dullness to percussion and crackles in the right lower zone. A chest X-ray is performed to assess for possible pneumonia, collapse or effusion.

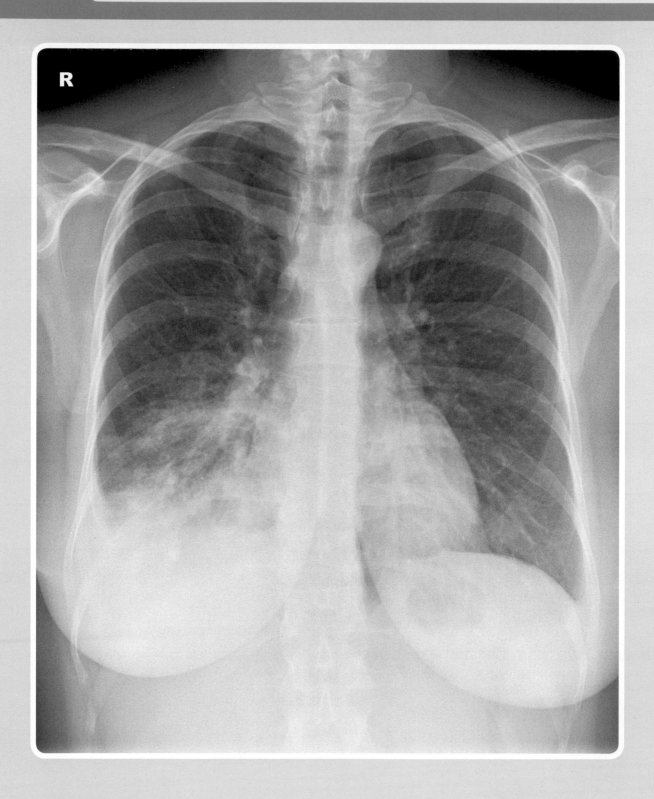

TECHNICAL INFORMATION

Patient ID: Anonymous
Projection: PA
Penetration: Adequate – vertebral bodies just visible behind heart
Inspiration: Adequate – seven anterior ribs visible
Rotation: The patient is slightly rotated to the left

● AIRWAY

The trachea is central.

● BREATHING

There is heterogeneous airspace opacification of the right lower zone consistent with consolidation. The lungs are otherwise clear. The lungs are not hyperinflated.

There is blunting of the right costophrenic angle in keeping with a small right pleural effusion. The left-sided pleural spaces are clear.

Normal pulmonary vascularity.

● CIRCULATION AND MEDIASTINUM

The heart is not enlarged.

The right heart border is largely clear, although its inferior margin is indistinct. Clear left heart border.

The aorta appears normal.

The mediastinum is central, not widened, with clear borders.

Normal size, shape and position of the hila.

● DIAPHRAGM AND DELICATES

The right hemidiaphragm is obscured by consolidation. Normal position and appearance of the left hemidiaphragm.

No pneumoperitoneum.

The imaged skeleton is intact with no fractures or destructive bony lesions visible.

The visible soft tissues are unremarkable.

● EXTRAS AND REVIEW AREAS

No vascular lines, tubes or surgical clips.
Lung apices: Normal.
Hila: Normal.
Behind heart: Normal.
Costophrenic angles: Blunted right costophrenic angle. Normal left costophrenic angle.
Below the diaphragm: Normal.

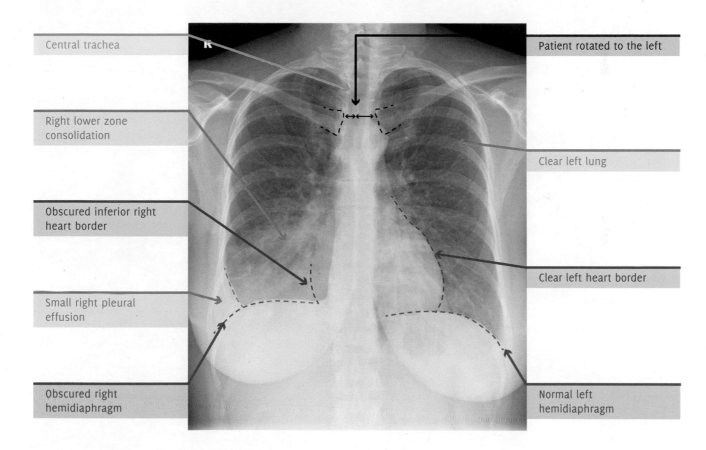

Central trachea	Patient rotated to the left
Right lower zone consolidation	Clear left lung
Obscured inferior right heart border	
	Clear left heart border
Small right pleural effusion	
Obscured right hemidiaphragm	Normal left hemidiaphragm

SUMMARY, INVESTIGATIONS AND MANAGEMENT

This X-ray demonstrates right lower zone consolidation which obscures the right hemidiaphragm, consistent with right lower lobe pneumonia. There may also be pneumonia affecting the right middle lobe, as the right heart border appears partially obscured. A small right parapneumonic effusion is also present.

Initial blood tests may include FBC, U&Es, CRP and blood cultures. A sputum culture may also be obtained.

The patient should be treated with appropriate antibiotics for community-acquired pneumonia, and a follow-up chest X-ray is performed to ensure resolution. The antibiotics may be oral or intravenous depending on the severity of pneumonia (CURB-65).

Ultrasound could be used to further assess the volume of the pleural effusion, particularly if a diagnostic pleural aspiration is being considered.

A 50-year-old female presents to ED with worsening abdominal pain. There is no significant past medical history. She is a nonsmoker. On examination, she has oxygen saturations of 92% in air, RR of 24, HR of 123 bpm, and is febrile with a temperature of 38.8°C. Lungs are resonant throughout with good bilateral air entry. The abdomen is extremely tender, with absent bowel sounds and percussion tenderness. An erect chest X-ray is requested to assess for possible perforation.

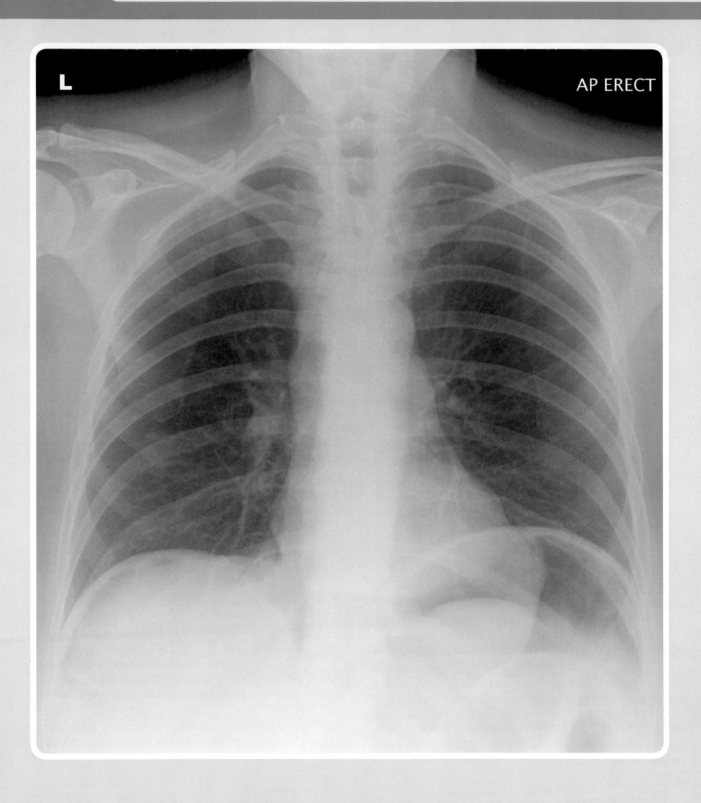

L
AP ERECT

TECHNICAL INFORMATION

Patient ID: Anonymous
Projection: AP erect
Penetration: Adequate – vertebral bodies just visible behind heart
Inspiration: Adequate – six anterior ribs visible
Rotation: Not rotated

● AIRWAY

The trachea is central.

● BREATHING

The lungs are clear. They are not hyperinflated.

The pleural spaces are clear.

Normal pulmonary vascularity.

● CIRCULATION AND MEDIASTINUM

The heart does not appear enlarged, although its size cannot be accurately assessed on an AP X-ray.

The heart borders are clear.

The aorta appears normal.

The mediastinum is central, not widened, with clear borders.

Normal size, shape and position of both hila.

● DIAPHRAGM AND DELICATES

Normal position and appearance of the hemidiaphragms.

There is a large lucency beneath the left hemidiaphragm, and a smaller lucency

beneath the right hemidiaphragm, in keeping with pneumoperitoneum.

The imaged skeleton is intact with no fractures or destructive bony lesions visible.

The visible soft tissues are unremarkable.

● EXTRAS AND REVIEW AREAS

No vascular lines, tubes or surgical clips.
Lung apices: Normal.
Hila: Normal.
Behind heart: Normal.
Costophrenic angles: Normal.
Below the diaphragm: Pneumoperitoneum.

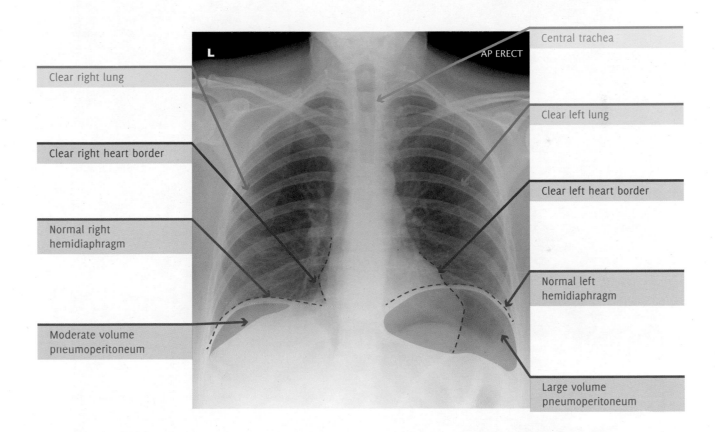

Central trachea

Clear right lung

L

AP ERECT

Clear left lung

Clear right heart border

Clear left heart border

Normal right hemidiaphragm

Normal left hemidiaphragm

Moderate volume pneumoperitoneum

Large volume pneumoperitoneum

SUMMARY, INVESTIGATIONS AND MANAGEMENT

This X-ray demonstrates a large-volume pneumoperitoneum in keeping with a perforated hollow viscus within the abdomen.

The patient should be urgently resuscitated using an ABCDE approach. Oxygen should be administered, wide-bore cannulae should be inserted, and a fluid bolus should be given, as well as broad-spectrum antibiotics. Initial blood tests

may include FBC, U&Es, LFTs, CRP, coagulation, group/save and blood cultures.

Urgent surgical review is required. Depending on the clinical picture, the patient may be taken straight to theatre, have an urgent CT abdomen/pelvis with IV contrast (to identify the site and cause of the perforation) or require further stabilization before any action.

A 50-year-old male presents to ED with worsening shortness of breath. He has a history of granulomatosis with polyangiitis (previously known as Wegener's granulomatosis) and is a nonsmoker. On examination, he has oxygen saturations of 90% in air and is afebrile. There is dullness to percussion and reduced air entry in the left middle and lower zones. A chest X-ray is requested to assess for possible pneumonia, collapse or pleural effusion.

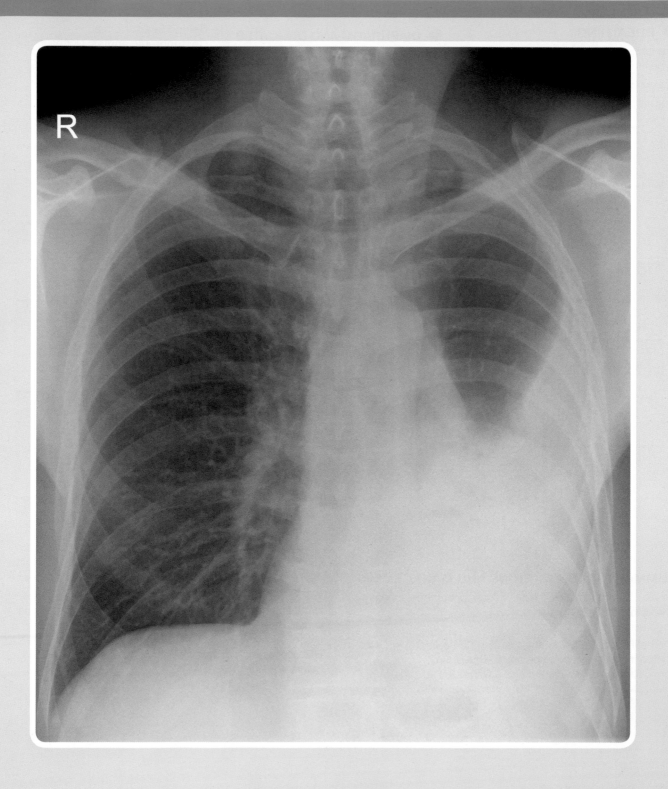

R

TECHNICAL INFORMATION

Patient ID: Anonymous
Projection: PA
Penetration: Adequate – vertebral bodies just visible behind heart
Inspiration: Adequate – six anterior ribs visible
Rotation: Not rotated

● AIRWAY

The trachea is central.

● BREATHING

There is homogenous opacification in the left mid and lower zones. A meniscus is present at the upper margin. The rest of the lungs are clear. The lungs are not hyperinflated.

The right pleural space is clear.

Normal pulmonary vascularity.

● CIRCULATION AND MEDIASTINUM

There is loss of the left heart border. It is therefore not possible to comment on cardiac size. The right heart border is clear.

The descending thoracic aortic contour is also obscured.

The mediastinum is central, not widened, with clear borders.

Normal size, shape and position of right hila. The left hilum is obscured.

● DIAPHRAGM AND DELICATES

The left hemidiaphragm is obscured. Normal position and appearance of the right hemidiaphragm.

No pneumoperitoneum.

The imaged skeleton is intact with no fractures or destructive bony lesions visible.

The visible soft tissues are unremarkable.

● EXTRAS AND REVIEW AREAS

No vascular lines, tubes or surgical clips.
Lung apices: Normal.
Hila: Left hilar region is obscured by opacification.
Behind heart: Obscured by opacification on the left.
Costophrenic angles: Loss of the left costophrenic angle, normal right costophrenic angle.
Below the diaphragm: Normal.

Central trachea

R

Clear right lung

Clear right heart border

Normal right hemidiaphragm

Large left pleural effusion

Obscured descending thoracic aorta

Obscured left heart border

Obscured left hemidiaphragm

SUMMARY, INVESTIGATIONS AND MANAGEMENT

This X-ray demonstrates a large left-sided pleural effusion. This may be directly related to the patient's granulomatous vasculitis, although other causes for effusions such as infection and malignancy are also possible.

Supplementary oxygen should be given.

Initial blood tests may include FBC, U&Es, LFTs, coagulation and CRP. An ultrasound-guided chest drain should be inserted, with pleural fluid sent for protein, albumin, glucose, microscopy, white cell count and cytology. A chest X-ray should be performed to ensure adequate positioning of the drain.

Further management will be guided by the underlying aetiology of the effusion. If the patient has recurrent pleural effusions, then referral to thoracic surgery with a view to pleurodesis may be considered.

A 52-year-old female presents to ED with a 12-week history of cough. She has a 30 pack-year smoking history. On examination, she has oxygen saturations of 99% in air and is afebrile. Lungs are resonant throughout, with good bilateral air entry. A chest X-ray is requested to assess for possible malignancy.

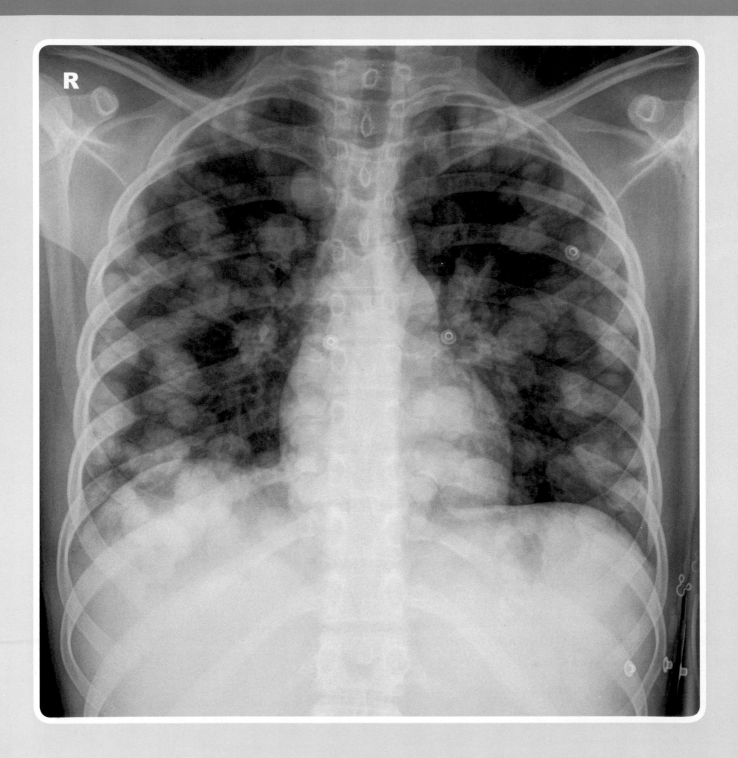

TECHNICAL INFORMATION

Patient ID: Anonymous
Projection: PA
Penetration: Adequate – vertebral bodies just visible behind heart
Inspiration: Adequate – six anterior ribs visible
Rotation: Not rotated

● AIRWAY

The trachea is central.

● BREATHING

There are innumerable, well-circumscribed round soft tissue opacities distributed throughout both lungs. The lungs are not hyperinflated.

The pleural spaces are clear.

Normal pulmonary vascularity.

● CIRCULATION AND MEDIASTINUM

The heart is not enlarged.

The heart borders are clear.

The aorta appears normal.

The mediastinum is central, not widened, with clear borders.

The hila appear bulky bilaterally.

● DIAPHRAGM AND DELICATES

Normal appearance and position of the hemidiaphragms.

No pneumoperitoneum.

The imaged skeleton is intact with no fractures or destructive bony lesions visible.

The visible soft tissues are unremarkable.

● EXTRAS AND REVIEW AREAS

There are ECG electrodes in situ.

No vascular lines, tubes or surgical clips.
Lung apices: Multiple masses.
Hila: Enlarged lobulated contours of the hilum bilaterally.
Behind heart: Multiple masses.
Costophrenic angles: Multiple masses.
Below the diaphragm: Normal.

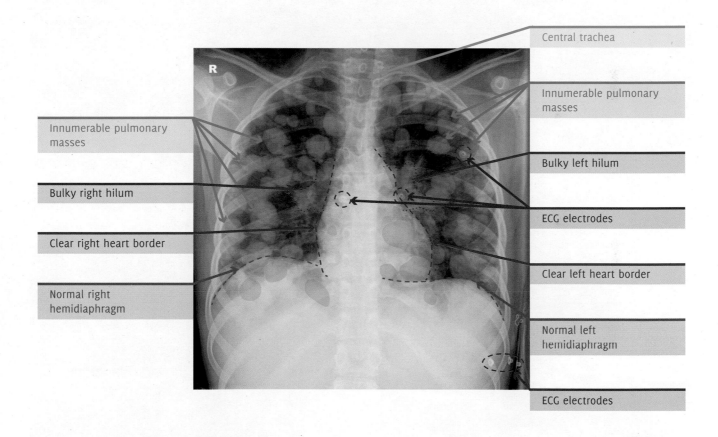

Central trachea

Innumerable pulmonary masses

Innumerable pulmonary masses

Bulky left hilum

Bulky right hilum

ECG electrodes

Clear right heart border

Clear left heart border

Normal right hemidiaphragm

Normal left hemidiaphragm

ECG electrodes

SUMMARY, INVESTIGATIONS AND MANAGEMENT

This X-ray demonstrates innumerable rounded pulmonary masses in keeping with metastases. The hila appear bulky – this could be due to pulmonary metastases projected over them or related to enlarged hilar lymph nodes. The differential diagnosis for 'cannonball' metastases includes breast cancer, renal cell carcinoma, choriocarcinoma and endometrial carcinoma.

The patient needs a thorough clinical examination, including the breasts. Initial blood tests may include FBC, U&Es, CRP, LFTs and bone profile.

A staging CT chest, abdomen and pelvis with IV contrast should be performed to identify the underlying primary and fully stage the cancer.

The patient should be referred to respiratory/oncology services for further management, which may include biopsy and MDT discussion. Treatment, which may include radiotherapy, chemotherapy or palliative treatment, will depend on the outcome of the MDT discussion, investigations and the patient's wishes.

A 55-year-old female develops a cough productive of 'nasty sputum'. She is in the gynaecology ward having undergone elective surgery 3 days earlier. There is no significant past medial history other than uterine fibroids. She is a nonsmoker. On examination, she has oxygen saturations of 91% in air and is febrile with a temperature of 38.5°C. There is dullness to percussion and coarse crackles in the right upper and mid zones. A chest X-ray is requested to assess for possible pneumonia or collapse.

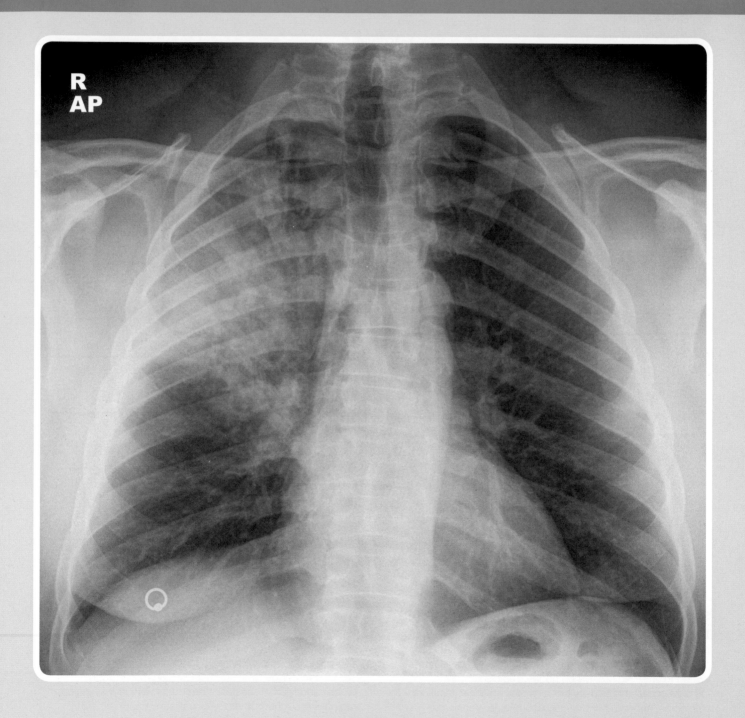

TECHNICAL INFORMATION

Patient ID: Anonymous
Projection: PA
Penetration: Adequate – vertebral bodies just visible behind heart
Inspiration: Adequate – eight anterior ribs visible
Rotation: Not rotated

● AIRWAY

The trachea is slightly deviated to the right.

● BREATHING

There is marked heterogeneous airspace opacification in the right upper zone with air bronchograms, in keeping with consolidation. It has a relatively sharp inferior margin which likely indicates a mildly elevated horizontal fissure. The remainder of the lungs are clear. The lungs are not hyperinflated.

The pleural spaces are clear.

Normal pulmonary vascularity.

● CIRCULATION AND MEDIASTINUM

The heart is not enlarged.

The heart borders are clear.

The aorta appears normal.

The mediastinum is central, not widened, with clear borders.

The right hilum is partially obscured by consolidation. Normal size, shape and position of the left hilum.

● DIAPHRAGM AND DELICATES

Normal position and appearance of the hemidiaphragms.

No pneumoperitoneum.

The imaged skeleton is intact with no fracture or destructive bony lesion visible.

The visible soft tissues are unremarkable.

● EXTRAS AND REVIEW AREAS

No vascular lines, tubes or surgical clips. A right-sided nipple ring is noted.
Lung apices: Heterogeneous right apical consolidation. Normal left apex.
Hila: Normal.
Behind heart: Normal.
Costophrenic angles: Normal.
Below the diaphragm: Normal.

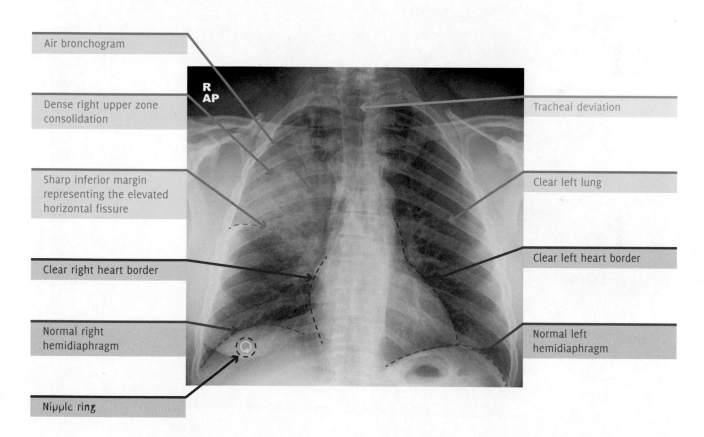

Air bronchogram

Dense right upper zone consolidation

Sharp inferior margin representing the elevated horizontal fissure

Clear right heart border

Normal right hemidiaphragm

Nipple ring

Tracheal deviation

Clear left lung

Clear left heart border

Normal left hemidiaphragm

SUMMARY, INVESTIGATIONS AND MANAGEMENT

This X-ray demonstrates extensive heterogeneous right upper zone consolidation in keeping with pneumonia. The consolidation has a relatively abrupt inferior margin which represents the horizontal fissure, indicating this is right upper lobe pneumonia. There is mild tracheal deviation and elevation of the horizontal fissure indicating concomitant volume loss/partial collapse.

Initial blood tests may include FBC, U&Es, blood cultures and CRP. A sputum culture may also be taken.

The patient should be treated with appropriate antibiotics for hospital-acquired pneumonia and a follow-up chest X-ray performed to ensure resolution. The antibiotics may be oral or intravenous depending on the severity of pneumonia.

A 60-year-old male presents with progressive shortness of breath. He has non-Hodgkin lymphoma. He is a nonsmoker. On examination, he has oxygen saturations of 90% in air and is afebrile. There is reduced air entry and dullness to percussion throughout the left side. A chest X-ray is requested to assess for possible pneumonia, effusion or collapse.

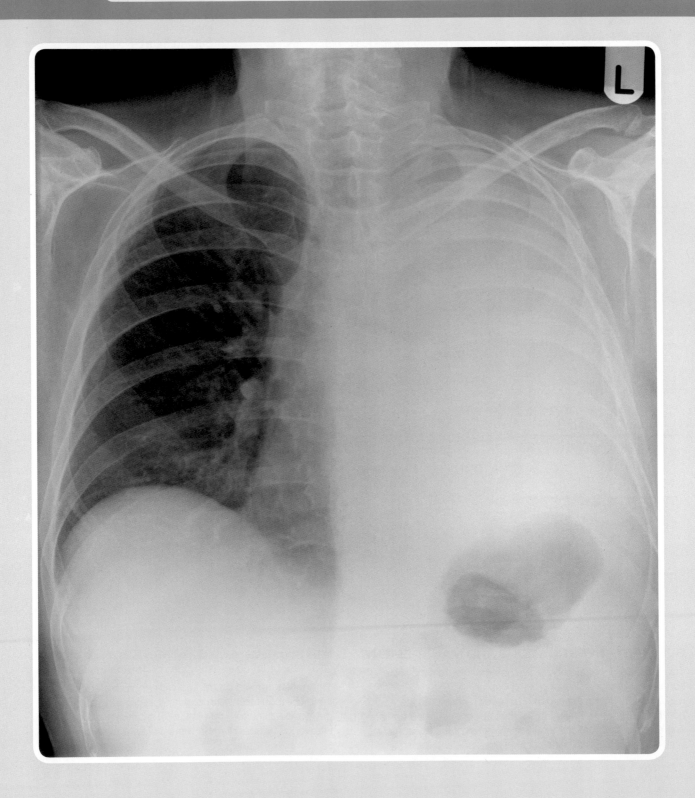

TECHNICAL INFORMATION

Patient ID: Anonymous
Projection: PA
Penetration: Adequate – vertebral bodies just visible behind heart
Inspiration: Limited – five anterior ribs visible
Rotation: The patient is rotated to the right

● AIRWAY

The trachea is displaced slightly to the right – this may be due to patient rotation or a mass effect.

● BREATHING

There is complete, homogeneous opacification of the left hemithorax, in keeping with a large pleural effusion.

The right lung is clear. The lungs are not hyperinflated.

The right pleural space is clear.

Normal pulmonary vascularity.

● CIRCULATION AND MEDIASTINUM

The left heart border is obscured by the effusion. The cardiac size cannot therefore be accurately assessed. The right heart border is clear.

The thoracic aorta is obscured.

The mediastinum is central, not widened, with a clear right border. The left border is obscured.

The left hilum is obscured by the effusion. Normal size, shape and position of the right hilum.

● DIAPHRAGM AND DELICATES

The left hemidiaphragm is obscured by the effusion. Normal position and appearance of the right hemidiaphragm.

The imaged skeleton is intact with no fractures or destructive bony lesions visible.

The visible soft tissues are unremarkable.

● EXTRAS AND REVIEW AREAS

No vascular lines, tubes or surgical clips.
Lung apices: The left apex is opacified. The right apex is clear.
Hila: Left hilum is obscured. Normal right hilum.
Behind heart: Left side obscured by the effusion.
Costophrenic angles: Obliteration of the left costophrenic angle. Right side clear.
Below the diaphragm: Normal.

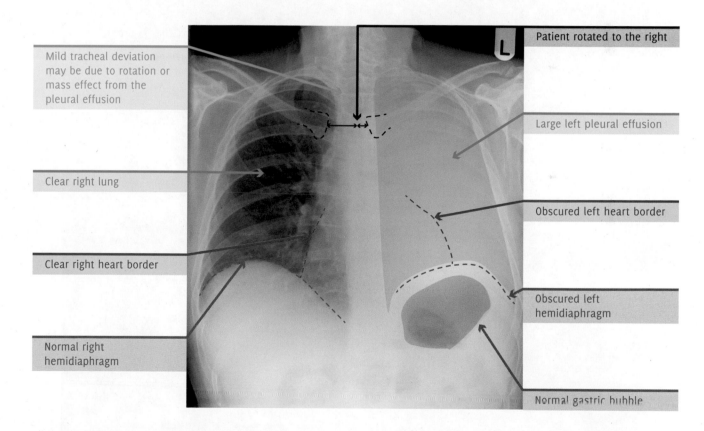

Mild tracheal deviation may be due to rotation or mass effect from the pleural effusion

Clear right lung

Clear right heart border

Normal right hemidiaphragm

Patient rotated to the right

Large left pleural effusion

Obscured left heart border

Obscured left hemidiaphragm

Normal gastric bubble

SUMMARY, INVESTIGATIONS AND MANAGEMENT

This X-ray demonstrates a large left-sided pleural effusion, which is likely related to the patient's known malignancy. Other causes of effusion, such as infection, are also possible.

Supplementary oxygen should be given.

Initial blood tests may include FBC, U&Es, LFTs, coagulation and CRP. An ultrasound-guided chest drain should be inserted, with pleural fluid sent for protein, albumin, glucose, microscopy, white cell count and cytology. A chest X-ray should be performed to ensure adequate positioning of the drain.

Further management will be guided by the underlying aetiology of the effusion. Previous imaging should be reviewed to assess for progression of the effusion. Referral to haematology for further management would be very helpful.

A 68-year-old male presents to preoperative assessment clinic prior to a cholecystectomy. He has a 60 pack-year smoking history. On examination, he has oxygen saturations of 100% in air and is afebrile. Lungs are resonant throughout, with good bilateral air entry. A routine preoperative chest X-ray is requested to assess for any underlying lung pathology.

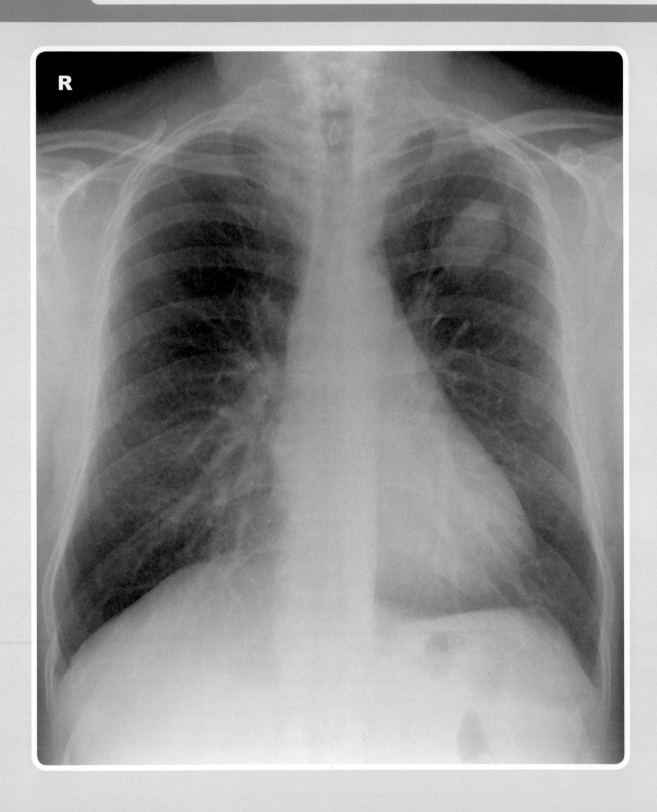

TECHNICAL INFORMATION

Patient ID: Anonymous
Projection: PA
Penetration: Adequate – vertebral bodies just visible behind heart
Inspiration: Adequate – eight anterior ribs visible
Rotation: Not rotated

● AIRWAY

The trachea is central.

● BREATHING

There is a well-defined oval opacity within the left upper zone.

The lungs are otherwise clear.

The lungs are not hyperinflated.

The pleural spaces are clear apart from mild biapical pleural thickening.

Normal pulmonary vascularity.

● CIRCULATION AND MEDIASTINUM

The heart is not enlarged.

The heart borders are clear.

The aorta appears normal.

The mediastinum is central, not widened, with clear borders.

Normal size, shape and position of both hila.

● DIAPHRAGM AND DELICATES

Normal appearance and position of the hemidiaphragms.

No pneumoperitoneum.

The imaged skeleton is intact with no fractures or destructive bony lesions visible.

The visible soft tissues are unremarkable.

● EXTRAS AND REVIEW AREAS

No vascular lines, tubes or surgical clips.
Lung apices: Mild biapical pleural thickening.
Hila: Normal.
Behind heart: Normal.
Costophrenic angles: Normal.
Below the diaphragm: Normal.

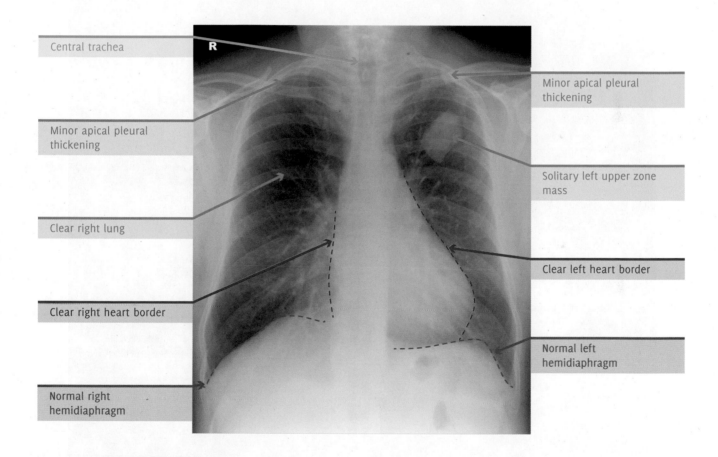

Central trachea

R

Minor apical pleural thickening

Minor apical pleural thickening

Solitary left upper zone mass

Clear right lung

Clear left heart border

Clear right heart border

Normal left hemidiaphragm

Normal right hemidiaphragm

SUMMARY, INVESTIGATIONS AND MANAGEMENT

This X-ray demonstrates a solitary mass in the left upper zone, which is highly suspicious for lung malignancy.

Initial tests will include FBC, U&Es, LFTs, bone profile and spirometry.

A staging CT chest and abdomen with IV contrast should be performed.

The patient should be referred to respiratory/oncology services for further management, which may include biopsy and MDT discussion. Treatment, which may include surgery, radiotherapy, chemotherapy or palliative treatment, will depend on the outcome of the MDT discussions, investigations and the patient's wishes. The patient's cholecystectomy should be postponed pending further investigations.

A 65-year-old female presents to ED with progressive shortness of breath. She has a history of breast cancer and is a nonsmoker. On examination, she has oxygen saturations of 99% in air and is afebrile. There is dullness to percussion and reduced air entry in the right middle and lower zones. A chest X-ray is requested to assess for possible pneumonia, collapse or effusion.

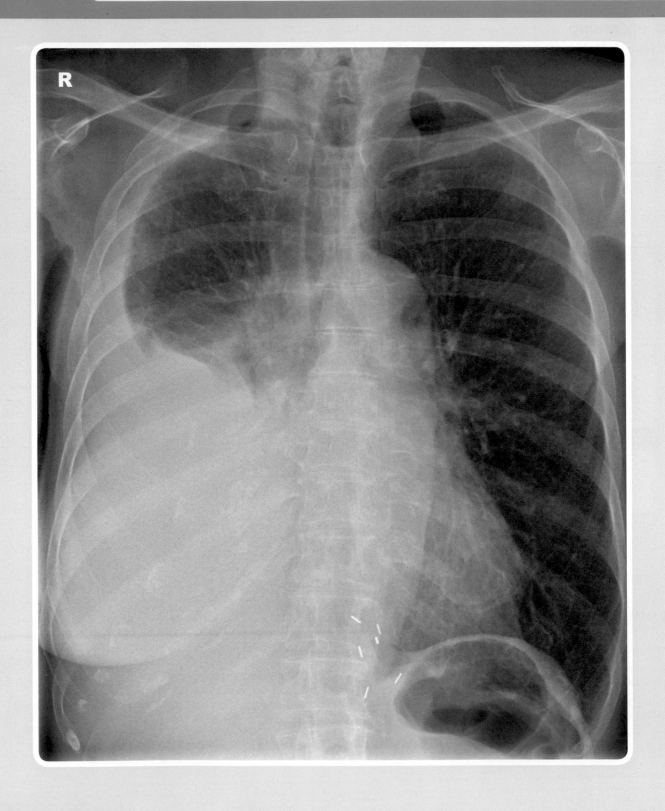

TECHNICAL INFORMATION

Patient ID: Anonymous
Projection: PA
Penetration: Adequate – vertebral bodies just visible behind heart
Inspiration: Adequate – eight anterior ribs visible
Rotation: The patient is rotated to the right

● AIRWAY

The trachea is central after factoring in patient rotation.

● BREATHING

There is homogeneous opacification over the right mid and lower zones. There is a meniscus present laterally tracking up to the right apex.

The lungs are not hyperinflated.

The left lung and pleural spaces are clear.

Normal pulmonary vascularity.

● CIRCULATION AND MEDIASTINUM

The right heart border is obscured, the heart size is therefore difficult to assess. Clear left heart border.

The aorta appears normal.

The mediastinum is central, not widened, with clear borders.

The right hilum is obscured. Normal size, shape and position of the left hilum.

● DIAPHRAGM AND DELICATES

The right hemidiaphragm is obscured. Normal position and appearance of the left hemidiaphragm.

No pneumoperitoneum.

The imaged skeleton is intact with no fractures or destructive bony lesions visible.

There has been a left-sided mastectomy. The visible soft tissues are otherwise unremarkable.

● EXTRAS AND REVIEW AREAS

Surgical clips are projected medially in the left lower zone. No vascular lines or tubes.
Lung apices: Opacification tracking up laterally to the right apex. Normal left apex.
Hila: Obscured right hilum, normal left hilum.
Behind heart: Right retrocardiac position obscured. Normal on the left.
Costophrenic angles: Obscured right costophrenic angle. Normal left costophrenic angle.
Below the diaphragm: Normal.

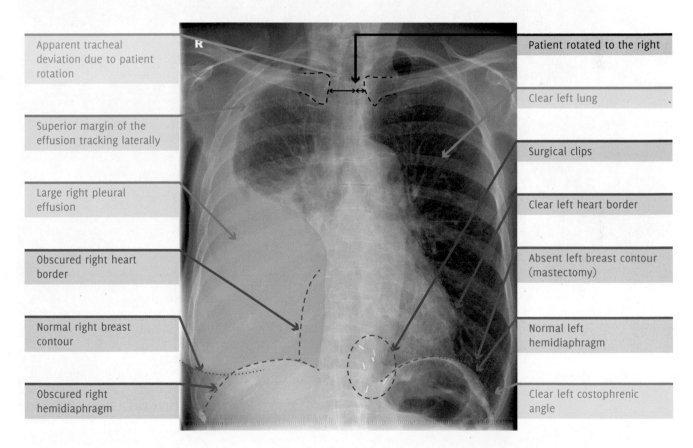

Apparent tracheal deviation due to patient rotation

Superior margin of the effusion tracking laterally

Large right pleural effusion

Obscured right heart border

Normal right breast contour

Obscured right hemidiaphragm

Patient rotated to the right

Clear left lung

Surgical clips

Clear left heart border

Absent left breast contour (mastectomy)

Normal left hemidiaphragm

Clear left costophrenic angle

SUMMARY, INVESTIGATIONS AND MANAGEMENT

This X-ray demonstrates a large right-sided pleural effusion, extending up towards the right apex. Given the previous left mastectomy, the findings are suspicious for a malignant pleural effusion. Other causes of an effusion such as infection are also possible.

Initial blood tests may include FBC, U&Es, LFTs, coagulation and CRP. An ultrasound-guided chest drain should be inserted, with pleural fluid sent for protein, albumin, glucose, microscopy, white cell count and cytology. A chest X-ray should be performed to ensure adequate positioning of the drain.

Further management will be guided by the underlying aetiology of the effusion. If this is a new finding, then the patient should undergo contrast enhanced CT of the chest, abdomen and pelvis for restaging. Referral to oncology for further management would be helpful.

A 72-year-old female currently admitted on the stroke ward has had an NG tube inserted for feeding. The nurses are unable to aspirate anything to confirm its position. She has recently suffered an ischaemic stroke. She has a past medical history of two myocardial infarctions and type II diabetes. She is a nonsmoker. On examination, she has oxygen saturations of 100% in air and is afebrile. Lungs are resonant throughout, with good bilateral air entry. A chest X-ray is requested to assess the position of the NG tube.

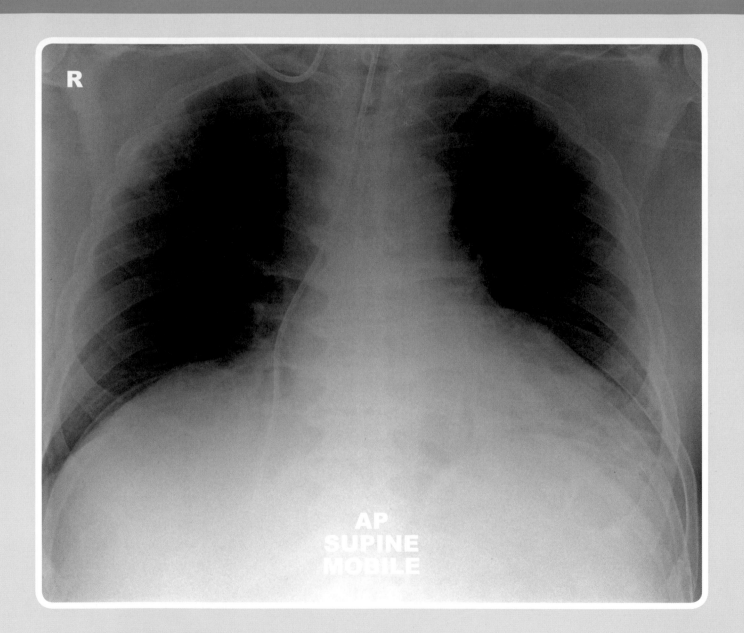

TECHNICAL INFORMATION

Patient ID: Anonymous
Projection: Portable AP supine
Penetration: Overpenetrated – vertebral bodies visible behind heart
Inspiration: Inadequate – five anterior ribs visible
Rotation: Not rotated

● AIRWAY

The trachea is central.

● BREATHING

There is minor linear atelectasis at the left costophrenic angle.

The lungs are otherwise clear.

The lungs are not hyperinflated.

The pleural spaces are clear.

Normal pulmonary vascularity.

● CIRCULATION AND MEDIASTINUM

The heart appears enlarged, although assessment of the size is difficult due to patient rotation.

The heart borders are clear.

There is mild unfolding of the thoracic aorta.

The mediastinum is central, not widened and with clear borders.

Normal size, shape and position of both hila.

● DIAPHRAGM AND DELICATES

Normal position and appearance of the hemidiaphragms.

No pneumoperitoneum, although this is difficult to assess on a supine chest X-ray.

There are multiple bridging osteophytes visible in the thoracic spine. No other bony changes.

The visible soft tissues are unremarkable.

● EXTRAS AND REVIEW AREAS

The NG tube is projected over the trachea and right main bronchus. The tip appears to be inferior to the diaphragm but on the right – it is therefore likely to be in the posterior inferior right lower lobe.
Lung apices: Normal.
Hila: Difficult to identify – no hilar mass visible.
Behind heart: Normal.
Costophrenic angles: Left basal atelectasis.
Below the diaphragm: Normal.

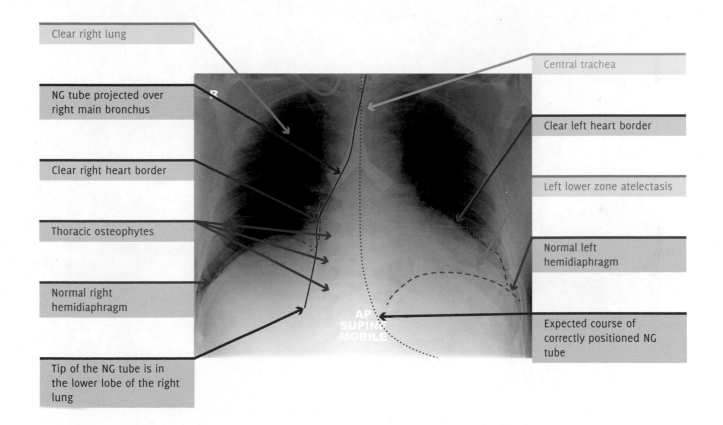

Clear right lung

NG tube projected over right main bronchus

Clear right heart border

Thoracic osteophytes

Normal right hemidiaphragm

Tip of the NG tube is in the lower lobe of the right lung

Central trachea

Clear left heart border

Left lower zone atelectasis

Normal left hemidiaphragm

Expected course of correctly positioned NG tube

SUMMARY, INVESTIGATIONS AND MANAGEMENT

This X-ray demonstrates the NG tube is misplaced in the right lower lobe. There is mild left basal atelectasis.

The NG tube needs to be removed and replaced. A repeat chest X-ray can be performed following reinsertion to confirm its position if necessary.

A 75-year-old female on the cardiology ward develops left-sided pleuritic chest pain after pacemaker insertion. She has a background of atrial fibrillation. She is a nonsmoker. On examination, she has oxygen saturations of 93% in air and is afebrile. There is increased resonance in the left upper zone, with reduced air entry. A chest X-ray is requested to assess for a possible pneumothorax.

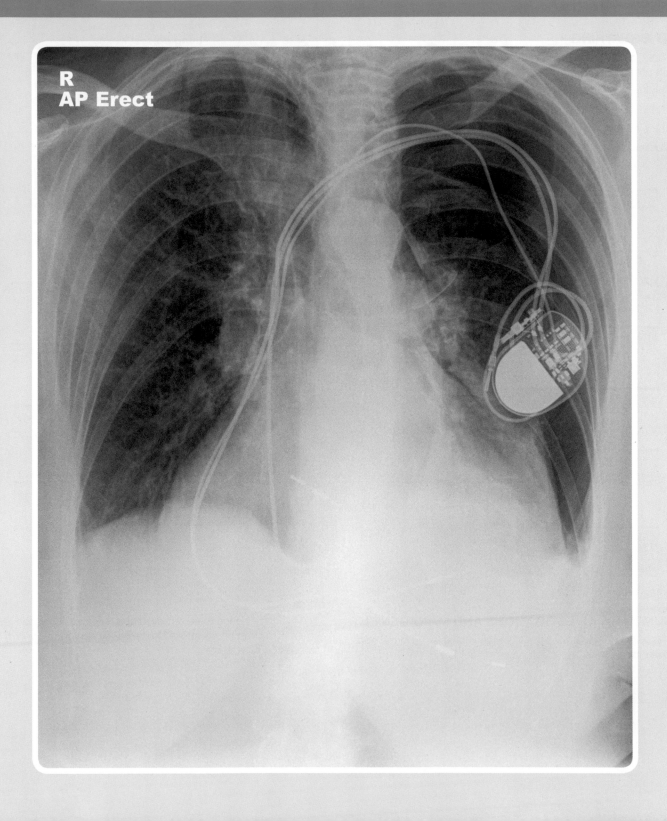

R
AP Erect

TECHNICAL INFORMATION

Patient ID: Anonymous
Projection: AP erect
Penetration: Adequate – vertebral bodies just visible behind heart
Inspiration: Limited – only five anterior ribs visible
Rotation: The patient is rotated to the left

● AIRWAY

The upper trachea is central after factoring in patient rotation. The lower trachea is displaced to the right around the aortic arch.

● BREATHING

A lung edge is visible in the left hemithorax, beyond which no lung markings are seen, consistent with a pneumothorax. There is possible left-sided retrocardic consolidation, although this may represent partially collapsed lung secondary to the pneumothorax. There is blunting of the left costophrenic angle, in keeping with a small effusion.

The right lung is not hyperexpanded.

The right pleural spaces are clear.

There is mild increased pulmonary vascularity evident in the right lung.

● CIRCULATION AND MEDIASTINUM

The heart appears enlarged, although its size cannot be accurately assessed given the AP projection and limited inspiratory achievement.

The heart borders are clear.

The aorta appears normal.

The mediastinum is displaced to the right, which is probably related to patient rotation. It is not widened, with clear borders.

Normal size, shape and position of both hila.

● DIAPHRAGM AND DELICATES

Normal appearance and position of the right hemidiaphragm. The left is difficult to identify.

No pneumoperitoneum.

The imaged skeleton is intact with no fractures or destructive bony lesions visible.

The visible soft tissues are unremarkable. Of note, there is no surgical emphysema.

● EXTRAS AND REVIEW AREAS

There is a triple-chamber pacemaker projected over the left mid zone. The tips of the pacing leads are appropriately sited, with one projected over the right atrium, one over the right ventricle and the third over the left ventricle. No vascular lines, tubes or surgical clips.
Lung apices: Left pneumothorax. Clear right apex.
Hila: Normal.
Behind heart: Normal.
Costophrenic angles: Blunted left costophrenic angle. Normal right.
Below the diaphragm: Normal.

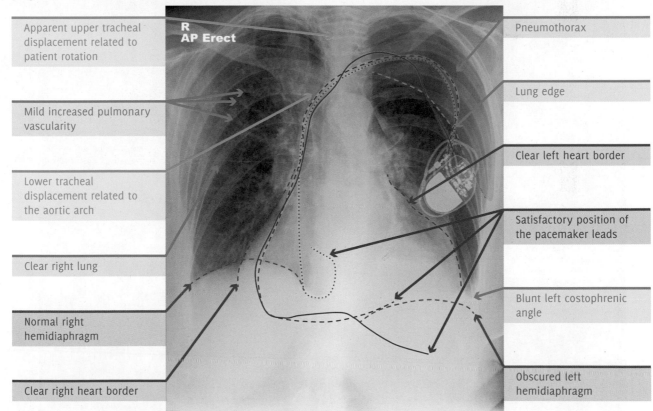

Apparent upper tracheal displacement related to patient rotation

Mild increased pulmonary vascularity

Lower tracheal displacement related to the aortic arch

Clear right lung

Normal right hemidiaphragm

Clear right heart border

R
AP Erect

Pneumothorax

Lung edge

Clear left heart border

Satisfactory position of the pacemaker leads

Blunt left costophrenic angle

Obscured left hemidiaphragm

SUMMARY, INVESTIGATIONS AND MANAGEMENT

This X-ray demonstrates a large, iatrogenic left-sided pneumothorax secondary to pacemaker insertion. The apparent mediastinal shift to the right is likely due to patient rotation; however, the patient should be assessed for clinical evidence of a tension pneumothorax. The heart appears enlarged. Although this cannot be assessed on an AP film, the patient probably has a background of heart failure given the triple-chamber pacemaker. There is mild increased

pulmonary vascularity on the right, and a small left pleural effusion, in keeping with pulmonary oedema.

Supplementary oxygen should be given.

The patient needs to be discussed with the respiratory team. Needle aspiration of the pneumothorax should be performed in the first instance. An intercostal chest drain may be required depending on the success of the aspiration. A follow-up chest X-ray is needed to ensure resolution post treatment.

An 18-year-old male presents to ED with sudden onset right-sided pleuritic chest pain and breathlessness. He has no significant past medical history and is a nonsmoker. On examination, he has oxygen saturations of 92% in air and is afebrile. HR is 90 bpm, and BP is 118/82 mmHg. There is increased resonance in the right hemithorax and reduced air entry. A chest X-ray is requested to assess for a possible pneumothorax.

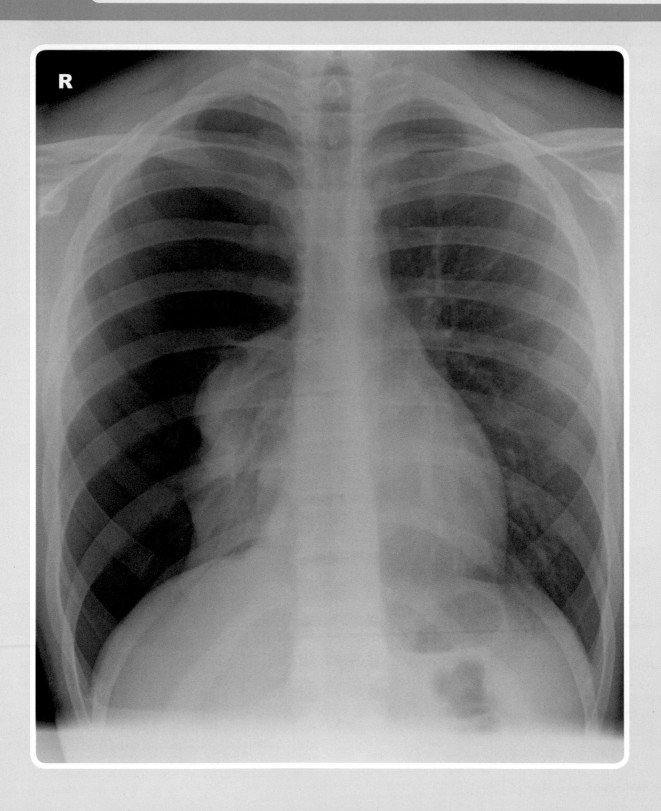

R

TECHNICAL INFORMATION

Patient ID: Anonymous
Projection: PA
Penetration: Adequate – vertebral bodies just visible behind heart
Inspiration: Adequate – seven anterior ribs visible
Rotation: Not rotated

● AIRWAY

The trachea is central.

● BREATHING

A lung edge is visible in the right hemithorax, beyond which no lung markings are seen, consistent with a large pneumothorax. The underlying right lung is almost completely collapsed (visible medially in the right mid and lower zones).

The left lung is clear, with normal expansion, clear pleural spaces and normal vascularity.

● CIRCULATION AND MEDIASTINUM

The heart is not enlarged.

The heart borders are clear.

The aorta appears normal.

The mediastinum is central, not widened, with clear borders.

The right hilum is difficult to identify because of the adjacent collapsed right lung. Normal size, shape and position of the left hilum.

● DIAPHRAGM AND DELICATES

Normal appearance and position of the hemidiaphragms.

No pneumoperitoneum.

The imaged skeleton is intact with no fractures or destructive bony lesions visible.

The visible soft tissues are unremarkable. Of note, there is no surgical emphysema.

● EXTRAS AND REVIEW AREAS

No vascular lines, tubes or surgical clips.
Lung apices: Right pneumothorax. Normal left apex.
Hila: Right is difficult to identify. Normal left hilum.
Behind heart: Normal.
Costophrenic angles: Radiolucent on right due to pneumothorax. Normal on left.
Below the diaphragm: Normal.

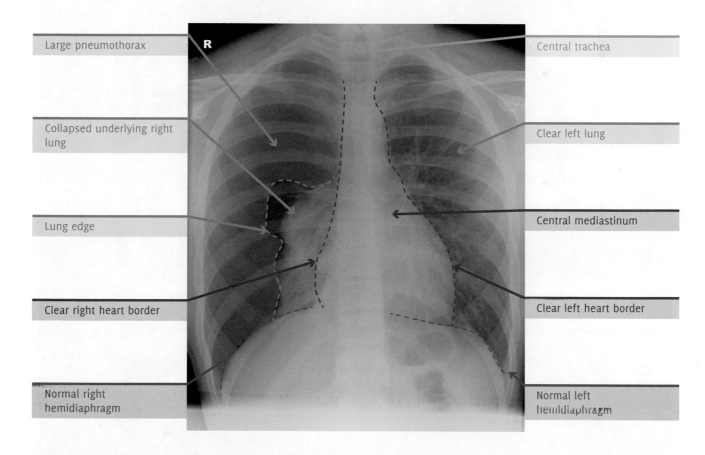

Large pneumothorax

Collapsed underlying right lung

Lung edge

Clear right heart border

Normal right hemidiaphragm

Central trachea

Clear left lung

Central mediastinum

Clear left heart border

Normal left hemidiaphragm

SUMMARY, INVESTIGATIONS AND MANAGEMENT

This X-ray demonstrates a large right-sided pneumothorax. The underlying right lung is almost completely collapsed. There is no mediastinal shift or flattening of the right hemidiaphragm to suggest a tension pneumothorax. No rib fracture is visible.

The patient should be given supplementary oxygen.

The pneumothorax will require active intervention due to its large size. Needle aspiration of the pneumothorax should be performed in the first instance. An intercostal chest drain may be required depending on the success of the aspiration.

The patient should be referred to the respiratory team, with follow-up chest X-rays performed until the pneumothorax has resolved.

An 80-year-old male on the cardiology ward develops left-sided pleuritic chest pain after pacemaker insertion. He has a background of sick sinus syndrome. He is a nonsmoker. On examination, he has oxygen saturations of 92% in air and is afebrile. There is increased resonance in the left upper zone, with reduced air entry. A chest X-ray is requested to assess for a possible pneumothorax.

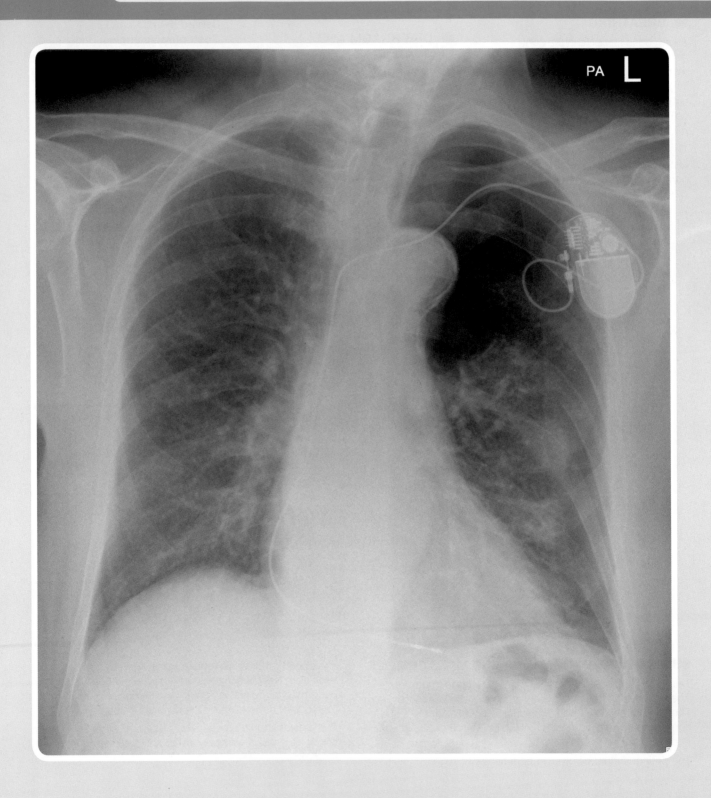

PA L

TECHNICAL INFORMATION

Patient ID: Anonymous
Projection: PA
Penetration: Adequate – vertebral bodies not clearly visible behind heart
Inspiration: Underpenetrated – seven anterior ribs visible
Rotation: The patient is rotated to the left

● AIRWAY

The trachea is central after factoring in patient rotation.

● BREATHING

A lung edge is visible in the left hemithorax, beyond which no lung markings are seen, consistent with a pneumothorax. Both lungs are otherwise clear. The right lung is not hyperinflated.

The right pleural spaces are clear.

There is normal pulmonary vascularity.

● CIRCULATION AND MEDIASTINUM

The heart is not enlarged.

The heart borders are clear.

The aorta appears normal.

The mediastinum is central, not widened, with clear borders.

Normal size, shape and position of both hila.

● DIAPHRAGM AND DELICATES

Normal appearance and position of the hemidiaphragms.

No pneumoperitoneum.

The imaged skeleton is intact with no fractures or destructive bony lesions visible.

The visible soft tissues are unremarkable. Of note, there is no surgical emphysema.

● EXTRAS AND REVIEW AREAS

A single-chamber cardiac pacemaker is projected over the upper left chest. The tip of the pacing lead is projected over the right ventricle. No vascular lines, tubes or surgical clips.
Lung apices: Left pneumothorax. Normal right apex.
Hila: Normal.
Behind heart: Normal.
Costophrenic angles: Normal.
Below the diaphragm: Normal.

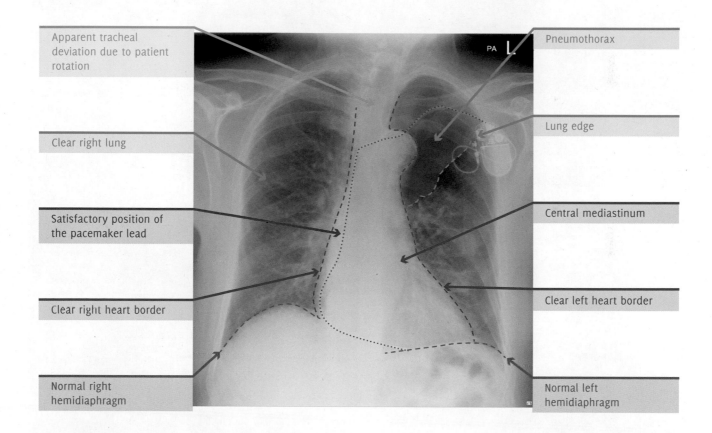

Apparent tracheal deviation due to patient rotation

Clear right lung

Satisfactory position of the pacemaker lead

Clear right heart border

Normal right hemidiaphragm

PA L

Pneumothorax

Lung edge

Central mediastinum

Clear left heart border

Normal left hemidiaphragm

SUMMARY, INVESTIGATIONS AND MANAGEMENT

This X-ray demonstrates a left-sided pneumothorax. This is likely to be an iatrogenic pneumothorax secondary to the recent pacemaker insertion. There is no mediastinal shift (allowing for patient rotation) or flattening of the left hemidiaphragm to suggest a tension pneumothorax.

Supplementary oxygen should be given.

Needle aspiration of the pneumothorax should be performed in the first instance. An intercostal chest drain may be required depending on the success of the aspiration. A follow-up chest X-ray is needed to ensure resolution posttreatment.

An 80-year-old male presents to his GP with a 2-month history of productive cough. He has a 40 pack-year smoking history. On examination, he has oxygen saturations of 100% in air and is afebrile. There are bibasal crackles in the lungs and finger clubbing. A chest X-ray is requested to assess for possible malignancy.

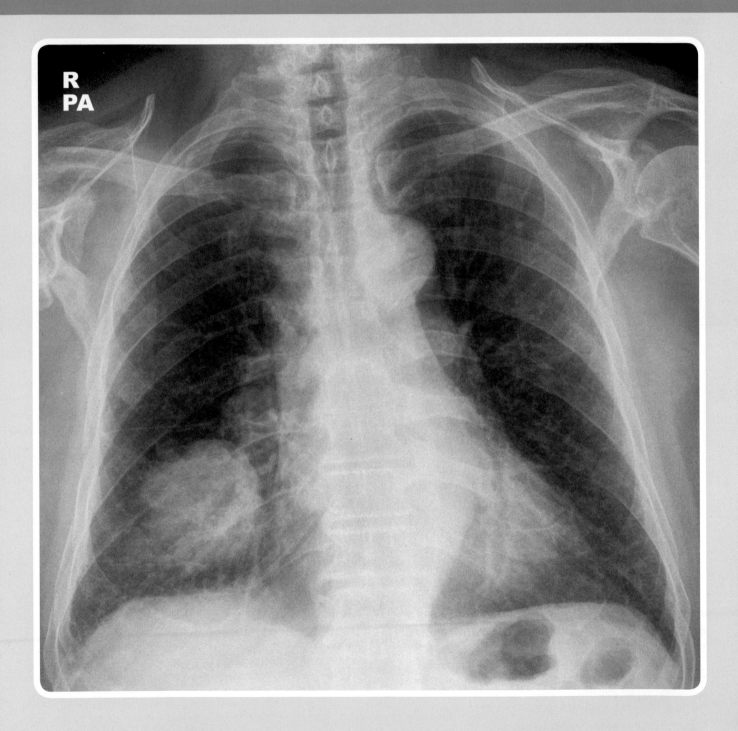

TECHNICAL INFORMATION

Patient ID: Anonymous
Projection: PA
Penetration: Adequate – vertebral bodies just visible behind heart
Inspiration: Adequate – seven anterior ribs visible
Rotation: The patient is slightly rotated to the left

● AIRWAY

The trachea is central after factoring in patient rotation.

● BREATHING

There is a large rounded mass within the right lower zone. A small dense nodule is present in the left upper zone.

The lungs are otherwise clear.

The lungs appear hyperinflated and there is coarsening of the lung markings which may represent background COPD.

The pleural spaces are clear.

Normal pulmonary vascularity.

● CIRCULATION AND MEDIASTINUM

The heart is not enlarged.

The heart borders are clear.

There is unfolding of the thoracic aorta.

The mediastinum is central, not widened, with clear borders.

The right hilum appears bulky. Normal size, shape and position of the left hilum.

● DIAPHRAGM AND DELICATES

Normal appearance and position of the hemidiaphragms.

No pneumoperitoneum.

Lateral osteophytes are present in the thoracic spine. The imaged skeleton is otherwise intact with no fracture or destructive bony lesion visible.

The visible soft tissues are unremarkable.

● EXTRAS AND REVIEW AREAS

No vascular lines, tubes or surgical clips.
Lung apices: Normal.
Hila: The right hilum appears bulky. Normal left hilum.
Behind heart: Normal.
Costophrenic angles: Normal.
Below the diaphragm: Normal.

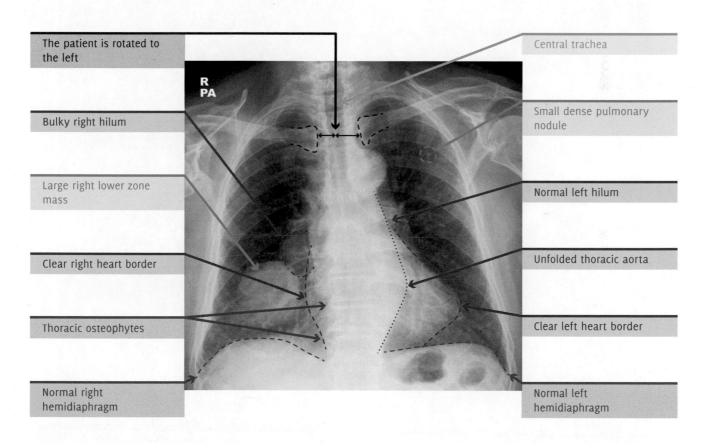

The patient is rotated to the left

Bulky right hilum

Large right lower zone mass

Clear right heart border

Thoracic osteophytes

Normal right hemidiaphragm

Central trachea

Small dense pulmonary nodule

Normal left hilum

Unfolded thoracic aorta

Clear left heart border

Normal left hemidiaphragm

R PA

SUMMARY, INVESTIGATIONS AND MANAGEMENT

This X-ray demonstrates a large mass in the right lower zone, which is highly suspicious for lung malignancy. The right hilum appears bulky, suggestive of hilar lymph node enlargement. There are background changes of COPD.

Initial tests will include FBC, U&Es, LFTs, bone profile and spirometry.

A staging CT chest and abdomen with IV contrast should be performed.

The patient should be referred to respiratory/oncology services for further management, which may include biopsy and MDT discussion. Treatment, which may include surgery, radiotherapy, chemotherapy or palliative treatment, will depend on the outcome of the MDT discussion, investigations and the patient's wishes.

An 81-year-old female presents to ED with a 2-week history of progressive shortness of breath. She also reports lethargy and weight loss. She has a 50 pack-year smoking history. On examination, she has oxygen saturations of 92% in 2 L of oxygen and is afebrile. There is scattered diffuse expiratory wheezing with reduced air entry in the right upper zone. In addition, a few crackles that quietened with deep coughing are heard in the right upper zone. A chest X-ray is requested to assess for possible pneumonia or malignancy.

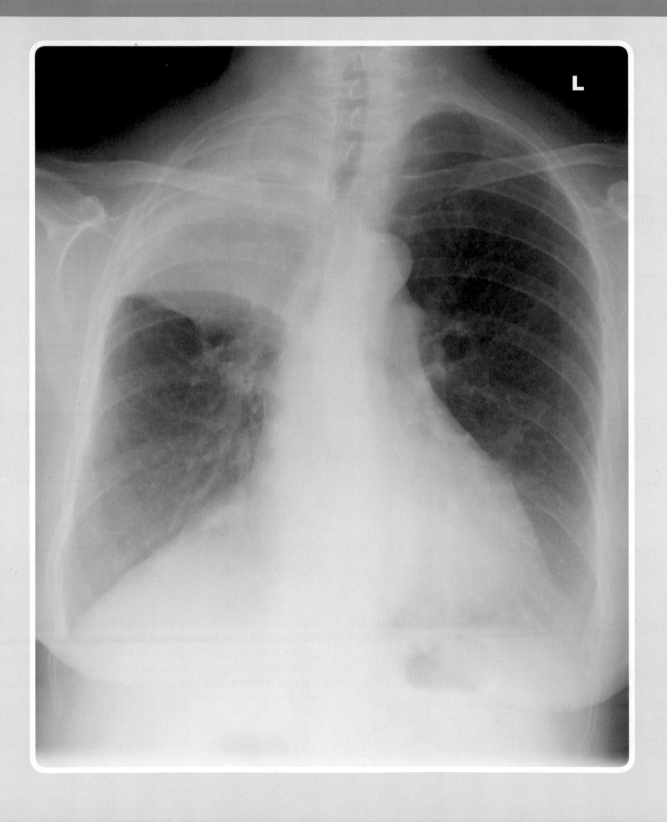

TECHNICAL INFORMATION

Patient ID: Anonymous
Projection: PA
Penetration: Underpenetrated – vertebral bodies not visible behind heart
Inspiration: Adequate – seven anterior ribs visible
Rotation: The patient is slightly rotated to the left

● AIRWAY

The trachea is deviated to the right.

● BREATHING

There is a well-defined homogeneous area of increased density in the right upper zone. It has a concave inferior border, in keeping with an elevated horizontal fissure.

The remainder of the lungs are clear. The lungs are not hyperinflated. The pleural spaces are clear.

Normal pulmonary vascularity.

● CIRCULATION AND MEDIASTINUM

The heart is not enlarged.

The heart borders are clear. There is a convex opacity at the right cardiophrenic angle consistent with an epicardial fat pad.

The aorta appears normal.

The mediastinum is central.

The right hilum is difficult to identify but appears elevated. No clear hilar mass visible. Normal size, shape and position of the left hilum.

● DIAPHRAGM AND DELICATES

The right hemidiaphragm is elevated. Its medial aspect is difficult to identify clearly due to an adjacent epicardial fat pad. Normal appearance and position of the left hemidiaphragm.

No pneumoperitoneum.

The imaged skeleton is intact with no fractures or destructive bony lesions visible.

The visible soft tissues are unremarkable.

● EXTRAS AND REVIEW AREAS

No vascular lines, tubes or surgical clips.
Lung apices: Increased density in the right upper zone. Normal left apex.
Hila: Right hilar elevation but no hilar mass visible. Normal left hilum.
Behind heart: Normal.
Costophrenic angles: Normal.
Below the diaphragm: Normal.

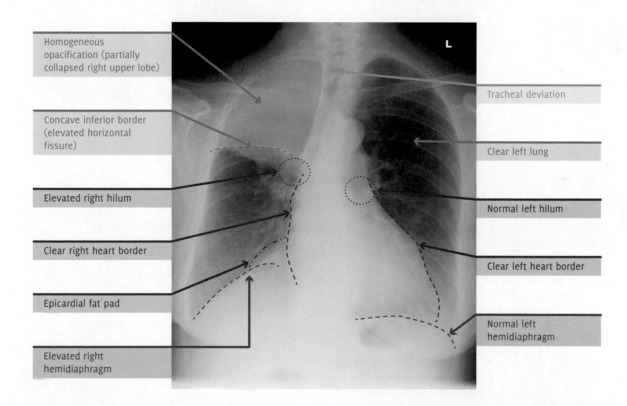

Homogeneous opacification (partially collapsed right upper lobe)

Concave inferior border (elevated horizontal fissure)

Elevated right hilum

Clear right heart border

Epicardial fat pad

Elevated right hemidiaphragm

Tracheal deviation

Clear left lung

Normal left hilum

Clear left heart border

Normal left hemidiaphragm

SUMMARY, INVESTIGATIONS AND MANAGEMENT

This X-ray demonstrates a right upper lobe collapse (homogeneous opacity in the right upper zone, concave inferior margin representing the displaced horizontal fissure) with resultant volume loss demonstrated by tracheal deviation and elevation of the right hilum and hemidiaphragm.

Given the history, the findings are suspicious for a proximal tumour compressing the right upper lobe bronchus. Other differentials include a mucus plug or an inhaled foreign body.

Supplementary oxygen should be continued.

Initial blood tests may include FBC, U&Es, LFTs, bone profile, CRP, ESR and TFTs. A CT chest with IV contrast should be performed to assess for an underlying tumour. A CT of the abdomen will usually also be acquired at the same time to enable lung cancer staging.

The patient should be referred to respiratory/oncology services for further management, which may include biopsy and MDT discussion. Treatment, which may include surgery, radiotherapy, chemotherapy or palliative treatment, will depend on the outcome of the further investigations and the patient's wishes.

An 88-year-old male presents to the ED with 3 weeks of progressive shortness of breath, cough and some haemoptysis. He has a 60 pack-year smoking history. On examination, he has oxygen saturations of 85% in air and is afebrile. There is dullness to percussion and reduced air entry in the left lower zone. A chest X-ray is requested to assess for possible pneumonia or malignancy.

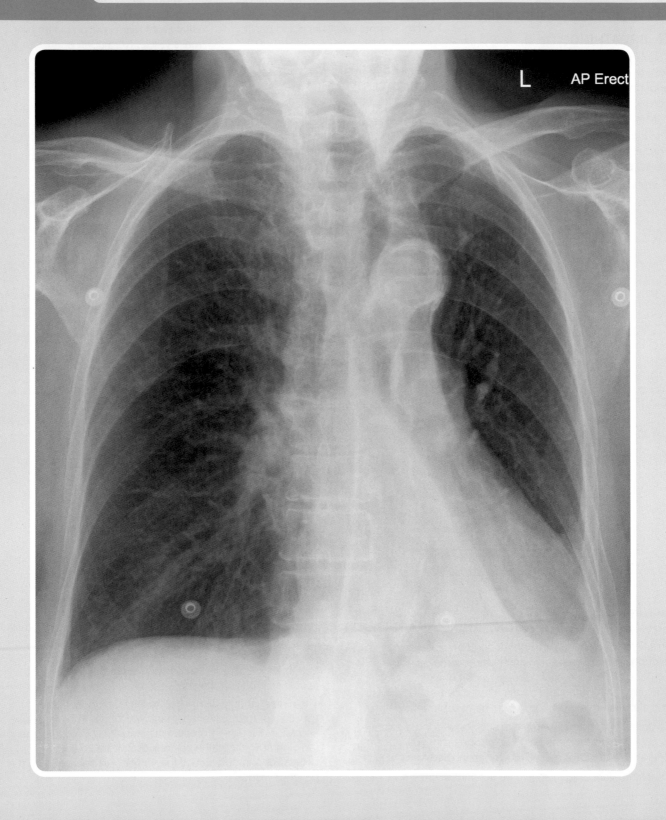

L   AP Erect

TECHNICAL INFORMATION

Patient ID: Anonymous
Projection: AP
Penetration: Adequate – vertebral bodies just visible behind heart
Inspiration: Adequate – six anterior ribs visible
Rotation: The patient is slightly rotated to the left

● AIRWAY

The trachea is deviated to the left, even when allowing for the patient rotation.

● BREATHING

The lungs appear hyperinflated with coarsening of the lung markings.

There is an abnormal triangular opacity projected over the medial aspect of the left middle and lower zones in keeping with the sail sign.

The right lung and pleural spaces are clear.

Normal pulmonary vascularity.

● CIRCULATION AND MEDIASTINUM

The heart does not appear enlarged, although its size cannot be accurately assessed on an AP X-ray.

There is an apparent double left heart border. The right heart border is difficult to assess as it is projected over the thoracic spine, but appears clear.

The descending thoracic aortic contour is not visible.

The mediastinum is displaced to the left.

Normal size and shape of both hila. There is mild depression of the left hilum.

● DIAPHRAGM AND DELICATES

The left hemidiaphragm is partially obscured indicating left lower lobe pathology. The right hemidiaphragm is flattened, in keeping with lung hyperinflation.

No pneumoperitoneum.

The imaged skeleton is intact with no fractures or destructive bony lesions visible.

The visible soft tissues are unremarkable.

● EXTRAS AND REVIEW AREAS

ECG clips in situ.

No vascular lines, tubes or surgical clips.
Lung apices: Normal.
Hila: Left hilum is depressed. Normal right hilum.
Behind heart: Sail sign with left double cardiac contour. Loss of outline of the descending thoracic aorta.
Costophrenic angles: Normal.
Below the diaphragm: Normal.

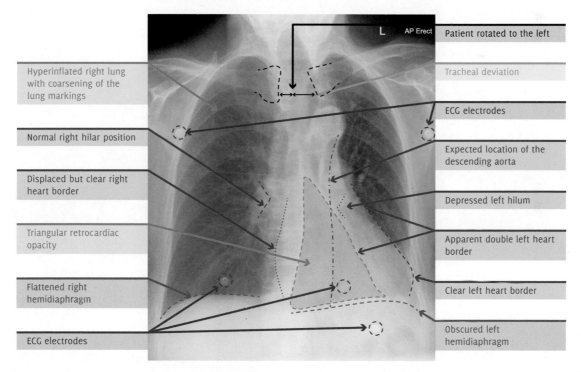

- L AP Erect
- Patient rotated to the left
- Hyperinflated right lung with coarsening of the lung markings
- Tracheal deviation
- ECG electrodes
- Normal right hilar position
- Expected location of the descending aorta
- Displaced but clear right heart border
- Depressed left hilum
- Triangular retrocardiac opacity
- Apparent double left heart border
- Flattened right hemidiaphragm
- Clear left heart border
- ECG electrodes
- Obscured left hemidiaphragm

SUMMARY, INVESTIGATIONS AND MANAGEMENT

This X-ray demonstrates a left lower lobe collapse (sail sign, apparent double left heart border and loss of descending aortic outline). Resultant volume loss in the left hemithorax is indicated by mediastinal deviation and depression of the left hilum.

Coarsening of the lung markings and hyperinflation of the right lung are in keeping with COPD.

Given the strong smoking history combined with 3 weeks of progressive symptoms, a proximal obstructing mass (tumour or hilar lymph node) is the most likely cause of the lobar collapse. Other differentials include a mucus plug or an inhaled foreign body.

Supplementary oxygen should be given.

Initial blood tests may include FBC, U&Es, LFTs, bone profile, CRP, ESR and TFTs. CT chest with IV contrast to assess for a proximal obstructing lesion, such as a tumour, should be performed. A CT of the abdomen will usually also be acquired at the same time to enable lung cancer staging.

The patient should be referred to respiratory/oncology services for further management, which may include biopsy and MDT discussion. Treatment, which may include surgery, radiotherapy, chemotherapy or palliative treatment, will depend on the outcome of the MDT investigations and the patient's wishes.

INTERMEDIATE CASES

A 75-year-old female presents to ED with increasing confusion, a cough that has lasted 2 weeks and increasing shortness of breath. There is no significant past medical history and she is a nonsmoker. On examination, she has oxygen saturations of 85% in air and is afebrile. There is dullness to percussion and reduced air entry at both lung bases. A chest X-ray is performed to assess for possible collapse, pneumonia or effusions.

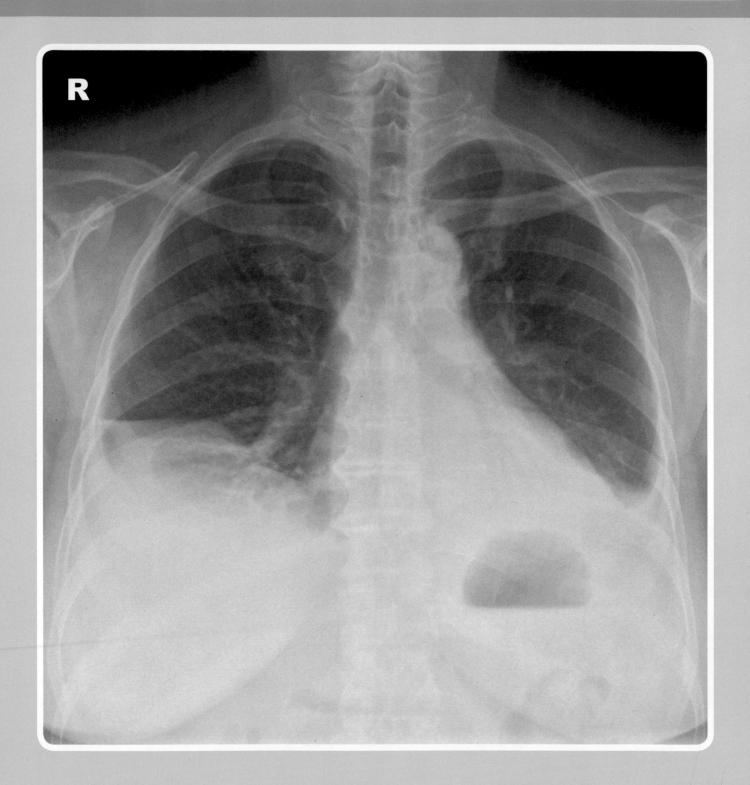

TECHNICAL INFORMATION

Patient ID: Anonymous
Projection: PA
Penetration: Adequate – vertebral bodies just visible behind heart
Inspiration: Limited – five anterior ribs visible
Rotation: The patient is slightly rotated to the right

● AIRWAY

The trachea is central after factoring in patient rotation.

● BREATHING

There is heterogeneous left retrocardiac opacification with air bronchograms, in keeping with consolidation. Further consolidation is visible at the right base. The remainder of the lungs are clear. The lungs are not hyperinflated.

There is blunting of both costophrenic angles in keeping with small pleural effusions.

Normal pulmonary vascularity.

● CIRCULATION AND MEDIASTINUM

The heart is not enlarged.

The heart borders are clear.

The aorta appears normal.

The mediastinum is central, not widened, with clear borders.

Normal size, shape and position of both hila.

● DIAPHRAGM AND DELICATES

The left hemidiaphragm and the lateral aspect of the right hemidiaphragm are obscured. Normal appearance of the medial aspect of the right hemidiaphragm.

No pneumoperitoneum.

There are osteophytes visible within the thoracic spine. The imaged skeleton is otherwise intact with no fractures or destructive bony lesions visible.

The visible soft tissues are unremarkable.

● EXTRAS AND REVIEW AREAS

No vascular lines, tubes or surgical clips.
Lung apices: Normal.
Hila: Normal.
Behind heart: Left retrocardiac consolidation.
Costophrenic angles: Bilateral blunting of the costophrenic angles.
Below the diaphragm: Normal.

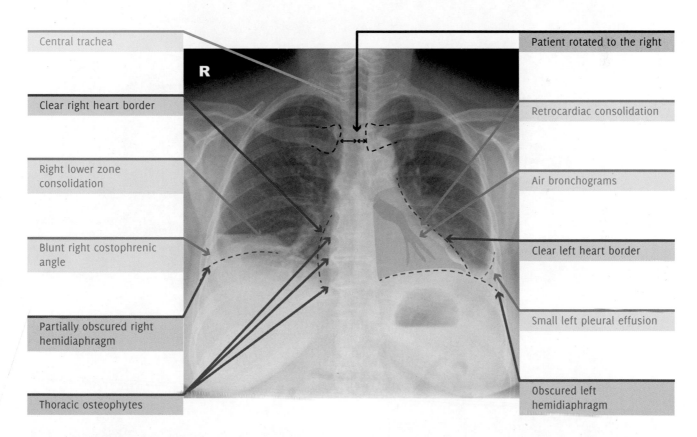

Labels (left)	Labels (right)
Central trachea	Patient rotated to the right
Clear right heart border	Retrocardiac consolidation
Right lower zone consolidation	Air bronchograms
Blunt right costophrenic angle	Clear left heart border
Partially obscured right hemidiaphragm	Small left pleural effusion
Thoracic osteophytes	Obscured left hemidiaphragm

SUMMARY, INVESTIGATIONS AND MANAGEMENT

This X-ray demonstrates left retrocardiac consolidation obscuring the left hemidiaphragm, consistent with left lower lobe pneumonia. The lateral aspect of the right hemidiaphragm is obscured by right lower lobe pneumonia. There are small bilateral pleural effusions.

Supplementary oxygen should be given. Initial blood tests may include FBC, U&Es, CRP and blood cultures. A sputum culture may also be obtained.

The patient should be treated with appropriate antibiotics for community-acquired pneumonia, and a follow-up chest X-ray performed in 4 to 6 weeks to ensure resolution. The antibiotics may be oral or intravenous depending on the severity of pneumonia (CURB-65).

Ultrasound could be used to further assess the volume of the pleural effusion, particularly if a diagnostic pleural aspiration is being considered.

A 65-year-old female presents to her GP with worsening shortness of breath. She has a 30 pack-year smoking history and has a background of recurrent pneumonia. On examination, she is pyrexial (38.5°C), and her oxygen saturations are 98% in air. There is reduced air entry in the right mid-lower zone, with dullness to percussion and occasional crackles. A chest X-ray is requested to assess for possible malignancy, collapse or consolidation.

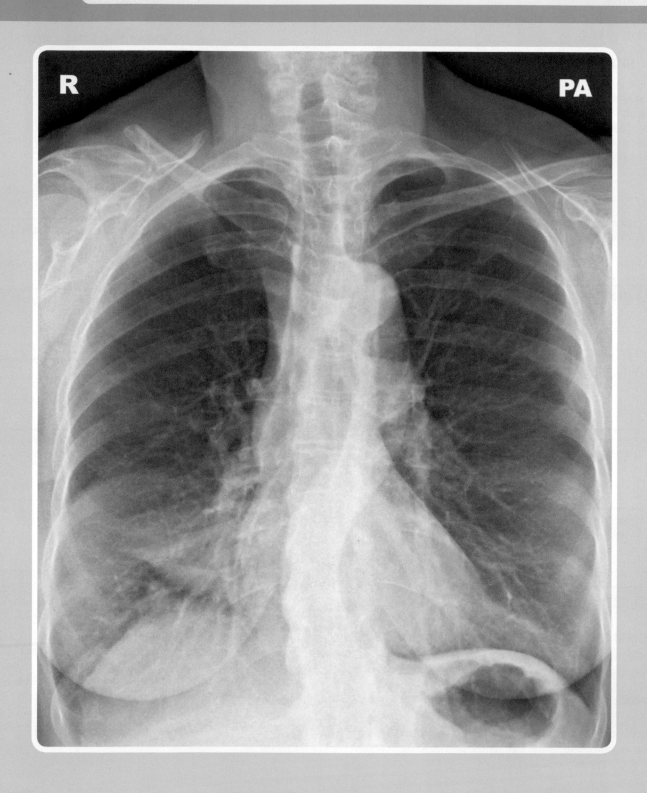

TECHNICAL INFORMATION

Patient ID: Anonymous
Projection: PA
Penetration: Adequate – vertebral bodies just visible behind heart
Inspiration: Adequate – eight anterior ribs visible
Rotation: The patient is rotated to the right

● AIRWAY

The trachea is central after factoring in patient rotation.

● BREATHING

There is a triangular area of opacification medially in the right lower zone adjacent to the right heart border. The horizontal fissure is not visible.

The remainder of the lungs are clear.

The lungs are not hyperinflated.

The pleural spaces are clear.

Normal pulmonary vascularity.

● CIRCULATION AND MEDIASTINUM

The heart is not enlarged.

The right heart border is slightly indistinct. The left heart border is normal.

The descending aorta is unfolded.

The mediastinum is central.

Normal size, shape and position of both hila.

● DIAPHRAGM AND DELICATES

Normal appearance and position of the hemidiaphragms.

No pneumoperitoneum.

There is an old displaced fracture of the distal right clavicle and an old fracture of the left 4th rib posteriorly. No other bony changes.

The visible soft tissues are unremarkable.

● EXTRAS AND REVIEW AREAS

No vascular lines, tubes or surgical clips.
Lung apices: Normal.
Hila: Normal.
Behind heart: Normal.
Costophrenic angles: Normal.
Below the diaphragm: Normal.

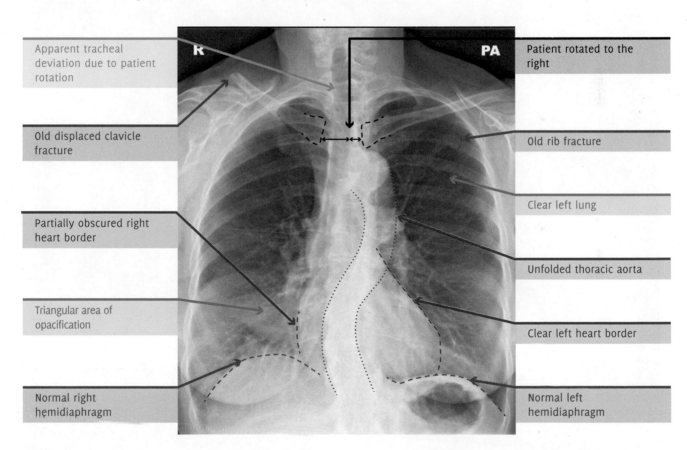

Apparent tracheal deviation due to patient rotation

Old displaced clavicle fracture

Partially obscured right heart border

Triangular area of opacification

Normal right hemidiaphragm

R   PA

Patient rotated to the right

Old rib fracture

Clear left lung

Unfolded thoracic aorta

Clear left heart border

Normal left hemidiaphragm

SUMMARY, INVESTIGATIONS AND MANAGEMENT

This X-ray demonstrates opacification medially in the right mid zone obscuring the right heart border. There is no definite volume loss visible.

The most likely differentials are right middle lobe pneumonia or collapse.

Initial blood tests may include FBC, U&Es, LFTs, bone profile, ESR and CRP.

Previous imaging should be reviewed to determine if this is a new finding. A CT of the chest would help differentiate between collapse and pneumonia and could demonstrate an underlying cause.

The management depends on the CT findings, although respiratory referral would be helpful. Appropriate antibiotics should be given to treat a community-acquired pneumonia, which may be oral or intravenous depending on the severity of pneumonia (CURB-65), with a follow-up chest X-ray to ensure resolution.

A 57-year-old female has had a PICC inserted in her right arm for long-term intravenous antibiotics (she has a persistent infected ulcer). She has a past medical history of multiple myeloma. She is a nonsmoker. On examination, she has oxygen saturations of 100% in air and is afebrile. Lungs are resonant throughout, with good bilateral air entry. A routine postprocedure chest X-ray is requested to assess PICC position.

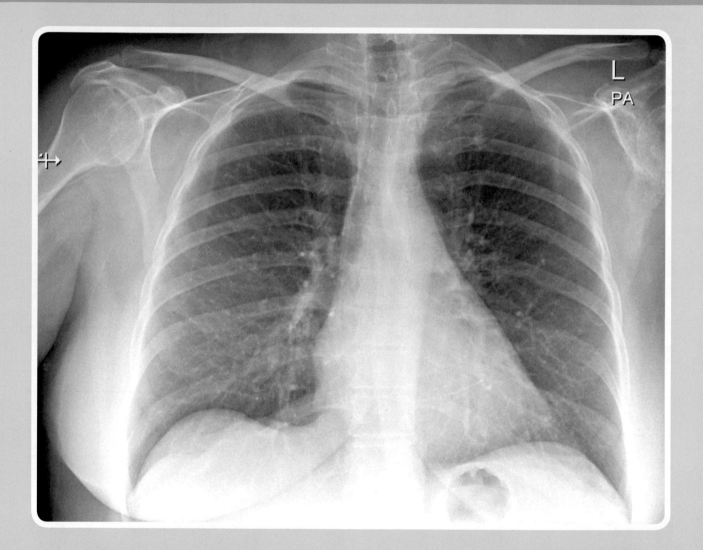

TECHNICAL INFORMATION

Patient ID: Anonymous
Projection: PA
Penetration: Adequate – vertebral bodies just visible behind heart
Inspiration: Adequate – seven anterior ribs visible
Rotation: The patient is rotated slightly to the right

● AIRWAY

The trachea is central after factoring in patient rotation.

● BREATHING

The lungs are clear.

The lungs are not hyperinflated.

The pleural spaces are clear. No pneumothorax.

Normal pulmonary vascularity.

● CIRCULATION AND MEDIASTINUM

The heart is not enlarged.

The heart borders are clear.

The aorta appears normal.

The mediastinum is central, not widened, with clear borders.

Normal size, shape and position of both hila.

● DIAPHRAGM AND DELICATES

Normal position and appearance of the diaphragm.

No pneumoperitoneum.

There is a partially imaged patchy sclerotic/lucent abnormality of the left glenoid. No fractures or other bony changes.

The visible soft tissues are unremarkable.

● EXTRAS AND REVIEW AREAS

The tip of the right PICC is projected over the right ventricle.
Lung apices: Normal.
Hila: Normal.
Behind heart: Tip of the misplaced right PICC.
Costophrenic angles: Normal.
Below the diaphragm: Normal.

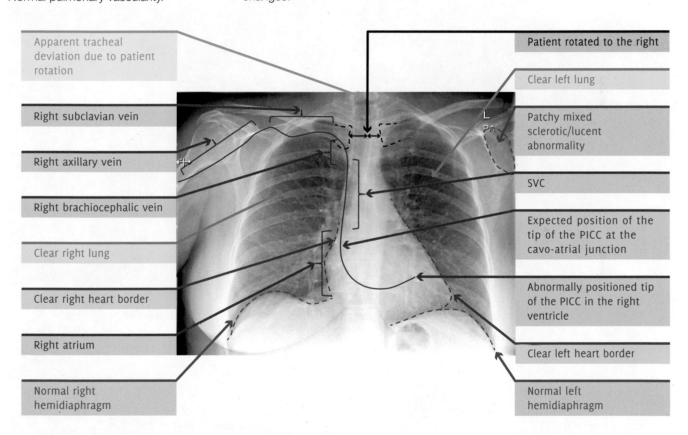

Apparent tracheal deviation due to patient rotation

Right subclavian vein

Right axillary vein

Right brachiocephalic vein

Clear right lung

Clear right heart border

Right atrium

Normal right hemidiaphragm

Patient rotated to the right

Clear left lung

Patchy mixed sclerotic/lucent abnormality

SVC

Expected position of the tip of the PICC at the cavo-atrial junction

Abnormally positioned tip of the PICC in the right ventricle

Clear left heart border

Normal left hemidiaphragm

SUMMARY, INVESTIGATIONS AND MANAGEMENT

This X-ray demonstrates the right PICC line is misplaced, with its tip in the right ventricle. In the context of myeloma, the left glenoid mixed sclerotic/lucent lesion may represent a plasmacytoma.

The right PICC should be resited (i.e. withdrawn by approximately 10 cm) and then reimaged.

Previous imaging should be reviewed to identify whether the left glenoid lesion is new or old, and any concerns should be discussed with the haematology team.

A 52-year-old male presents to ED with worsening shortness of breath. He has known inoperable small-cell lung carcinoma, having had palliative radiotherapy. He has a 60 pack-year smoking history. On examination, he has oxygen saturations of 83% in air. He is apyrexial and has a respiratory rate of 26. There is reduced air entry throughout the left lung, as well as dullness to percussion and reduced lung expansion. A chest X-ray is requested to assess for progression of the known lung tumour and possible secondary complications such as collapse or consolidation.

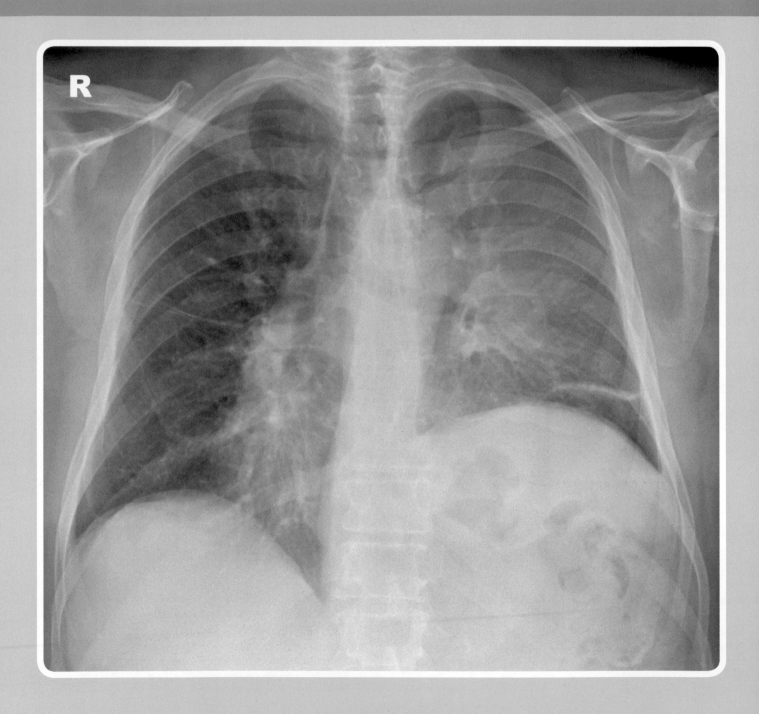

R

TECHNICAL INFORMATION

Patient ID: Anonymous
Projection: PA
Penetration: Adequate – vertebral bodies just visible behind heart
Inspiration: Adequate – six anterior ribs visible
Rotation: The patient is rotated to the right

● AIRWAY

The trachea is central after factoring in patient rotation.

● BREATHING

There is a hazy, veil-like opacity in the left hemithorax. A linear opacity is present in the left lower zone, consistent with atelectasis. There is left-sided volume loss.

The right lung is clear and not hyperinflated.

The pleural spaces are clear.

Normal pulmonary vascularity.

● CIRCULATION AND MEDIASTINUM

The heart size and cardiomediastinal contours are difficult to assess due to patient rotation.

The mediastinum is projected to the right, which is probably due to patient rotation. The aorta appears normal.

There is a rounded mass projected over the left hilum. The hilum itself is normally positioned. The right hilum appears bulky and abnormally dense, but in a normal position.

● DIAPHRAGM AND DELICATES

The left hemidiaphragm has a normal curvature but is markedly elevated.

Normal position and appearance of the right hemidiaphragm.

No pneumoperitoneum.

The imaged skeleton is intact with no fractures or destructive bony lesions visible.

The visible soft tissues are unremarkable.

● EXTRAS AND REVIEW AREAS

No vascular lines, tubes or surgical clips.
Lung apices: Left apical opacification. Normal right apex.
Hila: Left hilar mass. Bulky, dense right hilum.
Behind heart: Normal.
Costophrenic angles: Normal.
Below the diaphragm: Normal.

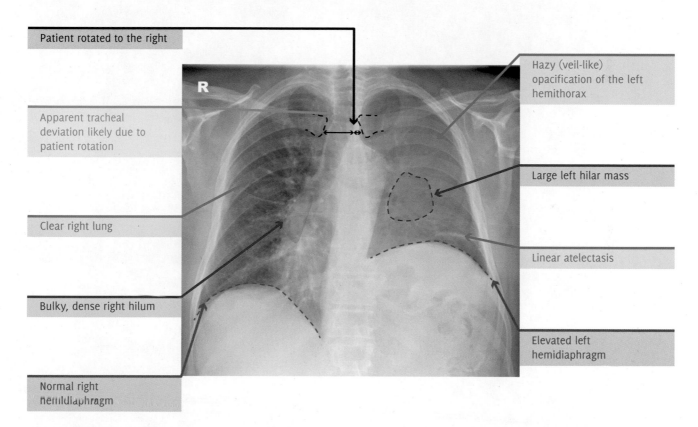

Patient rotated to the right

Apparent tracheal deviation likely due to patient rotation

Clear right lung

Bulky, dense right hilum

Normal right hemidiaphragm

Hazy (veil-like) opacification of the left hemithorax

Large left hilar mass

Linear atelectasis

Elevated left hemidiaphragm

SUMMARY, INVESTIGATIONS AND MANAGEMENT

This X-ray demonstrates a left upper lobe collapse (veil like opacity of the left hemithorax) likely secondary to the left hilar mass. There is associated volume loss demonstrated by the markedly elevated left hemidiaphragm. The right hilum is also abnormal. The apparent mediastinal shift to the right is probably due to patient rotation.

The most likely cause of the collapse is secondary to the left hilar mass. Other differentials for collapse, such as mucous plugging and an inhaled foreign body, are unlikely.

Supplementary oxygen should be given.

Initial blood tests may include FBC, U&Es, LFTs, bone profile and CRP. The X-ray should be compared with previous imaging to assess for progression. An up-to-date CT chest and abdomen with IV contrast may be needed for further assessment/restaging.

Discussion with respiratory and oncology for further palliative treatment will be necessary.

A 30-year-old female presents to the haematology ward because her Hickman line will no longer flush or aspirate. She has a history of leukaemia. She is a nonsmoker. On examination, she has oxygen saturations of 100% in air and is afebrile. Lungs are resonant throughout, with good bilateral air entry. A chest X-ray is requested to assess the Hickman line position.

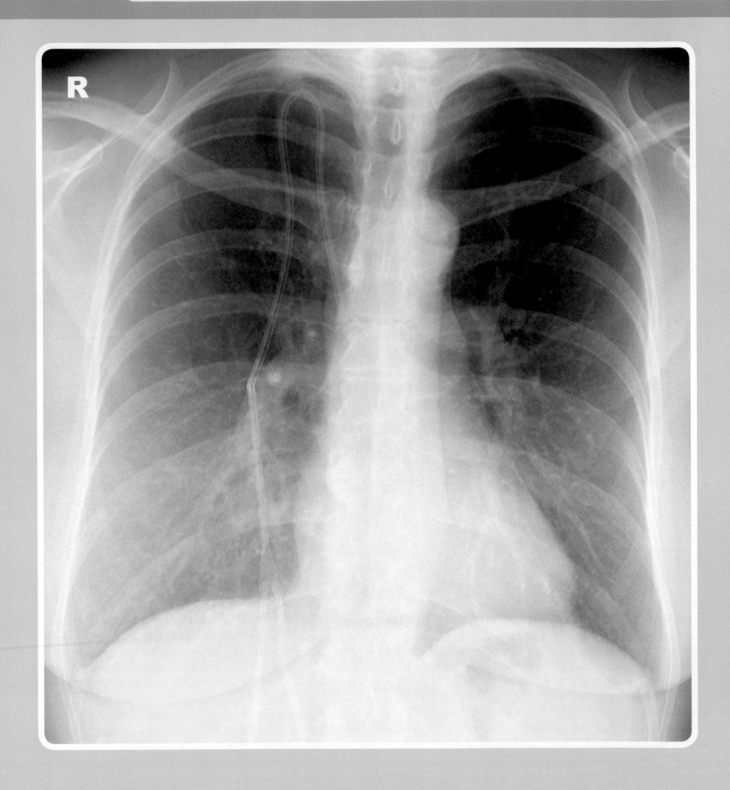

TECHNICAL INFORMATION

Patient ID: Anonymous
Projection: PA
Penetration: Adequate – vertebral bodies just visible behind heart
Inspiration: Adequate – six anterior ribs visible
Rotation: Not rotated

● AIRWAY

The trachea is central.

● BREATHING

The lungs are clear.

The lungs are not hyperinflated.

The pleural spaces are clear.

Normal pulmonary vascularity.

● CIRCULATION AND MEDIASTINUM

The heart is not enlarged.

The heart borders are clear.

The aorta appears normal.

The mediastinum is central, not widened, with clear borders.

Normal size, shape and position of both hila.

● DIAPHRAGM AND DELICATES

Normal position and appearance of the diaphragm.

No pneumoperitoneum.

The imaged skeleton is intact with no fractures or destructive bony lesions visible.

The visible soft tissues are unremarkable.

● EXTRAS AND REVIEW AREAS

A tunnelled right internal jugular (Hickman) line is visible. Its tip is appropriately sited, projected over the level of the mid superior vena cava. The line is kinked at the cutaneous entry site. The apex of the line (between the tunnelled portion and the intravenous portion) is rather tight. Careful inspection of this region reveals a fracture of the inferior wall of the line at its apex, just proximal to the site of entry into the right internal jugular vein.

Lung apices: Normal.
Hila: Normal.
Behind heart: Normal.
Costophrenic angles: Normal.
Below the diaphragm: Normal.

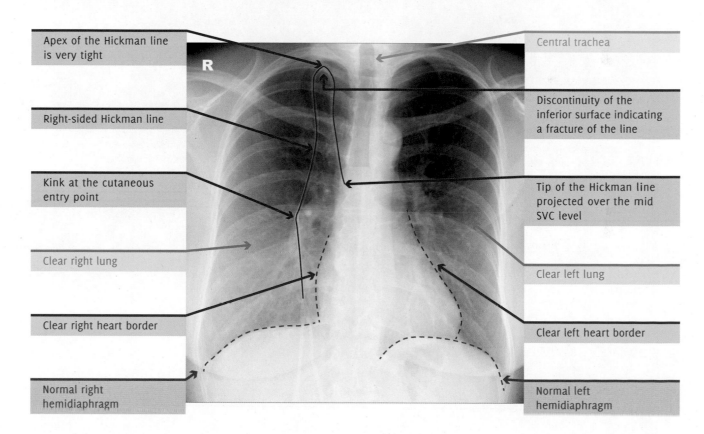

Apex of the Hickman line is very tight

Right-sided Hickman line

Kink at the cutaneous entry point

Clear right lung

Clear right heart border

Normal right hemidiaphragm

Central trachea

Discontinuity of the inferior surface indicating a fracture of the line

Tip of the Hickman line projected over the mid SVC level

Clear left lung

Clear left heart border

Normal left hemidiaphragm

SUMMARY, INVESTIGATIONS AND MANAGEMENT

This X-ray demonstrates a fracture of the apex of the right-sided Hickman line. There is also a kink at the cutaneous entry point.

The patient should be discussed with interventional radiology. A linogram (where contrast is injected through the line under fluoroscopy) may be performed to assess the Hickman line in more detail. However, it will likely need removing and replacing.

A 24-year-old female presents to her GP for a medical assessment as part of a visa application. She is asymptomatic. There is no significant past medical history. She is a nonsmoker. On examination, she has oxygen saturations of 100% in air and is afebrile. Lungs are resonant throughout, with good air entry bilaterally. A chest X-ray to assess for TB is requested as part of the visa application.

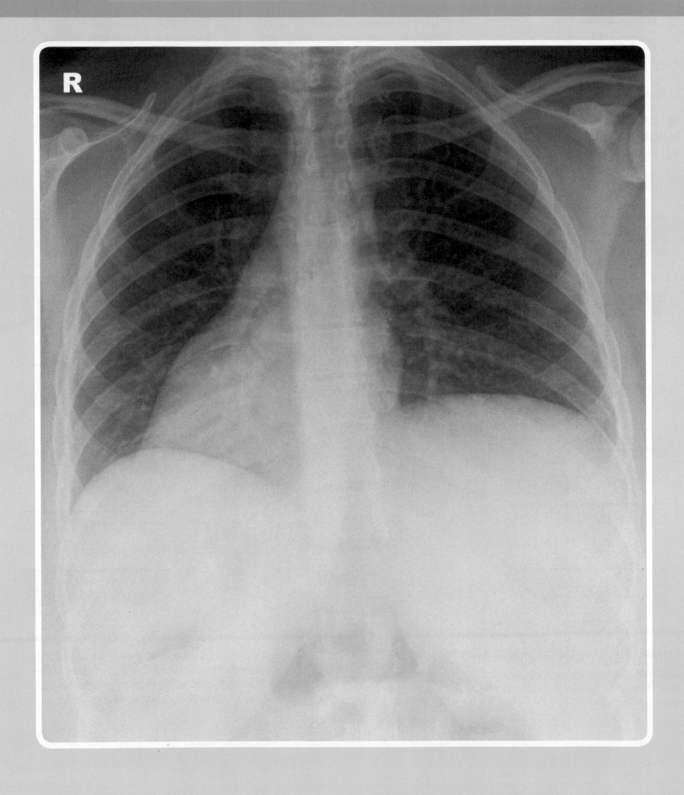

TECHNICAL INFORMATION

Patient ID: Anonymous
Projection: PA
Penetration: Adequate – vertebral bodies just visible behind heart
Inspiration: Adequate – six anterior ribs visible
Rotation: The patient is rotated to the left

● AIRWAY

The trachea is central after factoring in patient rotation.

● BREATHING

The lungs are clear.

The lungs are not hyperinflated.

The pleural spaces are clear.

Normal pulmonary vascularity.

● CIRCULATION AND MEDIASTINUM

The heart appears as a mirror image, located in the right hemithorax with a right-sided cardiac apex (dextrocardia).

The heart is not enlarged.

The heart borders are clear.

The aortic knuckle is difficult to identify but it is likely to also be right-sided as the descending aortic contour is right-sided.

The mediastinum is central, not widened, with clear borders.

Normal size, shape and position of both hila.

● DIAPHRAGM AND DELICATES

The left hemidiaphragm is higher than the right, consistent with a left-sided

liver. The gastric bubble appears more to the right of the midline.

No pneumoperitoneum.

The imaged skeleton is intact with no fractures or destructive bony lesions visible.

The visible soft tissues are unremarkable.

● EXTRAS AND REVIEW AREAS

No vascular lines, tubes or surgical clips.
Lung apices: Normal.
Hila: Normal.
Behind heart: Normal.
Costophrenic angles: Normal.
Below the diaphragm: Abdominal situs inversus.

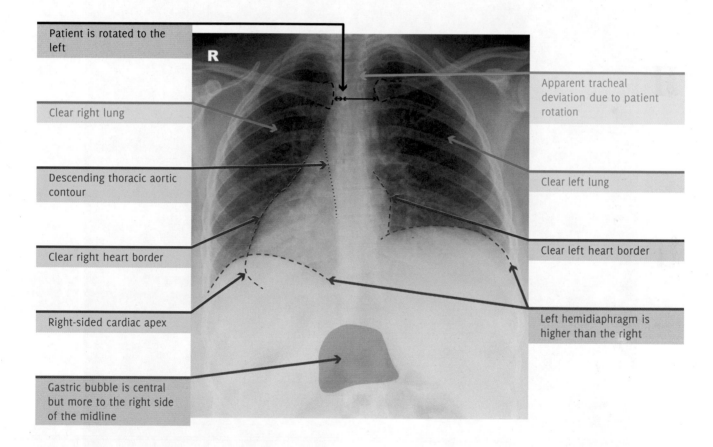

Patient is rotated to the left

R

Clear right lung

Descending thoracic aortic contour

Clear right heart border

Right-sided cardiac apex

Gastric bubble is central but more to the right side of the midline

Apparent tracheal deviation due to patient rotation

Clear left lung

Clear left heart border

Left hemidiaphragm is higher than the right

SUMMARY, INVESTIGATIONS AND MANAGEMENT

This X-ray demonstrates dextrocardia (the heart appears as a mirror image on the right side) with probable situs inversus (the abdominal organs such as the liver and stomach are mirrored). It is otherwise a normal X-ray with no evidence of pulmonary TB.

The patient will need to be clinically assessed for possible primary ciliary dyskinesia or heart defects. However, no specific investigation or treatment is required.

A 33-year-old female presents to ED with haemoptysis, chest pain and shortness of breath. She has recently returned from America. She is a nonsmoker. On examination, she has oxygen saturations of 95% in air and is afebrile. Her RR is 30 and HR is 85 bpm. Lungs are resonant throughout, with good bilateral air entry. A chest X-ray is requested to assess for possible pulmonary embolism or pneumonia.

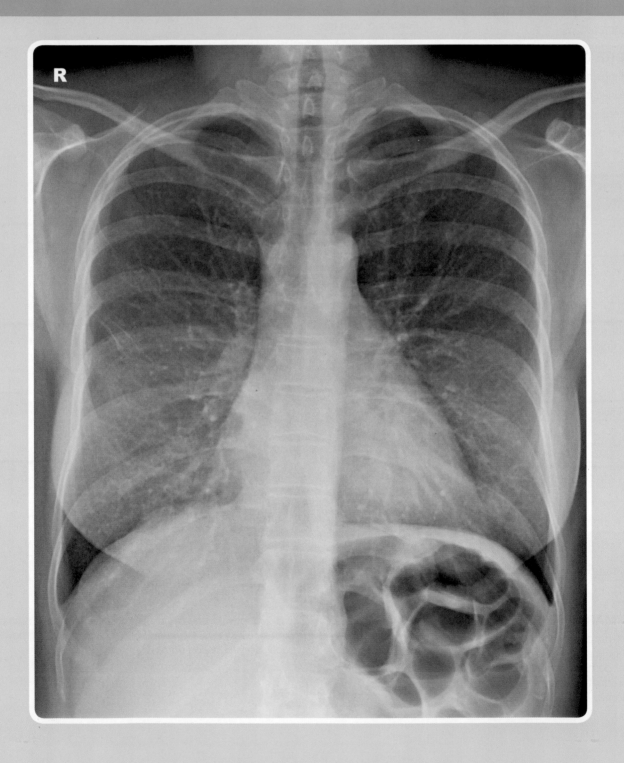

TECHNICAL INFORMATION

Patient ID: Anonymous
Projection: PA
Penetration: Adequate – vertebral bodies just visible behind heart
Inspiration: Adequate – six anterior ribs visible
Rotation: Not rotated

● AIRWAY

The trachea is central.

● BREATHING

There is increased symmetrical circular opacification in both mid and lower zones, extending below the diaphragm and lateral to the rib cage.

The underlying lungs are clear.

The lungs are not hyperinflated.

The pleural spaces are clear.

Normal pulmonary vascularity.

● CIRCULATION AND MEDIASTINUM

The heart is not enlarged.

The heart borders are clear.

The aorta appears normal.

The mediastinum is central, not widened, with clear borders.

Normal size, shape and position of both hila.

● DIAPHRAGM AND DELICATES

Normal appearance and position of the hemidiaphragms.

No pneumoperitoneum.

The imaged skeleton is intact with no fractures or destructive bony lesions visible.

The visible soft tissues are unremarkable.

● EXTRAS AND REVIEW AREAS

No vascular lines, tubes or surgical clips.
Lung apices: Normal.
Hila: Normal.
Behind heart: Normal.
Costophrenic angles: Normal.
Below the diaphragm: Normal.

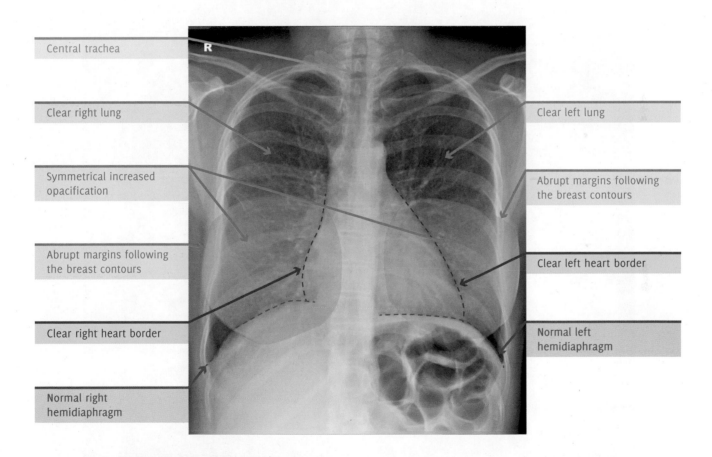

Central trachea
Clear right lung
Symmetrical increased opacification
Abrupt margins following the breast contours
Clear right heart border
Normal right hemidiaphragm

R

Clear left lung
Abrupt margins following the breast contours
Clear left heart border
Normal left hemidiaphragm

SUMMARY, INVESTIGATIONS AND MANAGEMENT

This X-ray demonstrates increased density projected over the mid and lower zones. The increased density follows the contours of the breasts and is consistent with bilateral breast prostheses. No causes for breathlessness are demonstrated.

Initial blood tests may include FBC, U&Es, CRP and D-Dimer. A blood gas and sputum culture may be helpful. The history is strongly suggested of a pulmonary embolism and so a CTPA or nuclear medicine perfusion scan would be indicated.

A 42-year-old female attends the cardiothoracic outpatient clinic for review 10 weeks post lung cancer surgery. Unfortunately her notes are unavailable. She says she has recovered well from the surgery. On examination, she is afebrile, and her oxygen saturations are 98% in air. There is reduced chest expansion on the right with no breath sounds and dullness to percussion. Examination of the left lung is normal. A chest X-ray is requested as part of the routine postoperative follow-up.

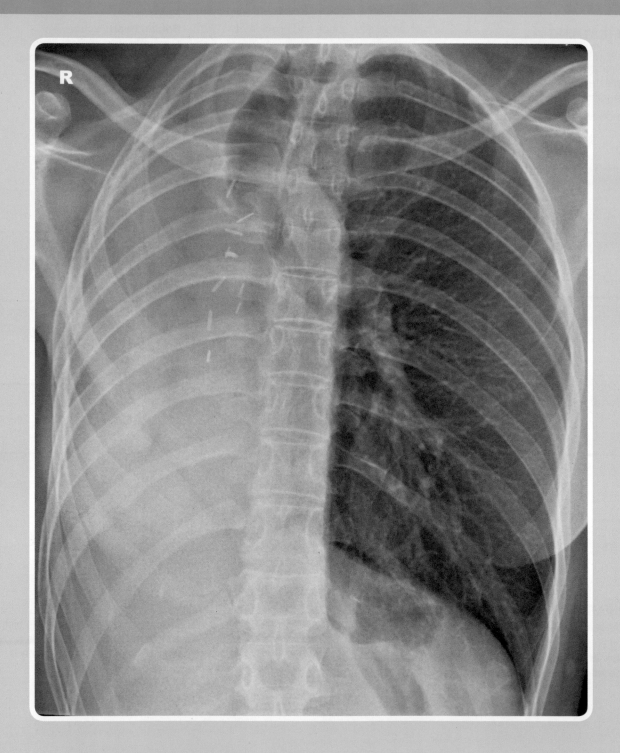

TECHNICAL INFORMATION

Patient ID: Anonymous
Projection: PA
Penetration: Adequate – vertebral bodies just visible behind heart
Inspiration: Adequate – eight anterior ribs visible
Rotation: Not rotated

● AIRWAY

The trachea is deviated to the right.

● BREATHING

There is a white out of the right hemithorax with a total absence of bronchovascular markings.

The left lung appears hyperexpanded but clear with normal pleural spaces and pulmonary vascularity.

● CIRCULATION AND MEDIASTINUM

The heart is difficult to identify. It is presumably displaced into the opacified right hemithorax.

The mediastinum is displaced to the right. The aorta is difficult to identify.

The right hilum is difficult to identify due to the opacification. Normal size, shape and position of the left hilum.

● DIAPHRAGM AND DELICATES

The right hemidiaphragm and costophrenic angle are obscured. Normal appearance and position of the left hemidiaphragm.

No pneumoperitoneum.

The imaged skeleton is intact with no fractures or destructive bony lesions visible.

The visible soft tissues are unremarkable.

● EXTRAS AND REVIEW AREAS

There are surgical clips projected medially over the right hemithorax, near the trachea and right main bronchus.

No vascular lines or tubes.
Lung apices: Opacification of the right apex. Normal left apex.
Hila: Right hilum difficult to see. Normal left hilum.
Behind heart: Difficult to assess.
Costophrenic angles: Obscured on the right. Preserved on the left.
Below the diaphragm: Normal.

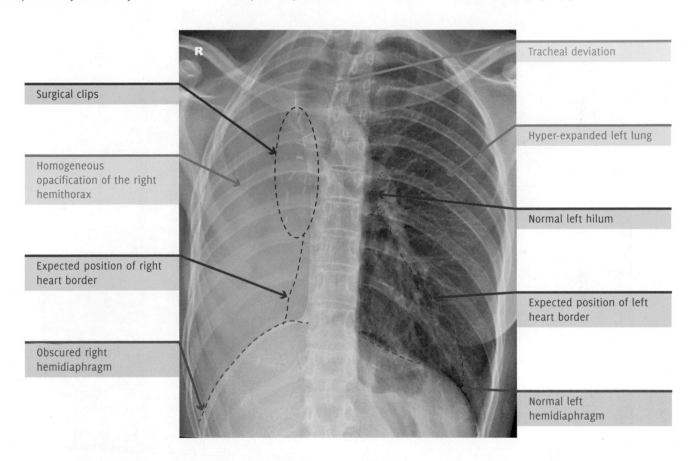

Surgical clips

Homogeneous opacification of the right hemithorax

Expected position of right heart border

Obscured right hemidiaphragm

Tracheal deviation

Hyper-expanded left lung

Normal left hilum

Expected position of left heart border

Normal left hemidiaphragm

SUMMARY, INVESTIGATIONS AND MANAGEMENT

This X-ray demonstrates a total white out of the right hemithorax with marked volume loss demonstrated by mediastinal deviation. There are surgical clips in the right mid and upper zones.

The findings are consistent with the normal appearance of a right pneumonectomy. The white out will be due to fluid filling the postpneumonectomy space. There is no air-fluid level (hydropneumothorax) to suggest a bronchopleural fistula.

It would be helpful to compare the current X-ray with previous imaging, but no specific investigation/action is required.

A 53-year-old male presents to ED with fever, productive cough and haemoptysis. He had a right-sided pneumonectomy 4 weeks earlier for lung cancer and had been recovering well until this point. He is a nonsmoker. On examination, he has oxygen saturations of 78% in air, has an HR of 90 bpm and is febrile with a temperature of 38.8°C. There are no breath sounds on the right, with hyperresonance in the right upper zone, and dullness to percussion in the right lower zone. A chest X-ray is requested to assess for possible pneumonia, or bronchopleural fistula.

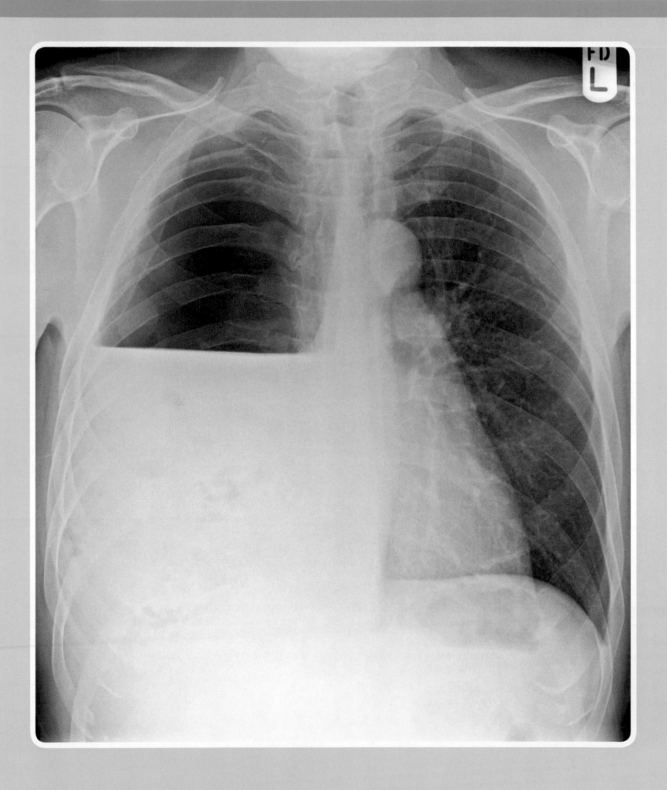

TECHNICAL INFORMATION

Patient ID: Anonymous
Projection: PA mobile erect
Penetration: Adequate – vertebral bodies just visible behind heart
Inspiration: Adequate – seven anterior ribs visible
Rotation: The patient is slightly rotated to the left

● AIRWAY

The trachea is central after factoring in patient rotation.

● BREATHING

There is homogeneous opacification of the right mid and lower zones. Its upper margin is horizontal and there is complete loss of bronchovascular markings in the right upper zone, consistent with an air-fluid level.

The left lung field and pleural spaces are clear. The lungs are not hyperinflated.

Normal left pulmonary vascularity.

● CIRCULATION AND MEDIASTINUM

The right heart border is not visible. The cardiac size therefore cannot be commented on. The left heart border is clear.

The aorta appears normal.

The mediastinum is central, not widened, with clear borders.

The right hilum is not visible. Normal size, shape and position of the left hilum.

● DIAPHRAGM AND DELICATES

The right hemidiaphragm is obscured. Normal position and appearance of the left hemidiaphragm.

No pneumoperitoneum.

The imaged skeleton is intact with no fractures or destructive bony lesions visible.

The visible soft tissues are unremarkable with no surgical emphysema.

● EXTRAS AND REVIEW AREAS

No vascular lines, tubes or surgical clips visible.
Lung apices: Right-sided pneumothorax. Normal left apex.
Hila: Right hilum not visible. Normal left hilum.
Behind heart: Right retrocardiac position obscured. Normal on the left.
Costophrenic angles: Right obscured. Normal left costophrenic angle.
Below the diaphragm: Normal.

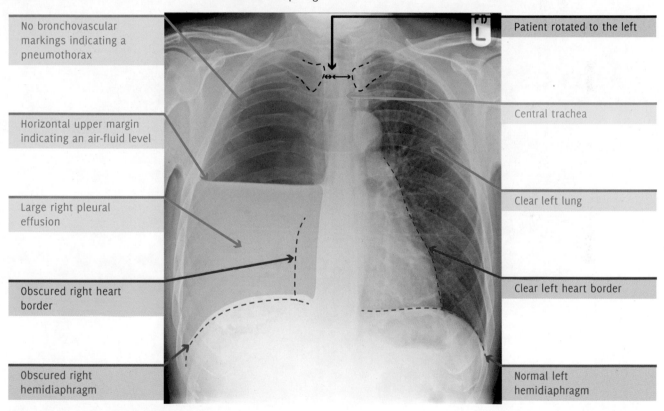

No bronchovascular markings indicating a pneumothorax

Horizontal upper margin indicating an air-fluid level

Large right pleural effusion

Obscured right heart border

Obscured right hemidiaphragm

Patient rotated to the left

Central trachea

Clear left lung

Clear left heart border

Normal left hemidiaphragm

SUMMARY, INVESTIGATIONS AND MANAGEMENT

This X-ray demonstrates a large right-sided hydropneumothorax, with an air-fluid level. The mediastinum appears central. This may be within normal limits 4 weeks postpneumonectomy. However, the patient is septic with haemoptysis and the amount of air in the right hemithorax is concerning. These features may indicate a bronchopleural fistula and empyema.

This is an acutely unwell patient who needs urgent resuscitation. 100% oxygen should be administered via a non-rebreathe mask and there should be a low threshold for escalation of respiratory support. Two points of intravenous access should be rapidly achieved, with an arterial blood gas sent, alongside venous bloods for FBC, U&Es, LFTs,

coagulation, CRP and blood cultures. Sputum cultures should be obtained if possible.

The patient should be given a fluid bolus and appropriate intravenous antibiotics. They should be urgently discussed with cardiothoracic surgery.

The current X-ray needs to be compared with the previous imaging to assess the change in size of the postpneumonectomy space (which should get progressively smaller as it is replaced by fluid). A significant increase in the amount of air in the right hemithorax is suspicious for a bronchopleural fistula +/− empyema. An ultrasound-guided pleural aspiration should be performed to assess for empyema.

A 60-year-old female presents to ED with a cough and mild shortness of breath. She has general flu-like symptoms. She has a history of severe epilepsy, for which a vagal nerve stimulator has been inserted. She is a nonsmoker. On examination, she has oxygen saturations of 95% in air and is afebrile. Lungs are resonant throughout, with good bilateral air entry. A chest X-ray is requested to assess for possible pneumonia or pulmonary embolism.

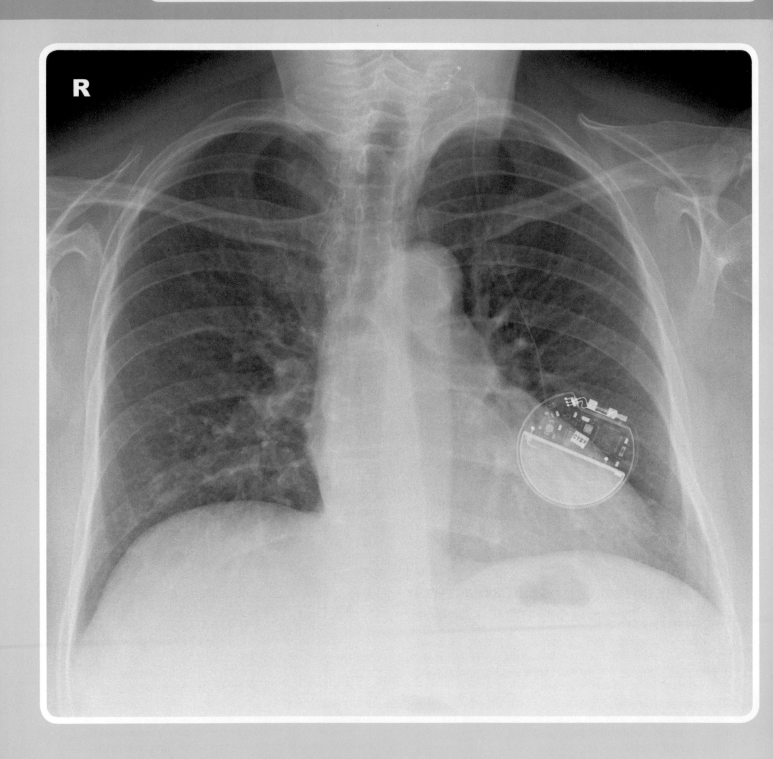

TECHNICAL INFORMATION

Patient ID: Anonymous
Projection: PA
Penetration: Adequate – vertebral bodies just visible behind heart
Inspiration: Adequate – six anterior ribs visible
Rotation: The patient is rotated to the left

● AIRWAY

The trachea is central after factoring in patient rotation.

● BREATHING

The lungs are clear.

The lungs are not hyperinflated.

The pleural spaces are clear.

Normal pulmonary vascularity.

● CIRCULATION AND MEDIASTINUM

The heart is not enlarged.

The heart borders are clear.

The aorta appears normal.

The mediastinum is central, not widened, with clear borders.

Normal size, shape and position of both hila.

● DIAPHRAGM AND DELICATES

Normal position and appearance of the diaphragm.

No pneumoperitoneum.

The imaged skeleton is intact with no fractures or destructive bony lesions visible.

The visible soft tissues are unremarkable.

● EXTRAS AND REVIEW AREAS

There is an electronic device projected over the left lower zone. A wire arises superiorly and travels over the left chest, terminating in the left side of the neck.
Lung apices: Normal.
Hila: Normal.
Behind heart: Normal.
Costophrenic angles: Normal.
Below the diaphragm: Normal.

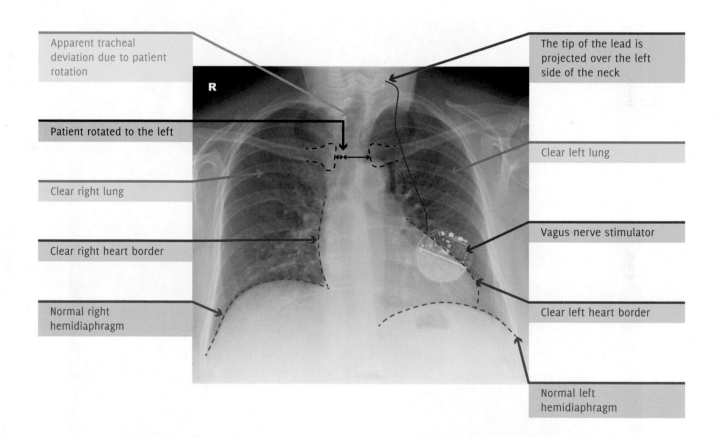

Apparent tracheal deviation due to patient rotation

Patient rotated to the left

Clear right lung

Clear right heart border

Normal right hemidiaphragm

R

The tip of the lead is projected over the left side of the neck

Clear left lung

Vagus nerve stimulator

Clear left heart border

Normal left hemidiaphragm

SUMMARY, INVESTIGATIONS AND MANAGEMENT

This X-ray demonstrates an electronic device, most likely a vagus nerve stimulator, used in patients to help alleviate intractable epilepsy. The wire tip within the left neck is connected to the left vagus nerve and is appropriately sited.

Initial blood tests may include FBC, U&Es and CRP. Further investigations and management will be guided by the clinical assessment. The history is suggestive of a viral infection. No specific further investigations or management is required based on the X-ray findings.

A 62-year-old male presents to ED with acute-on-chronic shortness of breath. He has a 50 pack-year smoking history. On examination, he has oxygen saturations of 86% in air and is afebrile. RR is 20 with an HR of 90 bpm. There are bilateral crackles and wheeze throughout the lungs. A chest X-ray is requested to assess for possible pneumonia, effusion or pulmonary oedema.

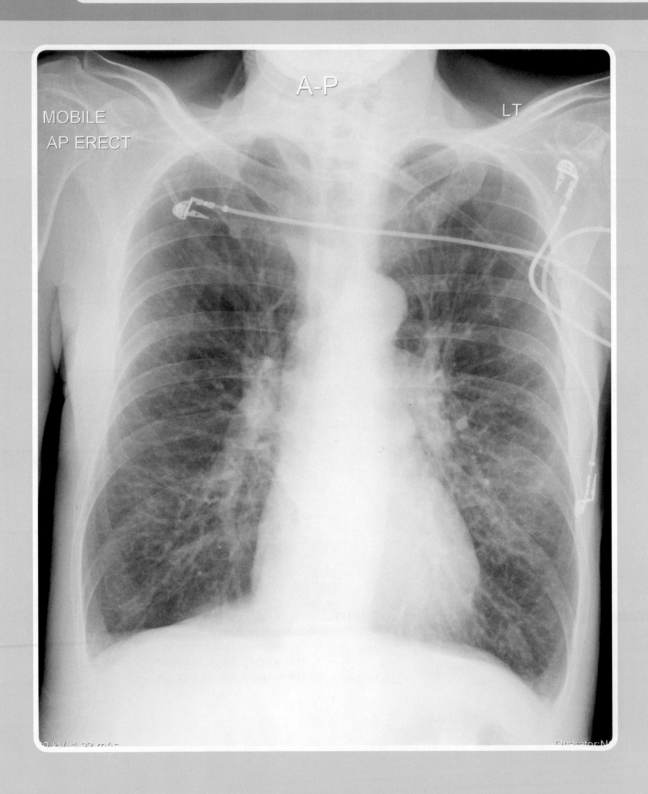

TECHNICAL INFORMATION

Patient ID: Anonymous
Projection: AP erect (mobile)
Penetration: Slightly underpenetrated – vertebral bodies not easily visible behind heart
Inspiration: Adequate – eight anterior ribs visible
Rotation: The patient is not rotated

● AIRWAY

The trachea is central.

● BREATHING

There is increased opacification in the left mid zone, with preservation of the left heart border, in keeping with consolidation. The lungs are hyperexpanded with flattening of the hemidiaphragms, and there is coarsening of the bronchovascular markings throughout the lungs, in keeping with COPD. The lungs are otherwise clear.

There is mild blunting of both costophrenic angles, but the pleural spaces are otherwise clear.

Normal pulmonary vascularity.

● CIRCULATION AND MEDIASTINUM

The heart does not appear enlarged, although its size cannot be accurately assessed on an AP X-ray.

The heart borders are clear.

The aorta appears normal.

The mediastinum is central, not widened, with clear borders.

Normal size, shape and position of both hila.

● DIAPHRAGM AND DELICATES

Bilateral flattening of the hemidiaphragms in keeping with lung hyperexpansion.

No pneumoperitoneum.

The imaged skeleton is intact with no fractures or destructive bony lesions visible.

The visible soft tissues are unremarkable.

● EXTRAS AND REVIEW AREAS

ECG monitoring leads and oxygen tubing in situ.

No vascular lines, tubes or surgical clips.
Lung apices: Normal.
Hila: Normal.
Behind heart: Normal.
Costophrenic angles: Bilateral blunting.
Below the diaphragm: Normal.

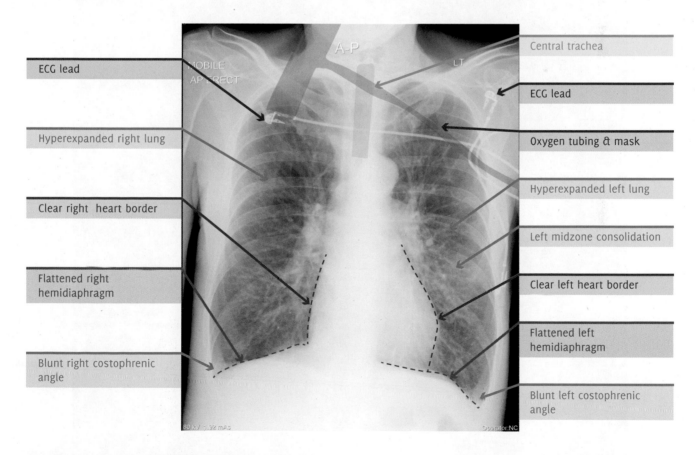

SUMMARY, INVESTIGATIONS AND MANAGEMENT

This X-ray demonstrates generalized increased bronchovascular markings associated with hyperinflated lungs, consistent with COPD. Increased left mid zone opacification is in keeping with consolidation. The blunted costophrenic angles may represent small effusions or pleural thickening. This is likely to be an infective exacerbation of COPD.

Supplementary oxygen should be titrated according to arterial blood gas results. Initial blood tests may include FBC, U&Es and CRP. A sputum culture may also be helpful.

Appropriate antibiotics should be commenced and a follow-up chest X-ray should be performed in 4 to 6 weeks to assess for resolution.

A 65-year-old female presents to ED with severe chest pain radiating to the back, and shortness of breath. There is no significant past medical history and she is a nonsmoker. On examination, she has oxygen saturations of 85% in air and is afebrile. Lungs are resonant throughout with good bilateral air entry. A chest X-ray is requested to assess for a possible aortic dissection, pneumonia or pulmonary oedema.

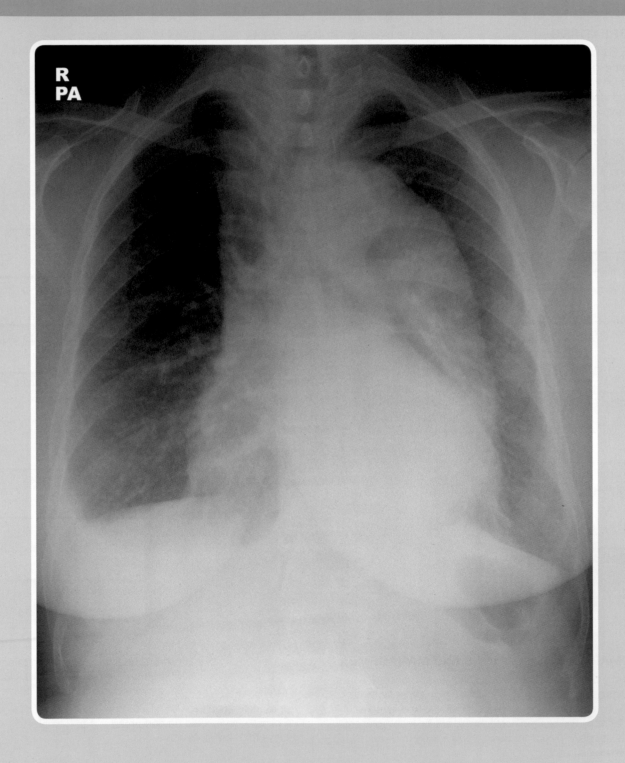

R
PA

TECHNICAL INFORMATION

Patient ID: Anonymous
Projection: PA
Penetration: Adequate – vertebral bodies just visible behind heart
Inspiration: Adequate – six anterior ribs visible
Rotation: Not rotated

● AIRWAY

Superiorly the trachea is central. Inferiorly it is displaced to the right by the aortic arch.

● BREATHING

There is increased left retrocardiac opacification, which may represent consolidation. The lungs are otherwise clear.

The lungs are not hyperinflated.

There is blunting of the right costophrenic angle in keeping with a small effusion.

Normal pulmonary vascularity.

● CIRCULATION AND MEDIASTINUM

The heart is enlarged (cardiothoracic ratio 0.6).

The heart borders are clear.

The aorta is widened and has an irregular contour.

The mediastinum is central, but widened (including the right paratracheal stripe), with clear borders.

Both hila are visible through the enlarged mediastinum but are difficult to assess.

● DIAPHRAGM AND DELICATES

The medial left hemidiaphragm is obscured. Clear right hemidiaphragm.

No pneumoperitoneum.

The imaged skeleton is intact with no fractures or destructive bony lesions visible.

The visible soft tissues are unremarkable.

● EXTRAS AND REVIEW AREAS

No vascular lines, tubes or surgical clips.
Lung apices: Normal.
Hila: Normal.
Behind heart: Left retrocardiac opacification.
Costophrenic angles: Right blunting in keeping with small effusions.
Below the diaphragm: Normal.

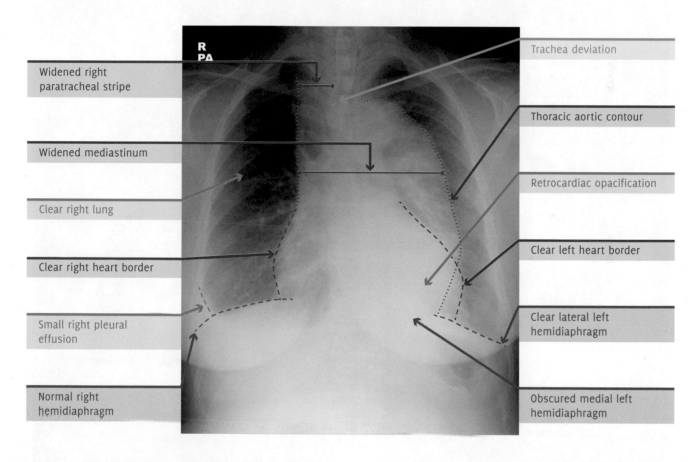

Labels (left): Widened right paratracheal stripe; Widened mediastinum; Clear right lung; Clear right heart border; Small right pleural effusion; Normal right hemidiaphragm.

Labels (right): Trachea deviation; Thoracic aortic contour; Retrocardiac opacification; Clear left heart border; Clear lateral left hemidiaphragm; Obscured medial left hemidiaphragm.

SUMMARY, INVESTIGATIONS AND MANAGEMENT

This X-ray shows widening of the mediastinum/thoracic aorta with a small right pleural effusion. Given the history aortic dissection is an important differential. The increased left retrocardiac opacification may be caused by the dissection or possible concomitant consolidation.

The patient requires urgent resuscitation using an ABCDE approach, with oxygen therapy and a fluid bolus given in the first instance.

Any previous imaging needs to be reviewed to assess whether this is a new finding. If it is, a CT of the aorta (noncontrast and arterial phases) should be performed to assess for an aortic dissection.

Management depends on the location and extent of dissection. Urgent discussion with cardiothoracic surgery and interventional radiology is required.

A 75-year-old female presents to ED with lethargy, shortness of breath and a cough. She has a background of breast cancer, treated with a left-sided mastectomy and axillary node clearance 8 years ago. She is a nonsmoker. On examination, she has oxygen saturations of 93% in air and is afebrile. Her RR is 20 with an HR of 90 bpm. There is dullness to percussion and reduced air entry in the right middle and lower zones. A chest X-ray is requested to assess for possible pneumonia, an effusion or collapse.

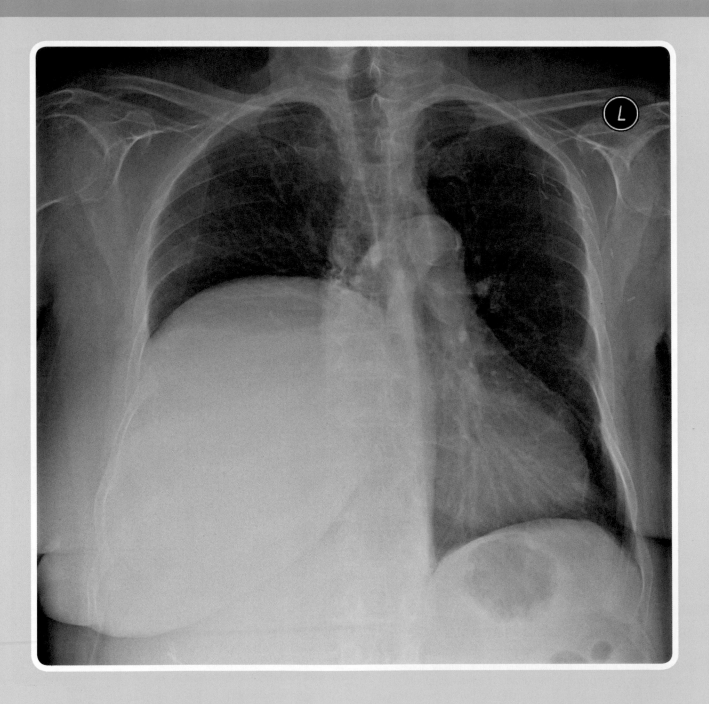

TECHNICAL INFORMATION

Patient ID: Anonymous
Projection: PA
Penetration: Adequate – vertebral bodies just visible behind heart
Inspiration: Adequate – eight anterior ribs visible
Rotation: The patient is slightly rotated to the right

● AIRWAY

The upper trachea is central allowing for patient rotation. The lower trachea is displaced to the left.

● BREATHING

There is a homogeneous opacity projected over the right mid and lower zones. This has a convex superior border and is consistent with elevation of the right hemidiaphragm. The lungs are otherwise clear.

The lungs are not hyperinflated.

The pleural spaces are clear.

Normal pulmonary vascularity.

● CIRCULATION AND MEDIASTINUM

The heart is displaced to the left. The right heart border is difficult to identify but the heart does not appear enlarged. The left heart border is clear.

The aorta appears normal.

The mediastinum is displaced to the left. It is not widened and has clear borders.

The right hilum is obscured. Normal size, shape and position of the left hilum.

● DIAPHRAGM AND DELICATES

The right hemidiaphragm is significantly elevated, causing mediastinal shift to the left. Normal appearance and position of the left hemidiaphragm.

No pneumoperitoneum.

The imaged skeleton is intact with no fractures or destructive bony lesions visible.

There has been a previous left-sided mastectomy. The visible soft tissues are otherwise unremarkable.

● EXTRAS AND REVIEW AREAS

There are multiple surgical clips projected over the left axilla consistent with previous axillary nodal clearance.

No vascular lines or tubes.
Lung apices: Normal.
Hila: The right hilum is obscured. Normal left hilum.
Behind heart: Normal.
Costophrenic angles: Normal.
Below the diaphragm: Elevated right hemidiaphragm.

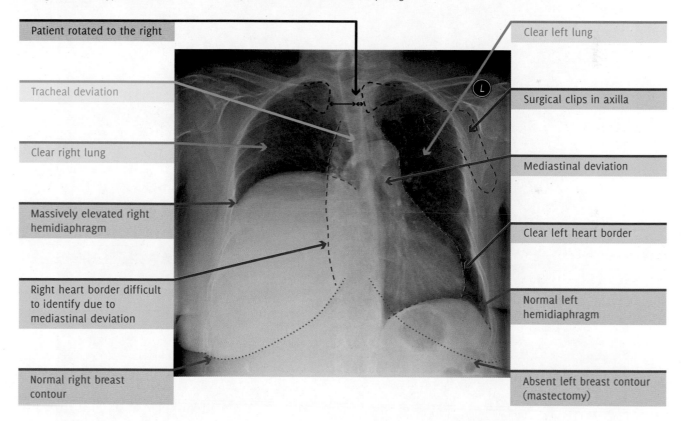

- Patient rotated to the right
- Clear left lung
- Tracheal deviation
- Surgical clips in axilla
- Clear right lung
- Mediastinal deviation
- Massively elevated right hemidiaphragm
- Clear left heart border
- Right heart border difficult to identify due to mediastinal deviation
- Normal left hemidiaphragm
- Normal right breast contour
- Absent left breast contour (mastectomy)

SUMMARY, INVESTIGATIONS AND MANAGEMENT

This X-ray demonstrates a markedly elevated right hemidiaphragm with mass effect on the right lung and mediastinum. This patient has had a previous left mastectomy and left axillary nodal clearance for breast malignancy.

The differential diagnoses for a raised right hemidiaphragm include mediastinal lymph node disease affecting the right phrenic nerve or multiple large liver metastases causing superior displacement of the diaphragm.

Previous imaging should be reviewed to ensure this is not a longstanding finding. Initial blood tests may include FBC, U&Es, LFTs and bone profile.

A contrast-enhanced CT of the chest, abdomen and pelvis is required to identify the underlying cause and restage the tumour. The patient should be referred to oncology.

A 25-year-old female presents to her GP with worsening shortness of breath. There is no significant past medical history and she is a nonsmoker. On examination, she has oxygen saturations of 98% in air and is afebrile. Lungs are resonant throughout with good bilateral air entry and occasional wheeze. A chest X-ray is requested to assess for possible pneumonia, collapse or pleural effusions.

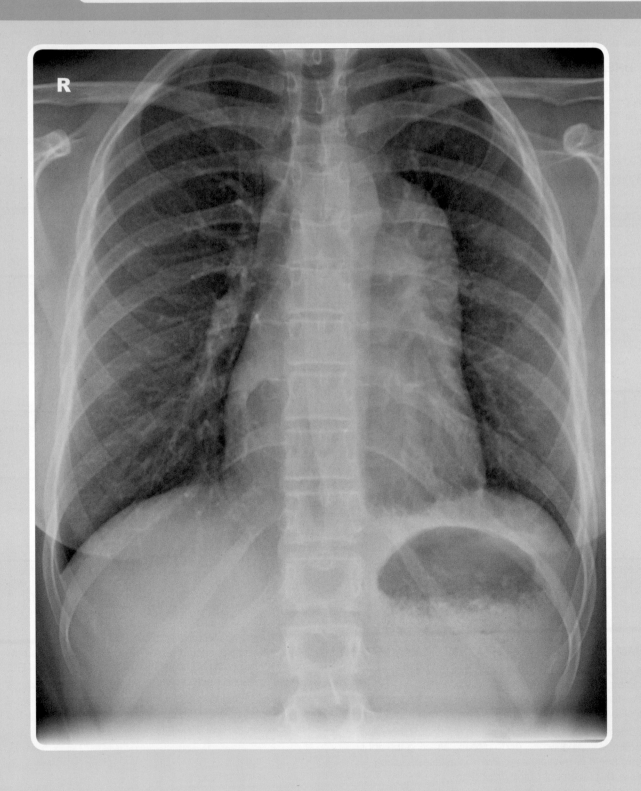

TECHNICAL INFORMATION

Patient ID: Anonymous
Projection: PA
Penetration: Adequate – vertebral bodies just visible behind heart
Inspiration: Adequate – seven anterior ribs visible
Rotation: Not rotated

● AIRWAY

The trachea is slightly deviated to the right.

● BREATHING

The lungs are clear.

The lungs are not hyperinflated.

The pleural spaces are clear.

Normal pulmonary vascularity.

● CIRCULATION AND MEDIASTINUM

There is a left-sided mediastinal mass, which is continuous with the left heart border. The left hilar structures can be seen through the mass (hilum overlay sign), indicating that the mass is not in the middle mediastinum. The aortic knuckle and descending thoracic aorta are also visible through the mass, and thus the mass is not in the posterior mediastinum.

The heart is not enlarged.

The right heart border is clear.

The aorta appears normal.

Normal size, shape and position of both hila.

● DIAPHRAGM AND DELICATES

Normal appearance and position of the hemidiaphragms.

No pneumoperitoneum.

The imaged skeleton is intact with no fractures or destructive bony lesions visible.

The visible soft tissues are unremarkable.

● EXTRAS AND REVIEW AREAS

No vascular lines, tubes or surgical clips.
Lung apices: Normal.
Hila: Normal (left hilum overlay sign).
Behind heart: Normal.
Costophrenic angles: Normal.
Below the diaphragm: Normal.

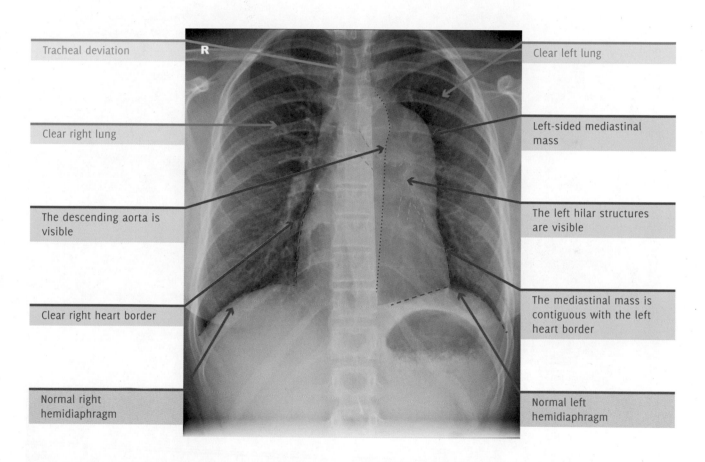

Tracheal deviation

Clear left lung

Clear right lung

Left-sided mediastinal mass

The descending aorta is visible

The left hilar structures are visible

Clear right heart border

The mediastinal mass is contiguous with the left heart border

Normal right hemidiaphragm

Normal left hemidiaphragm

SUMMARY, INVESTIGATIONS AND MANAGEMENT

This X-ray demonstrates a left-sided mediastinal mass. Loss of the left heart border indicates involvement of the anterior mediastinal compartment. The left hilum and descending thoracic aorta are visible separate to the mass, indicating the middle and posterior compartments are spared. The differentials include lymphoma, thyroid malignancy, thymoma (although usually in older patients) and teratoma.

A full examination to assess for lymph node enlargement should be undertaken. Initial blood tests may include FBC, U&Es, LFTs, bone profile and TFTs.

Further imaging in the form of contrast-enhanced CT of the chest should be performed. If lymphoma is suspected then the neck, abdomen and pelvis should also be included in the CT. A CT-guided anterior mediastinal mass biopsy may be required for a histological diagnosis.

The patient should be referred to respiratory/oncology services for further management, which may include biopsy and MDT discussion. Treatment, which may include surgery, radiotherapy, chemotherapy or palliative treatment, will depend on the outcome of the MDT discussion, investigations and the patient's wishes.

A 34-year-old male presents to ED after colliding with a truck while riding a bike. He has severe chest pain. There is no significant past medical history. He is a nonsmoker. On examination, he has oxygen saturations of 85% in air and is afebrile. His RR is 25, HR is 100 bpm and BP is 90/60 mmHg. There are crackles in both lungs. A chest X-ray is requested to assess for possible pneumothoraces and any other evidence of thoracic injury.

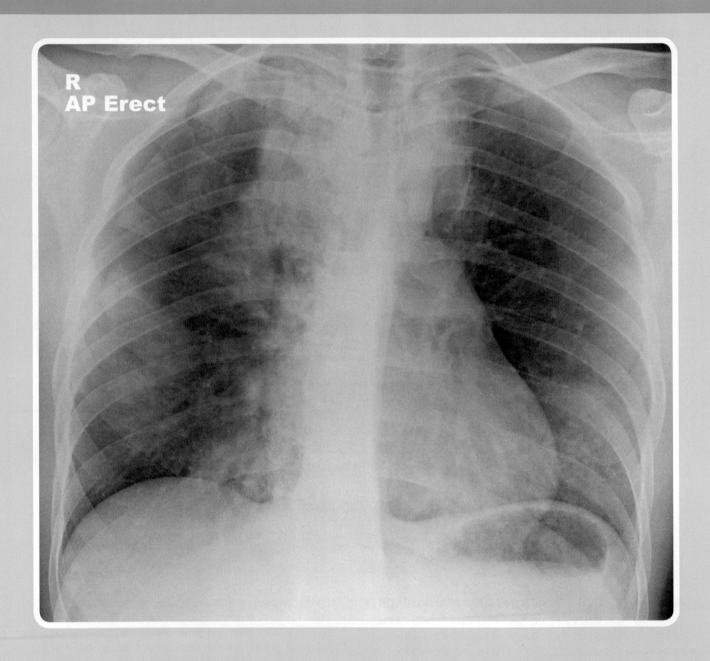

TECHNICAL INFORMATION

Patient ID: Anonymous
Projection: AP erect
Penetration: Adequate – vertebral bodies just visible behind heart
Inspiration: Adequate – eight anterior ribs visible
Rotation: The patient is slightly rotated to the left

● AIRWAY

The trachea is central after factoring in patient rotation.

● BREATHING

There are multiple areas of airspace opacification (medially in the right upper and lower zones, peripherally in the right mid zone, and in both lower zones) in keeping with consolidation.

A lung edge is visible in the right upper and mid zones with no lung markings seen beyond it, consistent with a small to moderate pneumothorax. there is a thin lucency projected over the posterior aspect of the 2nd left rib which may represent a tiny left apical pneumothorax. No pleural effusion/haemothorax.

The lungs are not hyperinflated.

Normal pulmonary vascularity.

● CIRCULATION AND MEDIASTINUM

The heart does not appear enlarged, although its size cannot be accurately assessed on an AP X-ray.

The right heart border is slightly indistinct, while the left heart border is clear.

The aorta is difficult to assess.

The superior mediastinum appears widened, although this is difficult to assess given the projection. there is increased associated density.

The right hilum is partially obscured by consolidation. normal size, shape and position of the left hilum.

● DIAPHRAGM AND DELICATES

Normal appearance and position of the hemidiaphragms.

No pneumoperitoneum.

The imaged skeleton is intact with no fractures or destructive bony lesions visible.

The visible soft tissues are unremarkable.

● EXTRAS AND REVIEW AREAS

No vascular lines, tubes or surgical clips.
Lung apices: Right apical pneumothorax and consolidation. Possible tiny left apical pneumothorax.
Hila: Partially obscured right hilum. Normal left hilum.
Behind heart: Bilateral lower zone consolidation.
Costophrenic angles: Normal.
Below the diaphragm: Normal.

Right pneumothorax

Right upper & mid zone consolidation

Obscured right heart border

Right lower zone consolidation

Normal right hemidiaphragm

R
AP Erect

Thin lucency may represent a tiny left pneumothorax

Central trachea

Superior mediastinal widening

Clear left heart border

Left lower zone consolidation

Normal left hemidiaphragm

SUMMARY, INVESTIGATIONS AND MANAGEMENT

This X-ray demonstrates multifocal consolidation, which in the context of trauma is in keeping with pulmonary contusions. There is a small to moderate right apical pneumothorax, and possibly a tiny left apical pneumothorax. The widened mediastinum with possible tracheal deviation is suspicious for mediastinal haematoma.

The patient needs to be assessed and resuscitated using the ATLS algorithm. Initial urgent bloods include FBC, U&Es and crossmatch. IV fluids and supplementary oxygen should be given. A low threshold for repeat X-ray of the chest and insertion of an intercostal drain should be applied in the case of a deterioration.

Early CT scanning of the chest, plus any other areas of concern (e.g. head, cervical spine, abdomen and/or pelvis) should be considered. The patient should be urgently referred to the cardiothoracic surgeons.

A 43-year-old male presents to ED after being found lying on the pavement by a passer-by. The patient is confused, has a cough and has left-sided chest pain. There is no significant past medical history. He is a nonsmoker. On examination, he has oxygen saturations of 99% in air and is afebrile. His RR is 22 with an HR of 90 bpm. Lungs are resonant throughout with good bilateral air entry. A chest X-ray is requested to assess for possible pneumonia.

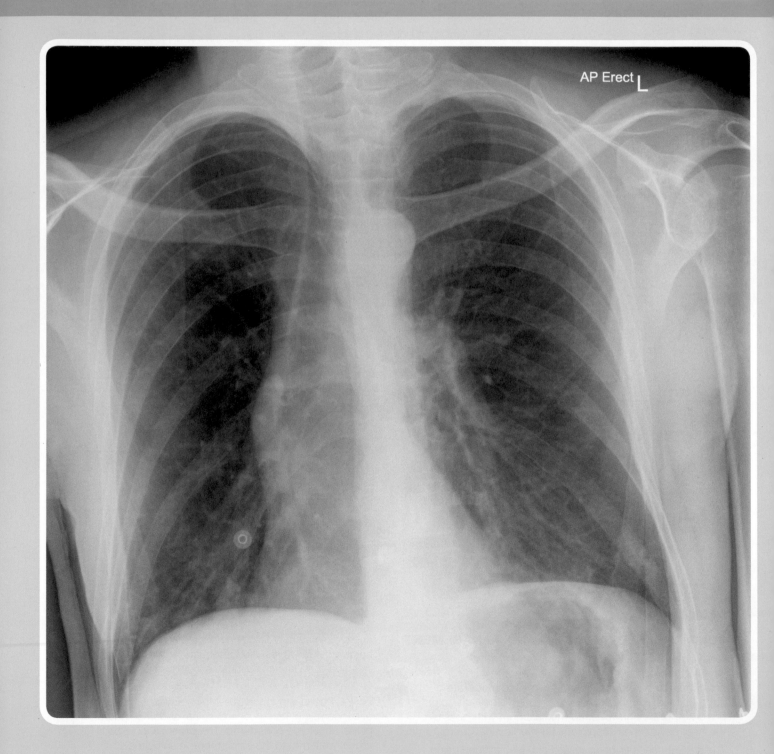

AP Erect L

TECHNICAL INFORMATION

Patient ID: Anonymous
Projection: AP erect
Penetration: Adequate – vertebral bodies just visible behind heart
Inspiration: Adequate – six anterior ribs visible
Rotation: The patient is rotated to the right

● AIRWAY

The trachea is projected to the right of the midline, which is likely due to patient rotation.

● BREATHING

The lungs are clear. The right hemithorax appears radiolucent compared to the left, which is likely due to patient rotation.

The lungs are not hyperinflated.

The pleural spaces are clear.

Normal pulmonary vascularity.

● CIRCULATION AND MEDIASTINUM

The heart does not appear enlarged, although its size cannot be accurately assessed on an AP X-ray.

The heart borders are clear.

The aorta appears normal.

The mediastinum is projected to the right of the midline, due to patient rotation. It is not widened and its visible borders are clear.

Normal size, shape and position of both hila, allowing for patient rotation.

● DIAPHRAGM AND DELICATES

Normal appearance and position of the hemidiaphragms.

No pneumoperitoneum.

There is a minimally displaced fracture through the lateral third of the left clavicle. The AC joint appears intact, although this is a nondedicated view. No other fractures or bony changes. The visible soft tissues are unremarkable.

● EXTRAS AND REVIEW AREAS

ECG electrodes in situ. No vascular lines, tubes or surgical clips.
Lung apices: Normal.
Hila: Normal.
Behind heart: Normal.
Costophrenic angles: Normal.
Below the diaphragm: Normal.

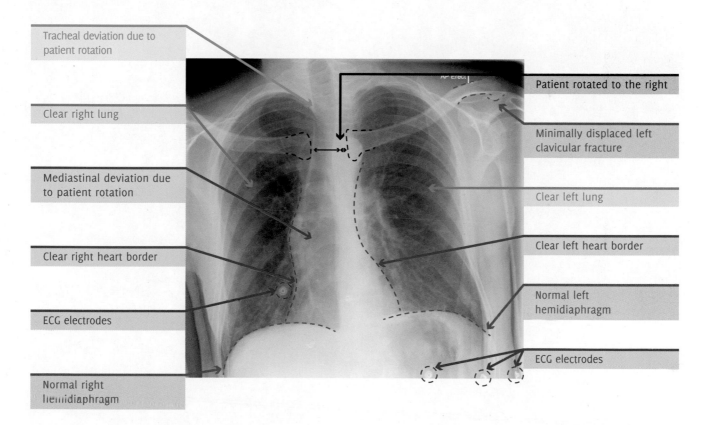

Tracheal deviation due to patient rotation

Clear right lung

Mediastinal deviation due to patient rotation

Clear right heart border

ECG electrodes

Normal right hemidiaphragm

Patient rotated to the right

Minimally displaced left clavicular fracture

Clear left lung

Clear left heart border

Normal left hemidiaphragm

ECG electrodes

SUMMARY, INVESTIGATIONS AND MANAGEMENT

This X-ray demonstrates a minimally displaced fracture of the lateral left clavicle. The patient is significantly rotated to the right. Allowing for this the lungs and mediastinal structures are normal.

Dedicated views of the left AC joint would be useful to ensure no AC joint disruption. A broad-arm sling should be applied to manage the clavicular fracture.

Initial blood tests may include FBC, U&Es and CRP. A urine dipstick may also be helpful to assess for causes of confusion. If clinical suspicion remains about a lung pathology, a repeat well-centred chest X-ray should be performed.

A 45-year-old female presents to ED with right-sided pleuritic chest pain and breathlessness. She has no significant past medical history and is a nonsmoker. On examination, she has oxygen saturations of 91% in air and is afebrile. There is increased resonance in the right upper zone, with reduced air entry. A chest X-ray is requested to assess for a possible pneumothorax.

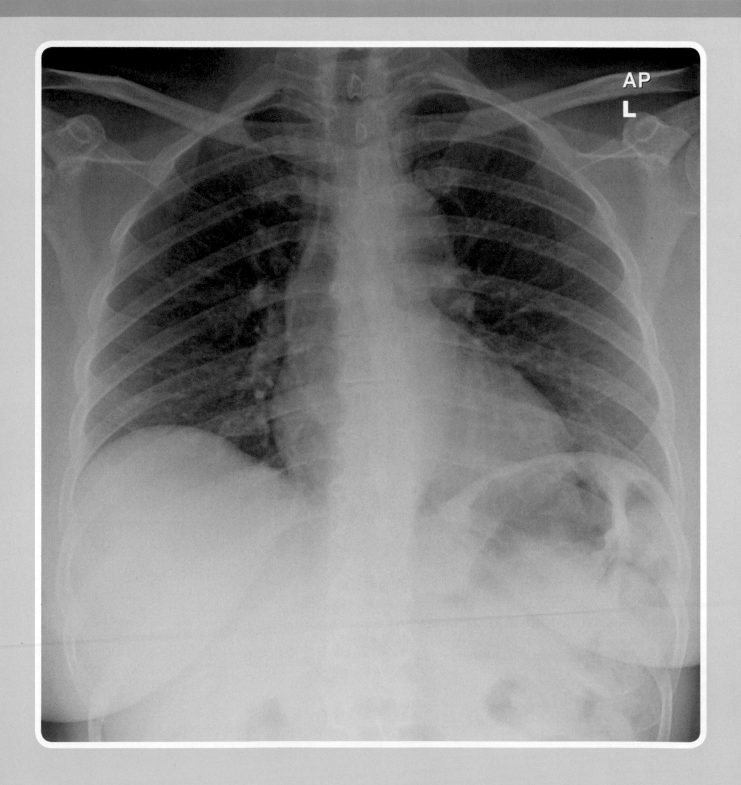

TECHNICAL INFORMATION

Patient ID: Anonymous
Projection: AP
Penetration: Adequate – vertebral bodies just visible behind heart
Inspiration: Limited – five anterior ribs visible
Rotation: Not rotated

● AIRWAY

The trachea is slightly deviated to the right.

● BREATHING

There is a subtle line in the right apex beyond which no lung markings are visible, consistent with a small pneumothorax.

The lungs are clear. The left lung is not hyperinflated.

The left-sided pleural spaces are clear.

Normal pulmonary vascularity.

● CIRCULATION AND MEDIASTINUM

The heart does not appear enlarged, although its size cannot be accurately assessed on an AP X-ray.

The heart borders are clear.

There is minor unfolding of the thoracic aorta.

The mediastinum is central, not widened, with clear borders.

Normal size, shape and position of both hila.

● DIAPHRAGM AND DELICATES

Normal appearance and position of the hemidiaphragms.

No pneumoperitoneum.

Thoracic vertebral osteophytes are visible. The imaged skeleton is otherwise intact with no fractures or destructive bony lesions visible.

The visible soft tissues are unremarkable. Of note, there is no surgical emphysema.

● EXTRAS AND REVIEW AREAS

No vascular lines, tubes or surgical clips.
Lung apices: Small right apical pneumothorax. Normal left apex.
Hila: Normal.
Behind heart: Normal.
Costophrenic angles: Normal.
Below the diaphragm: Normal.

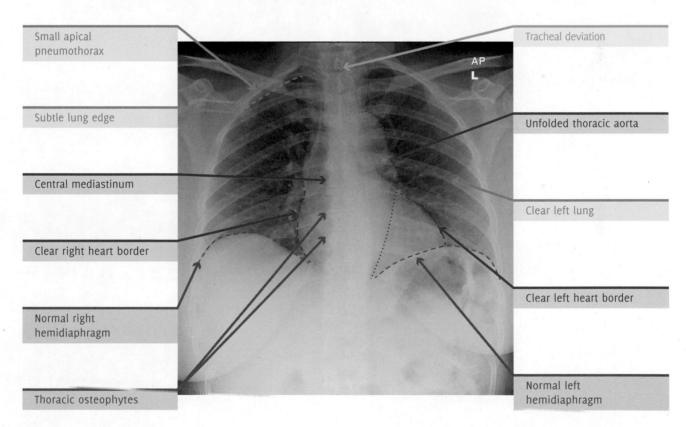

Small apical pneumothorax

Subtle lung edge

Central mediastinum

Clear right heart border

Normal right hemidiaphragm

Thoracic osteophytes

Tracheal deviation

Unfolded thoracic aorta

Clear left lung

Clear left heart border

Normal left hemidiaphragm

AP L

SUMMARY, INVESTIGATIONS AND MANAGEMENT

This X-ray demonstrates a small right apical pneumothorax. There is no mediastinal shift or flattening of the right hemidiaphragm to suggest a tension pneumothorax (the tracheal deviation may be related to unfolding of the thoracic aorta). No rib fracture is visible.

Management of a symptomatic small primary pneumothorax involves admission for supplementary oxygen, analgesia and monitoring. Active intervention is usually not required. It may be possible to discharge the patient quickly if the oxygen saturations improve. The patient should have a follow-up chest X-ray to ensure resolution.

A 50-year-old male is in the ICU following an oesophagectomy, for oesophageal cancer. Over the last 24 hours he has become increasingly difficult to ventilate through his tracheostomy. A chest X-ray the previous day to assess line position showed clear lungs. A further chest X-ray is requested to look for possible reasons for this deterioration such as pneumonia or a pneumothorax.

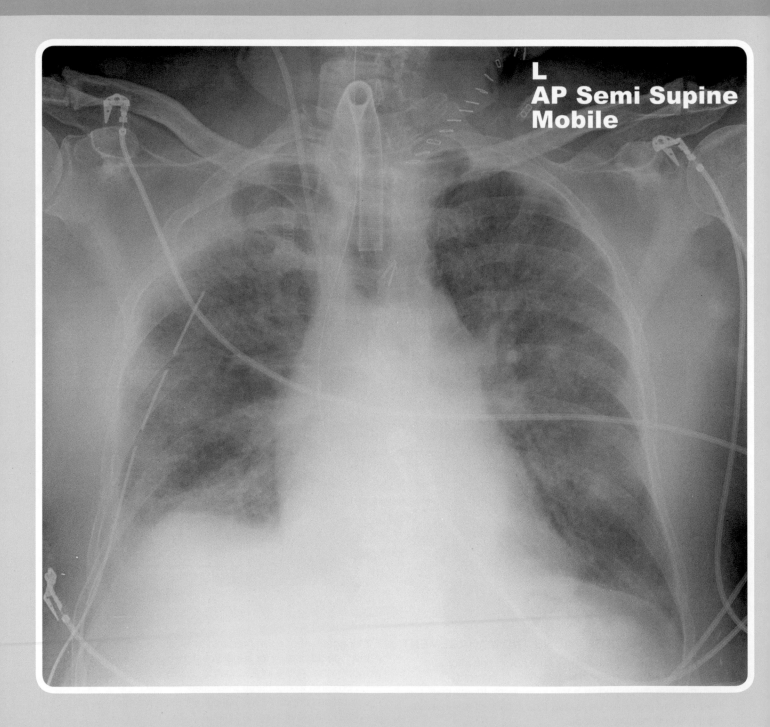

L
AP Semi Supine
Mobile

TECHNICAL INFORMATION

Patient ID: Anonymous
Projection: Portable AP semisupine
Penetration: Slightly underpenetrated – vertebral bodies not visible behind heart
Inspiration: Adequate – six anterior ribs visible
Rotation: Not rotated

● AIRWAY

The trachea is central.

● BREATHING

There is diffuse heterogeneous airspace opacification throughout both lungs. Bilateral interstitial opacification is also present.

The lungs are not hyperinflated.

The pleural spaces are clear.

Normal pulmonary vascularity.

● CIRCULATION AND MEDIASTINUM

The heart is not enlarged, even allowing for the magnification caused by the AP projection.

The heart borders are clear.

The aorta appears normal.

The mediastinum is central, not widened, with clear borders.

Normal size, shape and position of both hila.

● DIAPHRAGM AND DELICATES

The lateral aspect of the right hemidiaphragm is partially obscured by consolidation. Normal appearance and position of the left hemidiaphragm.

No pneumoperitoneum visible, although this is difficult to assess on a semisupine X-ray.

The imaged skeleton is intact with no fractures or destructive bony lesions visible.

The visible soft tissues are unremarkable.

● EXTRAS AND REVIEW AREAS

Tracheostomy in situ, with its tip projected above the carina. An external device, likely related to the ventilator, is also visible. The tip of the right internal jugular line is projected over the mid-SVC level. NG tube in situ, although the position of its tip is difficult to identify. Right intercostal chest drain, the tip of which is projected over the right upper zone.

ECG monitoring leads in situ.

There are surgical clips projected over the mediastinum and extending from the sternoclavicular joint up towards the neck in keeping with the recent surgery.
Lung apices: Interstitial opacification of the lung apices.
Hila: Normal.
Behind heart: Normal.
Costophrenic angles: Consolidation at right costophrenic angle.
Below the diaphragm: Normal.

Right internal jugular line

ECG lead

Tracheostomy

Subtle lace-like interstitial opacification

Intercostal chest drain

Clear right heart border

Patchy airspace opacification

Lateral part of right hemidiaphragm is obscured

L
AP Semi Supine Mobile

Surgical clips

Subtle lace-like interstitial opacification

Central trachea

Surgical clips

No evidence of cardiomegally

Patchy airspace opacification

Clear left heart border

Normal left hemidiaphragm

Nasogastric tube

SUMMARY, INVESTIGATIONS AND MANAGEMENT

This X-ray demonstrates patchy airspace consolidation and interstitial opacification. The differential diagnosis includes ARDS, pulmonary oedema and atypical/severe pneumonia. Considering the rapid appearance of the changes, the distribution of findings, the recent surgery and the lack of cardiomegaly or pleural effusions, ARDS is the most likely diagnosis.

The patient needs supportive care including ventilator support. The patient's oxygenation and ventilation status should be monitored with regular arterial blood gas sampling. Initial blood tests may include FBC, U&Es and CRP. Antibiotics should be given if infection is suspected or confirmed. An ECHO may be useful to assess left ventricular function. Serial chest X-rays should be performed to assess response to treatment.

A 50-year-old male presents to ED with severe central chest pain and breathlessness. There is no significant past medical history and he is a nonsmoker. On examination, he has oxygen saturations of 88% in air and is afebrile. Lung fields are resonant throughout with good bilateral air entry. He is hypotensive and has asymmetrical blood pressure recordings in the left and right arms. There is a diastolic murmur. A chest X-ray is requested to assess for possible pulmonary oedema, aortic dissection, pneumonia, collapse or pleural effusions.

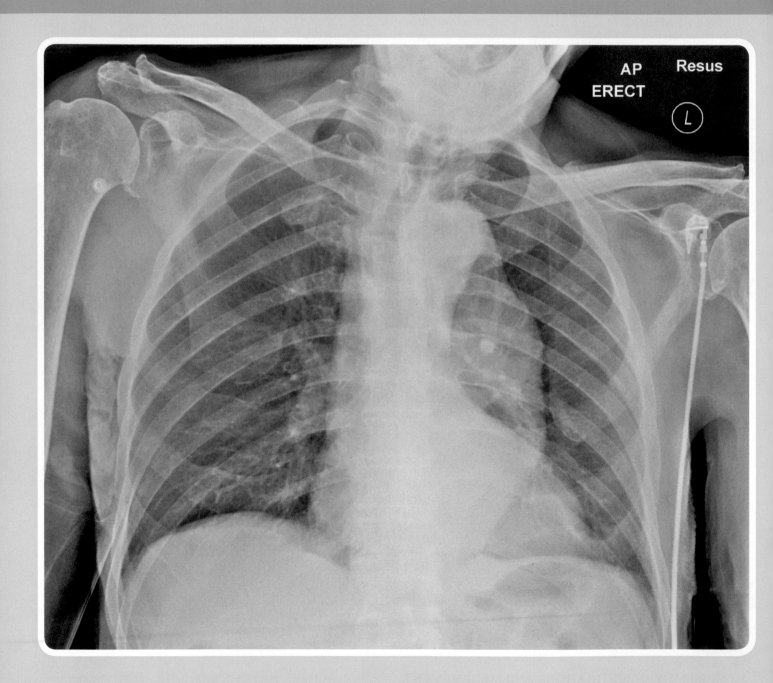

TECHNICAL INFORMATION

Patient ID: Anonymous
Projection: AP erect
Penetration: Adequate – vertebral bodies just visible behind heart
Inspiration: Adequate – six anterior ribs seen
Rotation: The patient is rotated to the left

● AIRWAY

The upper trachea is central after factoring in patient rotation. The lower trachea is displaced to the right by the aorta.

● BREATHING

The lungs are clear.

The lungs are not hyperinflated.

The pleural spaces are clear.

Normal pulmonary vascularity.

● CIRCULATION AND MEDIASTINUM

The heart is not enlarged.

The heart borders are clear.

The aorta appears widened.

The mediastinum is central, but widened. It has clear borders.

Normal size, shape and position of both hila.

● DIAPHRAGM AND DELICATES

Normal appearance and position of the hemidiaphragms.

No pneumoperitoneum.

The imaged skeleton is intact with no fracture or destructive bony lesion visible.

The visible soft tissues are unremarkable.

● EXTRAS AND REVIEW AREAS

Two ECG monitors are visible.

No vascular lines, tubes or surgical clips.
Lung apices: Normal.
Hila: Normal.
Behind heart: Normal.
Costophrenic angles: Normal.
Below the diaphragm: Normal.

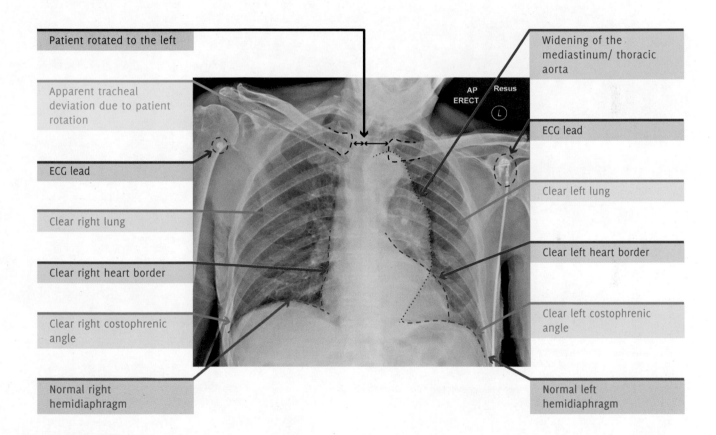

Patient rotated to the left

Apparent tracheal deviation due to patient rotation

ECG lead

Clear right lung

Clear right heart border

Clear right costophrenic angle

Normal right hemidiaphragm

Widening of the mediastinum/ thoracic aorta

ECG lead

Clear left lung

Clear left heart border

Clear left costophrenic angle

Normal left hemidiaphragm

AP ERECT   Resus   (L)

SUMMARY, INVESTIGATIONS AND MANAGEMENT

This X-ray demonstrates apparent widening of the mediastinum/thoracic aorta. This appearance may be related to the AP projection and unfolding of the thoracic aorta, but given the history, there should be a high index of suspicion for an aortic dissection.

The patient requires urgent resuscitation using an ABCDE approach, with oxygen therapy and a fluid bolus given in the first instance.

Any previous imaging needs to be reviewed to assess whether this is a new finding. If it is, a CT of the aorta (noncontrast and arterial phases) should be performed to assess for an aortic dissection.

Management depends on the location and extent of dissection. Urgent discussion with cardiothoracic surgery and interventional radiology is required.

A 51-year-old male presents to ED after falling down the escalators at the underground station. He is in severe pain and is breathless. He has no significant past medical history. He is a nonsmoker. On examination, he has oxygen saturations of 86% in air and is haemodynamically stable. There is increased resonance in the right hemithorax and reduced air entry. A chest X-ray is requested to assess for a possible pneumothorax.

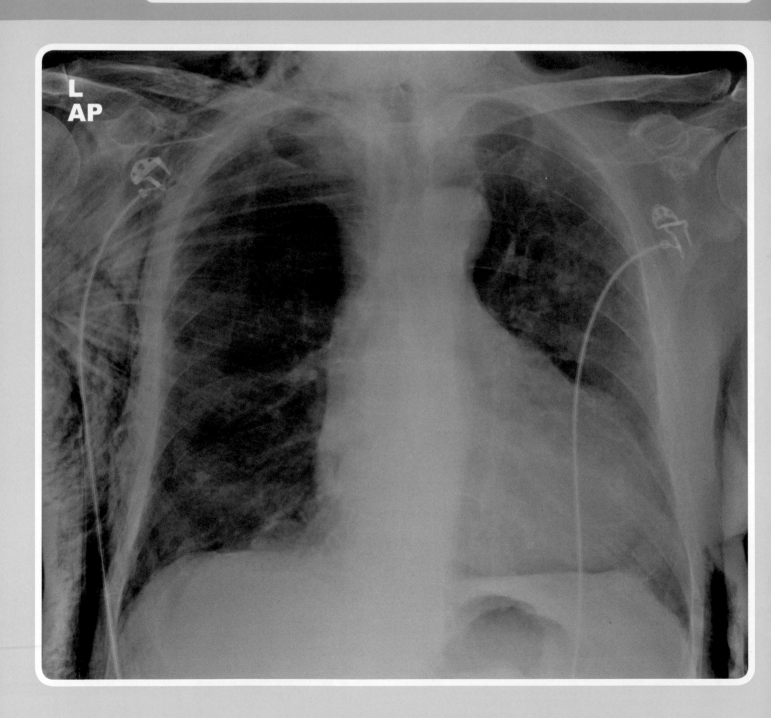

L
AP

TECHNICAL INFORMATION

Patient ID: Anonymous
Projection: AP
Penetration: Adequate – vertebral bodies just visible behind heart
Inspiration: Adequate – six anterior ribs visible
Rotation: Not rotated

● AIRWAY

The trachea is central.

● BREATHING

A lung edge is visible in the right hemithorax, beyond which no lung markings are seen, consistent with a pneumothorax. In the left apex another curvilinear line is visible, with no lung markers beyond it, representing a second pneumothorax.

The lungs are otherwise clear. Normal pulmonary vascularity.

● CIRCULATION AND MEDIASTINUM

The heart size cannot be accurately assessed due to the AP projection. The heart borders are clear.

The aorta appears normal.

The mediastinum is central, not widened, with clear borders.

Normal size, shape and position of both hila.

● DIAPHRAGM AND DELICATES

Normal appearance and position of the hemidiaphragms.

No pneumoperitoneum.

The imaged skeleton is intact with no fractures or destructive bony lesions visible.

There are extensive streaky, linear lucencies projected over the right axilla, chest wall and neck, consistent with surgical emphysema.

● EXTRAS AND REVIEW AREAS

ECG monitoring leads in situ. No vascular lines, tubes or surgical clips.
Lung apices: Bilateral apical lucencies consistent with pneumothoraces.
Hila: Normal.
Behind heart: Normal.
Costophrenic angles: Normal.
Below the diaphragm: Normal.

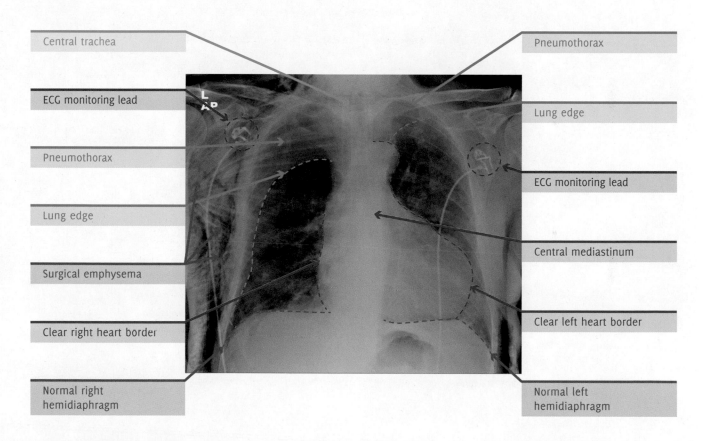

Central trachea
ECG monitoring lead
Pneumothorax
Lung edge
Surgical emphysema
Clear right heart border
Normal right hemidiaphragm

Pneumothorax
Lung edge
ECG monitoring lead
Central mediastinum
Clear left heart border
Normal left hemidiaphragm

SUMMARY, INVESTIGATIONS AND MANAGEMENT

This X-ray demonstrates a large, traumatic, right-sided pneumothorax associated with extensive right-sided surgical emphysema. There should be a high suspicion for an underlying rib fracture even though none are visible on the chest X-ray. There is no evidence of associated haemothorax.

A smaller left apical pneumothorax is also visible.

The patient needs to be assessed and resuscitated using the ATLS algorithm. Cardiothoracic surgery should be involved and bilateral chest drains will be required.

Imaging with contrast enhanced CT will provide more accurate assessment of the thoracic injuries (pneumothoraces, surgical emphysema, rib fractures and lung parenchymal/mediastinal injuries). Other parts of the body (head, cervical spine, abdomen or pelvis) can also be imaged with CT depending on the clinical assessment.

A 54-year-old male presents to his GP with weight loss, worsening shortness of breath and a chronic cough. He has COPD and a 60 pack-year smoking history. On examination, he has oxygen saturations of 94% in air and is afebrile. Lungs are resonant throughout with good bilateral air entry. A chest X-ray is requested to assess for worsening COPD changes or malignancy.

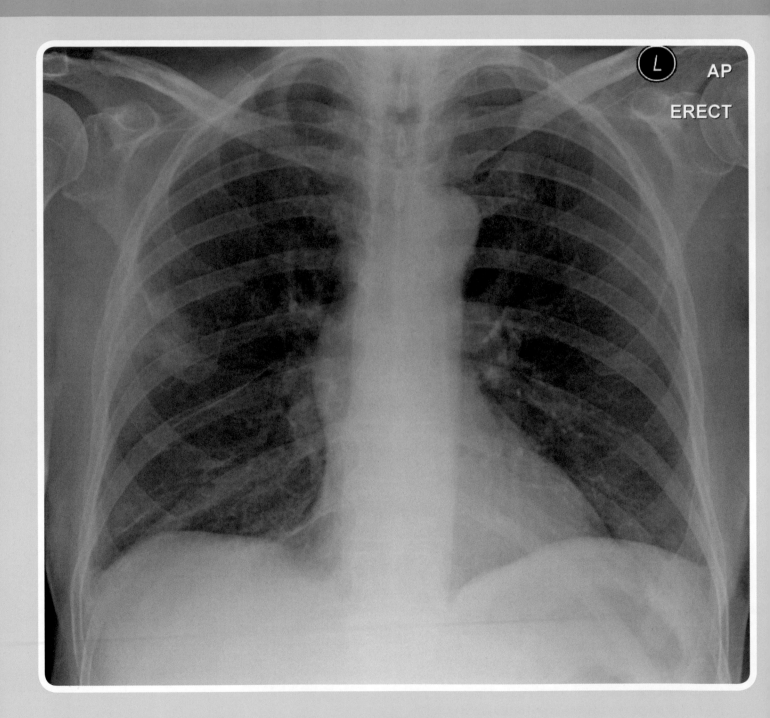

TECHNICAL INFORMATION

Patient ID: Anonymous
Projection: AP erect
Penetration: Adequate – vertebral bodies just visible behind heart
Inspiration: Adequate – six anterior ribs visible
Rotation: Not rotated

● AIRWAY

The trachea is central.

● BREATHING

There is a peripheral area of ill-defined opacification in the right mid zone. There is a small subtle nodule at the right costophrenic angle. A further small nodule is present at the left costophrenic angle.

The lungs are otherwise clear.

The lungs are not hyperinflated.

There is minor blunting of the costophrenic angles bilaterally, in keeping with small effusions.

Normal pulmonary vascularity.

● CIRCULATION AND MEDIASTINUM

The heart is not enlarged.

The heart borders are clear.

The aorta appears normal.

The mediastinum is central, not widened, with clear borders. There is a well-defined mediastinal bulge to the right side at the level of the right hilum, which is probably vascular in origin.

Normal size, shape and position of both hila.

● DIAPHRAGM AND DELICATES

Normal appearance and position of the hemidiaphragms.

No pneumoperitoneum.

The anterior aspect of the right 4th rib is difficult to identify. There are osteophytes visible in the thoracic spine. The imaged skeleton is otherwise intact with no fractures or other destructive bony lesions visible. The soft tissues are unremarkable.

● EXTRAS AND REVIEW AREAS

No vascular lines, tubes or surgical clips.
Lung apices: Normal.
Hila: Normal.
Behind heart: Normal.
Costophrenic angles: Bilateral blunting.
Below the diaphragm: Normal.

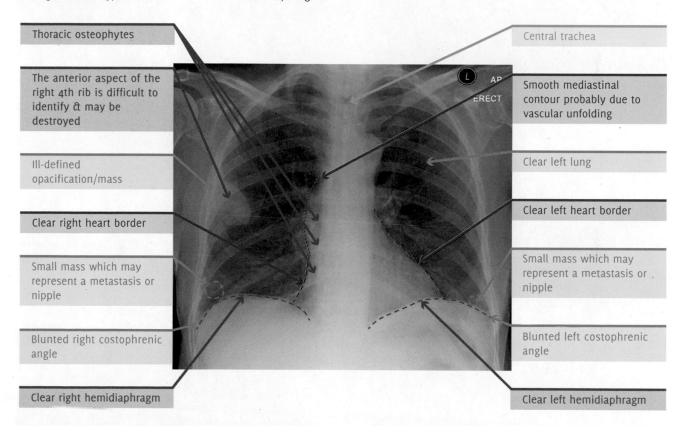

Thoracic osteophytes

The anterior aspect of the right 4th rib is difficult to identify & may be destroyed

Ill-defined opacification/mass

Clear right heart border

Small mass which may represent a metastasis or nipple

Blunted right costophrenic angle

Clear right hemidiaphragm

Central trachea

Smooth mediastinal contour probably due to vascular unfolding

Clear left lung

Clear left heart border

Small mass which may represent a metastasis or nipple

Blunted left costophrenic angle

Clear left hemidiaphragm

SUMMARY, INVESTIGATIONS AND MANAGEMENT

This X-ray demonstrates an area of peripheral ill-defined opacification, which may represent consolidation, although given the history of weight loss and a chronic cough in a smoker, a malignant pulmonary mass is an important concern. The overlying right 4th rib is difficult to identify and may be destroyed. The small masses at the costophrenic angles could represent metastases or nipple shadows. There are small pleural effusions.

Initial blood tests may include FBC, U&Es, CRP, LFTs and bone profile.

A staging CT chest and abdomen with IV contrast should be performed.

The patient should be referred to respiratory/oncology services for further management, which may include biopsy and MDT discussion. Treatment, which may include surgery, radiotherapy, chemotherapy or palliative treatment, will depend on the outcome of the MDT discussion, investigations and the patient's wishes.

A 55-year-old female presents to ED generally unwell with worsening headaches. She has a long history of hydrocephalus. She is a nonsmoker. On examination, she has oxygen saturations of 90% in air and is afebrile. Lungs are resonant throughout, with good bilateral air entry. A chest X-ray is requested to assess for possible pneumonia.

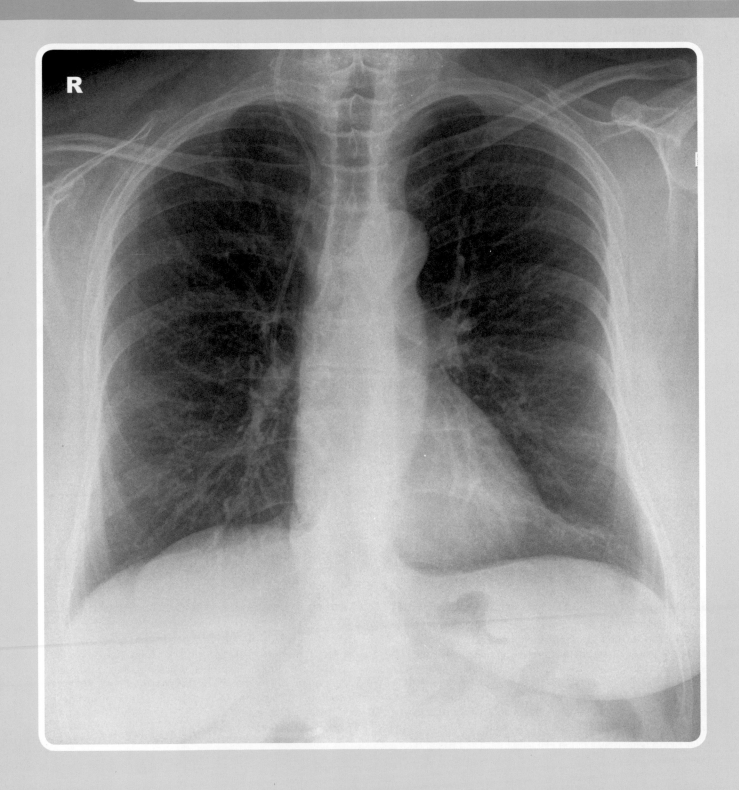

TECHNICAL INFORMATION

Patient ID: Anonymous
Projection: PA
Penetration: Adequate – vertebral bodies just visible behind heart
Inspiration: Adequate – six anterior ribs visible
Rotation: Not rotated

● AIRWAY

The trachea is central.

● BREATHING

The lungs are clear.

The lungs are not hyperinflated.

The pleural spaces are clear.

Normal pulmonary vascularity.

● CIRCULATION AND MEDIASTINUM

The heart is not enlarged.

The heart borders are clear.

The aorta appears normal.

The mediastinum is central, not widened, with clear borders.

Normal size, shape and position of both hila.

● DIAPHRAGM AND DELICATES

Normal position and appearance of the diaphragm.

No pneumoperitoneum.

The imaged skeleton is intact with no fractures or destructive bony lesions visible.

The visible soft tissues are unremarkable.

● EXTRAS AND REVIEW AREAS

There is a line that is projected over the right hemithorax. It runs caudally from the right side of the neck. The distal end of the line appears to be over the right atrium. The line appears intact with no apparent defects.

Lung apices: Normal.
Hila: Normal.
Behind heart: Normal.
Costophrenic angles: Normal.
Below the diaphragm: Normal.

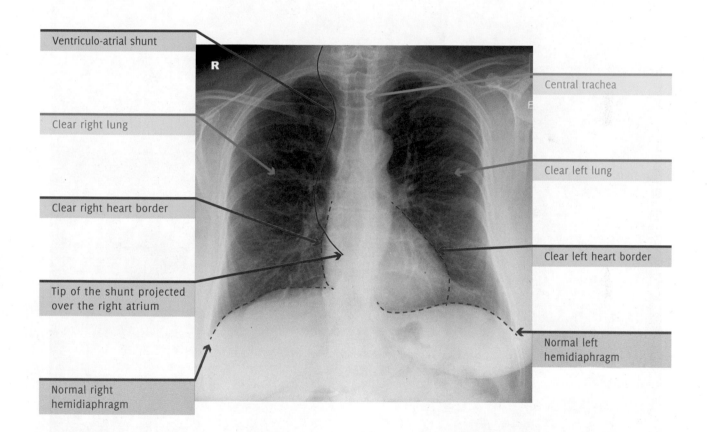

Labels: Ventriculo-atrial shunt; Clear right lung; Clear right heart border; Tip of the shunt projected over the right atrium; Normal right hemidiaphragm; Central trachea; Clear left lung; Clear left heart border; Normal left hemidiaphragm

SUMMARY, INVESTIGATIONS AND MANAGEMENT

In the context of the history, and given the position and course of this line, it is consistent with a ventriculoatrial shunt. The thoracic component appears intact. These lines are usually tunnelled subcutaneously and allow the excess cerebrospinal fluid to drain into the right atrium (as in this case) or peritoneal cavity (ventriculoperitoneal shunt).

Supplementary oxygen should be given.

Initial blood tests may include FBC, U&Es, CRP and blood cultures.

The patient should be referred to neurosurgery for further assessment. The shunt reservoir/valve can be compressed to see if it empties or worsens the headache. The remainder of the shunt needs to be imaged to check it is not fractured or kinked – this will require X-rays of the skull and neck. A CT head may be performed to assess for changes in the degree of hydrocephalus.

A 55-year-old male is admitted via ED to the coronary care unit after an acute presentation of shortness of breath. He has a history of dilated cardiomyopathy. Initial chest X-ray showed evidence of heart failure, and he is therefore being treated with oxygen and diuretics. A repeat chest X-ray is requested following 2 days of treatment to assess for any radiological response to treatment.

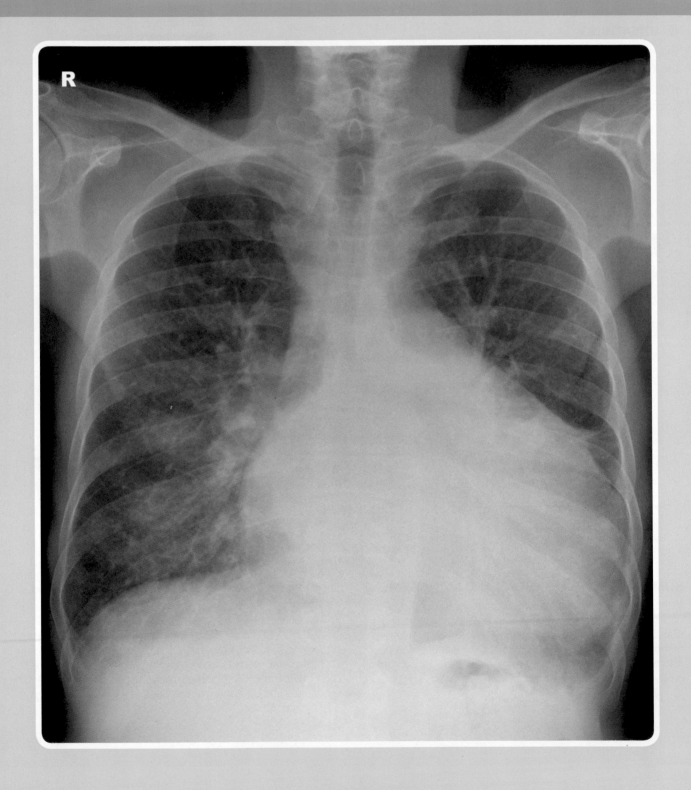

TECHNICAL INFORMATION

Patient ID: Anonymous
Projection: PA
Penetration: Adequate – vertebral bodies just visible behind heart
Inspiration: Adequate – seven anterior ribs visible
Rotation: Not rotated

● AIRWAY

The trachea is central.

● BREATHING

There is interstitial opacification in both lungs and perihilar opacification around the right hilum. A couple of peripheral septal lines are visible in the right lower zone, in keeping with Kerley B lines. Prominent pulmonary vessels within the upper lobes are in keeping with upper lobe venous diversion. There is minor blunting of the costophrenic angles, suggestive of small pleural effusions.

The lungs are not hyperinflated.

● CIRCULATION AND MEDIASTINUM

The heart is enlarged with a cardiothoracic ratio of 0.69.

The heart borders are clear.

The aorta is difficult to clearly identify.

The mediastinum is central, not widened, with clear borders.

Normal size, shape and position of the right hilum. The left hilum is obscured by the heart.

● DIAPHRAGM AND DELICATES

Normal appearance and position of the hemidiaphragms.

No pneumoperitoneum.

The imaged skeleton is intact with no fractures or destructive bony lesions visible.

The visible soft tissues are unremarkable.

● EXTRAS AND REVIEW AREAS

No vascular lines, tubes or surgical clips.
Lung apices: Upper lobe venous diversion.
Hila: Normal right hilum, the left is obscured.
Behind heart: Normal.
Costophrenic angles: Blunting consistent with small effusions.
Below the diaphragm: Normal.

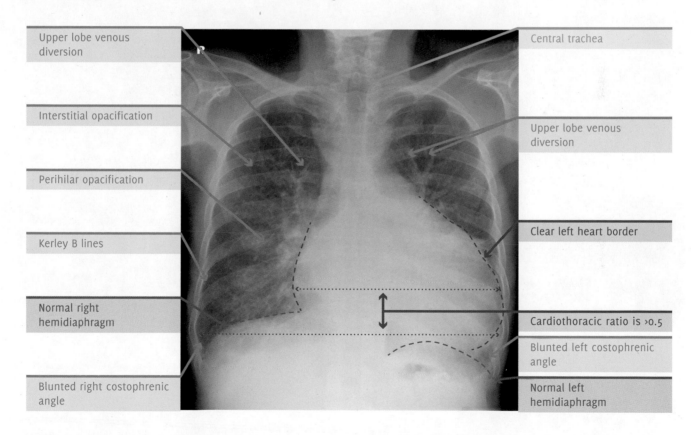

Labels (left, top to bottom): Upper lobe venous diversion · Interstitial opacification · Perihilar opacification · Kerley B lines · Normal right hemidiaphragm · Blunted right costophrenic angle

Labels (right, top to bottom): Central trachea · Upper lobe venous diversion · Clear left heart border · Cardiothoracic ratio is >0.5 · Blunted left costophrenic angle · Normal left hemidiaphragm

SUMMARY, INVESTIGATIONS AND MANAGEMENT

This X-ray demonstrates cardiomegaly in keeping with the known history of dilated cardiomyopathy. The upper lobe venous blood diversion, interstitial markings and small pleural effusions are in keeping with pulmonary oedema.

The X-ray needs to be compared with the previous imaging to assess for interval change to treatment. This should be correlated with the clinical assessment as well as an ECHO. His cardiac medication, including diuretic therapy, may need to be adjusted if the pulmonary oedema is worsening.

A 60-year-old female presents to ED after being stabbed in the right lateral chest wall. There is no significant past medical history. She is a nonsmoker. On examination, she has oxygen saturations of 99% in air, is haemodynamically stable and afebrile. The lungs are resonant throughout, with good bilateral air entry. The base of the stab wound is not visible. A chest X-ray is requested to assess for underlying thoracic injuries such as a pneumothorax.

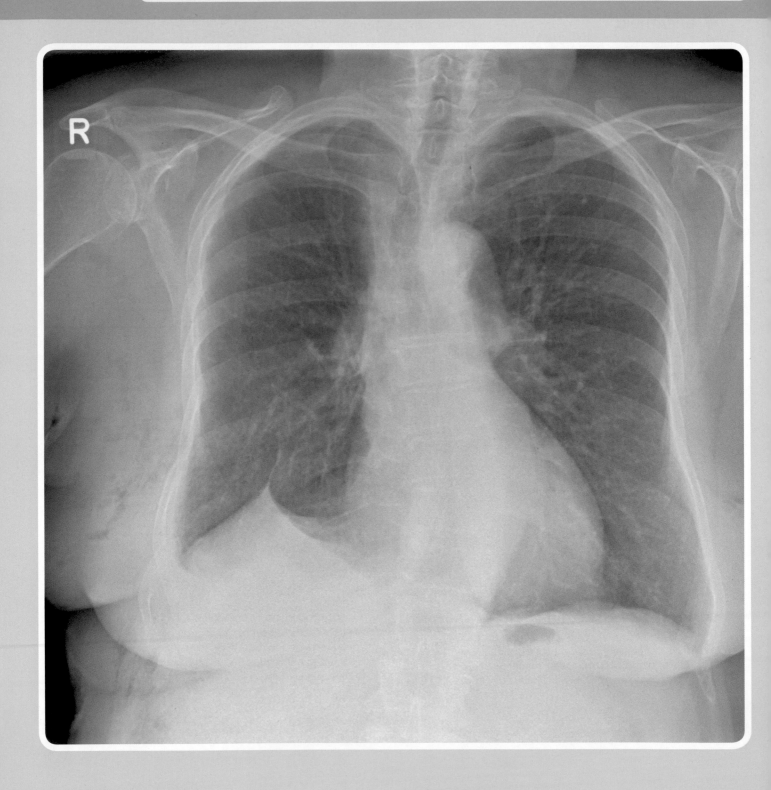

TECHNICAL INFORMATION

Patient ID: Anonymous
Projection: PA
Penetration: Adequate – vertebral bodies just visible behind heart
Inspiration: Adequate – seven anterior ribs visible
Rotation: The patient is not rotated

● AIRWAY

The upper trachea is central. The lower trachea is displaced slightly to the right.

● BREATHING

There is a tiny dense opacity in the left upper zone projected between the anterior ends of the 1st and 2nd ribs, consistent with a calcified granuloma. The lungs are otherwise clear.

The lungs are not hyperinflated.

The pleural spaces are clear.

Normal pulmonary vascularity.

● CIRCULATION AND MEDIASTINUM

The heart is not enlarged.

The heart borders are clear.

There is mild unfolding of the thoracic aorta.

The mediastinum is central, not widened with clear borders.

Normal size, shape and position of both hila.

● DIAPHRAGM AND DELICATES

There is tenting of the right hemidiaphragm, consistent with incidental eventration of the hemidiaphragm. Normal appearance and position of the left hemidiaphragm.

No pneumoperitoneum.

A mid and lower thoracic scoliosis is present. The imaged skeleton is otherwise intact with no fractures or destructive bony lesions visible.

There is surgical emphysema within the soft tissues of the right axilla/ lateral chest wall.

● EXTRAS AND REVIEW AREAS

No vascular lines, tubes or surgical clips.
Lung apices: Normal.
Hila: Normal.
Behind heart: Normal.
Costophrenic angles: Normal.
Below the diaphragm: Normal.

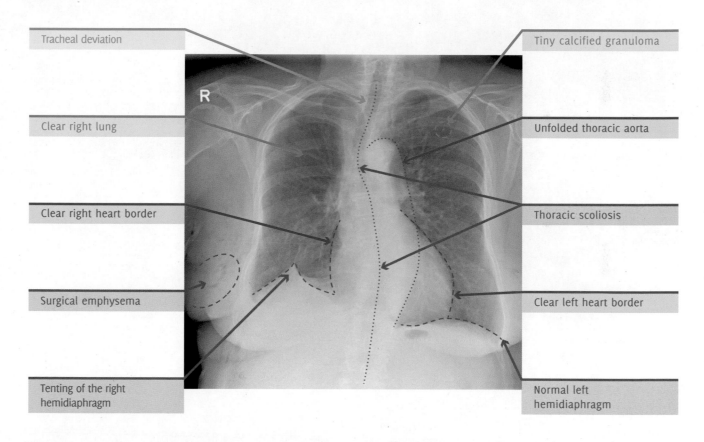

Tracheal deviation

Tiny calcified granuloma

Clear right lung

Unfolded thoracic aorta

Clear right heart border

Thoracic scoliosis

Surgical emphysema

Clear left heart border

Tenting of the right hemidiaphragm

Normal left hemidiaphragm

SUMMARY, INVESTIGATIONS AND MANAGEMENT

This X-ray demonstrates surgical emphysema in the right lateral chest wall/axilla. This presumably corresponds with the stab wound. There is no evidence of intrathoracic injury in the form of a pneumothorax, haemothorax or rib fracture. The displacement of the lower trachea is likely related to the thoracic scoliosis.

The patient should be assessed for other injuries using the ATLS algorithm.

The stab wound needs to be thoroughly assessed and managed based on clinical appearance. This may include a wash-out and suturing. It will also be important to look for any other associated injuries.

A 60-year-old female presents to ED with general fatigue, fever and a productive cough. There is no significant past medical history. She is a nonsmoker. On examination, she has oxygen saturations of 85% in air and is febrile with a temperature of 39.5°C. There are scattered crackles throughout the lungs. A chest X-ray is requested to assess for possible pneumonia.

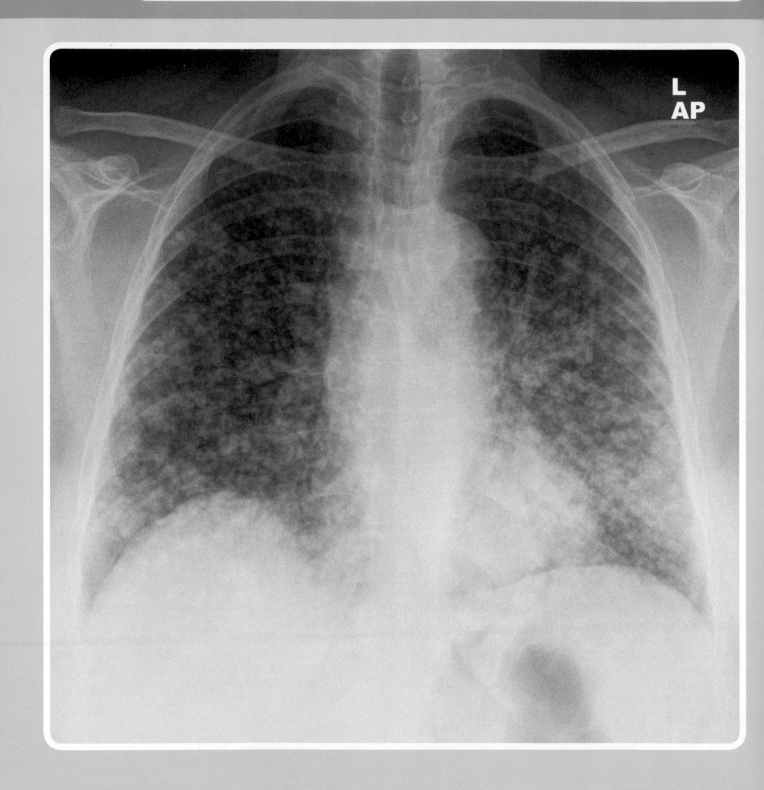

TECHNICAL INFORMATION

Patient ID: Anonymous
Projection: PA
Penetration: Adequate – vertebral bodies just visible behind heart
Inspiration: Adequate – six anterior ribs visible
Rotation: Not rotated

● AIRWAY

The trachea is central.

● BREATHING

There are diffuse nodular opacities spread throughout the lungs. The nodules are small (1–2 mm) and noncalcified. There is no evidence of cavitation.

The lungs are not hyperinflated.

The pleural spaces are clear.

Normal pulmonary vascularity.

● CIRCULATION AND MEDIASTINUM

The heart is not enlarged.

The heart borders are clear.

There is mild unfolding of the thoracic aorta.

The mediastinum is central, not widened, with clear borders.

Normal size, shape and position of both hila.

● DIAPHRAGM AND DELICATES

Normal appearance and position of the hemidiaphragms.

No pneumoperitoneum.

The imaged skeleton is intact with no fractures or destructive bony lesions visible.

The visible soft tissues are unremarkable.

● EXTRAS AND REVIEW AREAS

No vascular lines, tubes or surgical clips.
Lung apices: Multiple small pulmonary nodules.
Hila: Normal.
Behind heart: Multiple small pulmonary nodules.
Costophrenic angles: Normal.
Below the diaphragm: Normal.

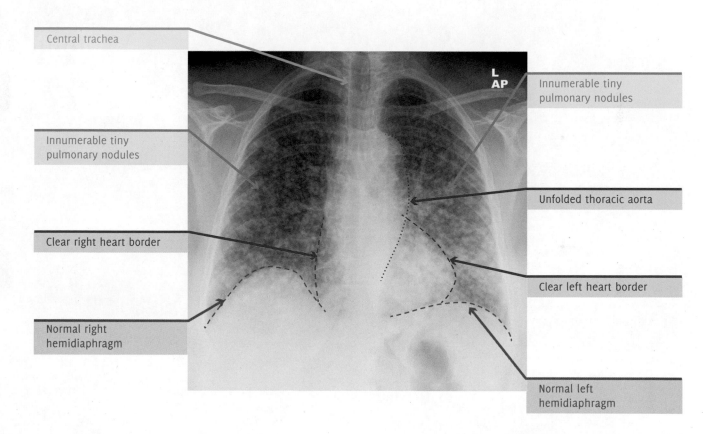

Central trachea

Innumerable tiny pulmonary nodules

Innumerable tiny pulmonary nodules

Clear right heart border

Unfolded thoracic aorta

Clear left heart border

Normal right hemidiaphragm

Normal left hemidiaphragm

SUMMARY, INVESTIGATIONS AND MANAGEMENT

This X-ray demonstrates innumerable small noncalcified pulmonary (miliary) nodules throughout both lungs. The patient is unwell making metastases or infection, such as TB (miliary TB) or fungal infections, most likely. If the patient was well the differential would include sarcoidosis and silicosis.

Supplementary oxygen should be given. Initial blood tests may include FBC, U&Es, LFTs, bone profile, CRP, ESR, TFTs, HIV and blood/mycobacterial cultures. Sputum culture and a Tuberculin skin prick test may also be helpful.

The patient should be considered to have active TB until proven otherwise and nursed appropriately in a single room. Anti-TB medication should be commenced (e.g. rifampicin, isoniazid, pyrazinamide and ethambutol).

A contrast-enhanced CT of the chest, abdomen and pelvis should be performed to assess for evidence of malignancy.

Specialist input may be required from respiratory, infectious disease and/or oncology.

A 65-year-old male has just had an NG tube inserted. He is currently in ITU post laparotomy for a perforated duodenal ulcer. He has previously had a CABG. On examination, he has oxygen saturations of 98% in 5L of facemask oxygen and is afebrile. Lungs are resonant throughout with good bilateral air entry. A chest X-ray is requested to assess the position of the NG tube.

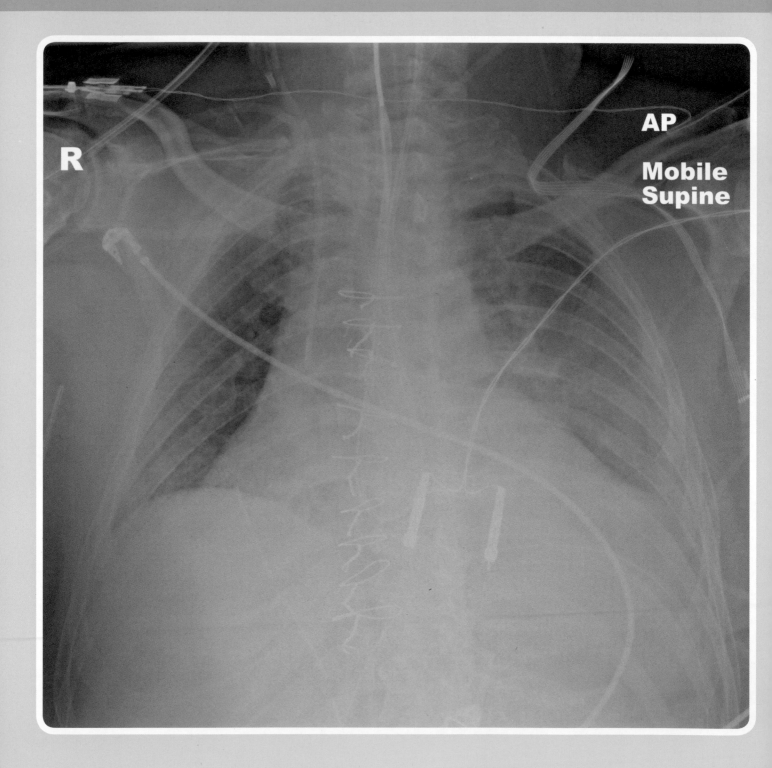

TECHNICAL INFORMATION

Patient ID: Anonymous
Projection: Portable supine AP
Penetration: Adequate – vertebral bodies just visible behind heart
Inspiration: Inadequate – four anterior ribs visible
Rotation: The patient is rotated to the right

● AIRWAY

The trachea is central after factoring in patient rotation.

● BREATHING

There is heterogeneous airspace opacification in the left lower zone, consistent with consolidation or atelectasis.

The lungs are otherwise clear. They are not hyperinflated.

The pleural spaces are clear.

Normal pulmonary vascularity.

● CIRCULATION AND MEDIASTINUM

The cardiac size cannot be accurately assessed given the projection and limited inspiratory achievement.

The heart borders are clear.

The aorta appears normal.

The mediastinum is central, not widened, with clear borders.

The hila are difficult to identify but no hilar mass is visible.

● DIAPHRAGM AND DELICATES

Normal appearance and position of the right hemidiaphragm. The left is difficult to identify and partially obscured.

No pneumoperitoneum visible, although this is difficult to assess on a supine X-ray.

The imaged skeleton is intact with no fractures or destructive bony lesions visible.

The visible soft tissues are unremarkable.

● EXTRAS AND REVIEW AREAS

The NG tube is looped within the oesophagus, with its tip coiled back up into the pharynx.

There is a central venous catheter in the right internal jugular vein with its tip projected over the lower superior vena cava.

Midline sternotomy wires are visible. There are two lines projected over the upper abdomen in keeping with surgical drains.

External lead monitoring wires are also noted.
Lung apices: Normal.
Hila: Difficult to identify.
Behind heart: Increased left retrocardiac opacification.
Costophrenic angles: Normal.
Below the diaphragm: Normal.

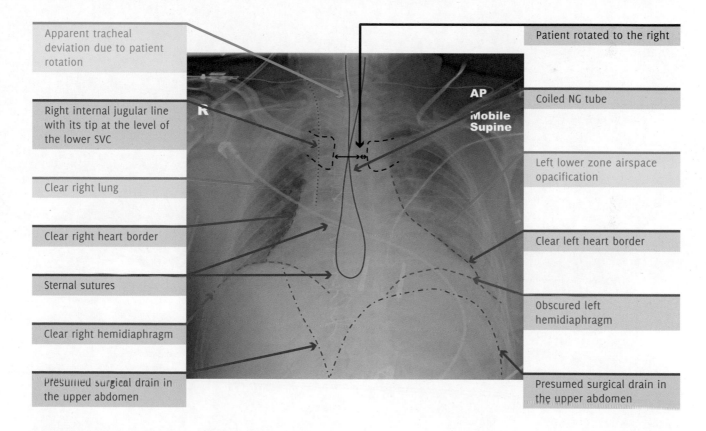

Apparent tracheal deviation due to patient rotation

Right internal jugular line with its tip at the level of the lower SVC

Clear right lung

Clear right heart border

Sternal sutures

Clear right hemidiaphragm

Presumed surgical drain in the upper abdomen

Patient rotated to the right

Coiled NG tube

AP
Mobile Supine

Left lower zone airspace opacification

Clear left heart border

Obscured left hemidiaphragm

Presumed surgical drain in the upper abdomen

R

SUMMARY, INVESTIGATIONS AND MANAGEMENT

This X-ray demonstrates an NG tube coiled within the oesophagus, with its tip looped back up into the pharynx. The other lines and drains are appropriately sited. Left lower zone changes are consistent with consolidation or atelectasis.

The NG tube needs to be removed and reinserted. A repeat X-ray will be required to confirm its position prior to feeding.

Ideally this X-ray would be an erect X-ray, with good inspiratory effort, as this would permit better assessment of the left lower zone. The patient is likely to be on antibiotics already, but if there is a strong clinical suspicion of pneumonia it would be reasonable to repeat bloods, particularly FBC and CRP, send sputum/blood cultures and start treatment for a postoperative pneumonia.

A 65-year-old male presents to ED with palpitations. He has recently had a pacemaker inserted for atrioventricular block. He is a nonsmoker. On examination, he has oxygen saturations of 98% in air, is tachycardic (regular, good-volume pulse at 130 bpm) and is afebrile. Lungs are resonant throughout with good air entry bilaterally. A chest X-ray is requested to assess lead position and exclude a pneumothorax.

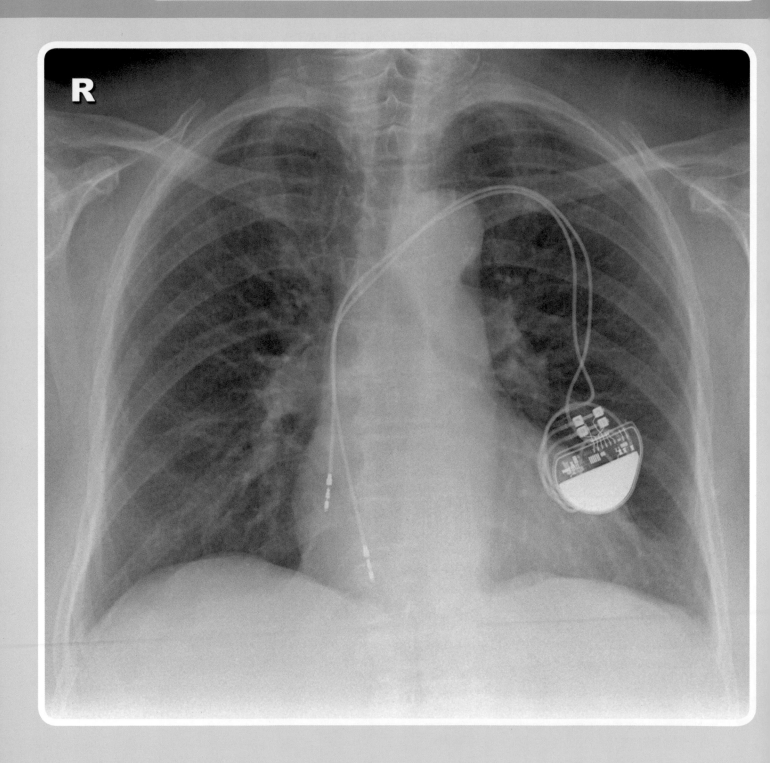

TECHNICAL INFORMATION

Patient ID: Anonymous
Projection: PA
Penetration: Adequate – vertebral bodies just visible behind
Inspiration: Adequate – six anterior ribs visible
Rotation: Not rotated

● AIRWAY

The trachea is central.

● BREATHING

The lungs are clear. They are not hyperinflated.

The pleural spaces are clear. No pneumothorax.

Normal pulmonary vascularity.

● CIRCULATION AND MEDIASTINUM

The heart is not enlarged.

The heart borders are clear.

The aorta appears normal.

The mediastinum is central, not widened, with clear borders.

Normal size, shape and position of both hila.

● DIAPHRAGM AND DELICATES

Normal position and appearance of the diaphragm.

No pneumoperitoneum.

The imaged skeleton is intact with no fractures or destructive bony lesions visible.

The visible soft tissues are unremarkable.

● EXTRAS AND REVIEW AREAS

There is a dual-chamber pacemaker in situ. Both electrode tips are projected over the right atrium. Only one should be projecting over in the right atrium, the other over the right ventricular apex. No fracture/break of the electrodes is visible.

Lung apices: Normal.
Hila: Normal.
Behind heart: Normal.
Costophrenic angles: Normal.
Below the diaphragm: Normal.

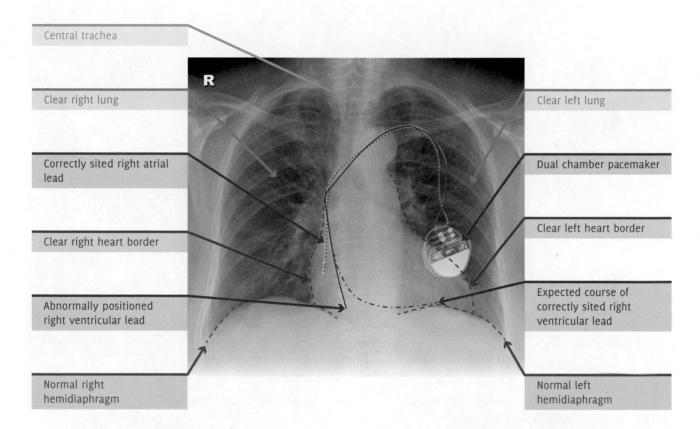

Central trachea

Clear right lung

Correctly sited right atrial lead

Clear right heart border

Abnormally positioned right ventricular lead

Normal right hemidiaphragm

Clear left lung

Dual chamber pacemaker

Clear left heart border

Expected course of correctly sited right ventricular lead

Normal left hemidiaphragm

SUMMARY, INVESTIGATIONS AND MANAGEMENT

This X-ray demonstrates an unsatisfactory positioning of the right ventricular pacemaker lead. There is no pneumothorax.

An ECG should be performed. The patient should be referred to cardiology for management of any acute arrhythmias and for pacemaker testing. Repositioning of the pacemaker is likely to be required.

A 65-year-old male presents to ED with worsening shortness of breath. He has a 60 pack-year smoking history. An initial chest X-ray showed bronchiectasis, and after acutely deteriorating he was admitted to ICU, intubated and had a central venous catheter inserted. Broad-spectrum antibiotics have already been commenced and the respiratory team are on route to review. On examination, he has oxygen saturations of 100% in 40% oxygen with minimal ventilator support. He is afebrile. Lungs are resonant throughout, with coarse crackles bilaterally throughout the lung fields. A chest X-ray is performed to assess the position of the ET tube and the central venous line.

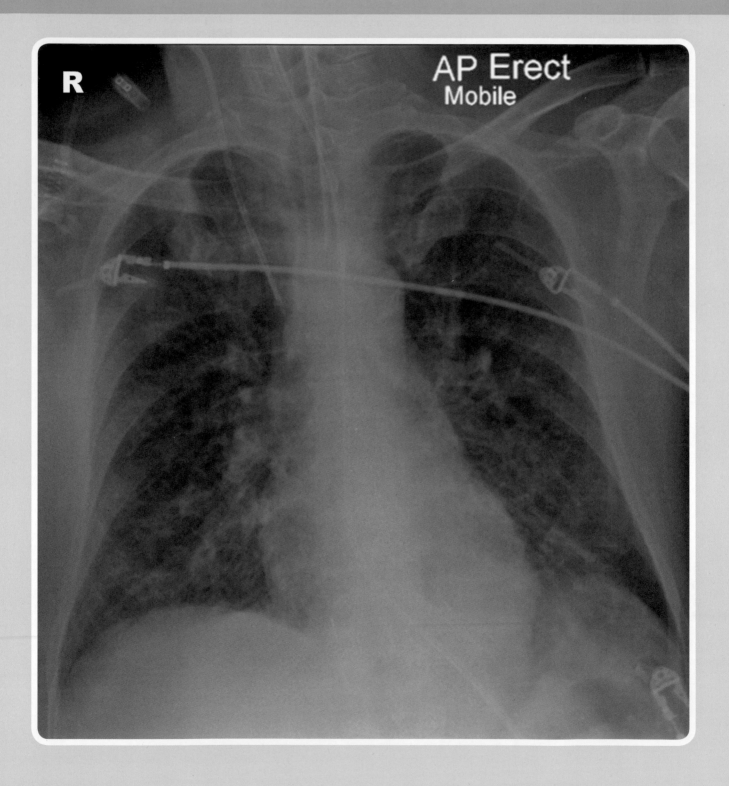

TECHNICAL INFORMATION

Patient ID: Anonymous
Projection: AP erect mobile
Penetration: Adequate – vertebral bodies just visible behind heart
Inspiration: Adequate – six anterior ribs visible
Rotation: The patient is slightly rotated to the right

● AIRWAY

The trachea is central allowing for patient rotation.

● BREATHING

There are bilateral coarse bronchovascular lung markings seen, particularly in the lower zones. Some ring shadows are also present. No focal consolidation is visible.

The lungs are not hyperinflated.

The pleural spaces are clear.

Normal pulmonary vascularity.

● CIRCULATION AND MEDIASTINUM

The heart does not appear enlarged, although its size cannot be accurately assessed on an AP X-ray.

The heart borders are clear.

The aorta appears normal.

The mediastinum is central, not widened, with clear borders.

Normal size, shape and position of both hila.

● DIAPHRAGM AND DELICATES

Normal position and appearance of the hemidiaphragms.

No pneumoperitoneum.

The imaged skeleton is intact with no fractures or destructive bony lesions visible.

The visible soft tissues are unremarkable.

● EXTRAS AND REVIEW AREAS

The ET tube tip is appropriately sited, with its tip a few centimetres above the carina.

There is a central venous catheter in the right internal jugular vein with its tip projected over the upper superior vena cava.

The NG tube is appropriately sited, with its tip below the level of the diaphragm on the left.

There are ECG monitoring leads in situ.
Lung apices: Normal.
Hila: Normal.
Behind heart: Normal.
Costophrenic angles: Normal.
Below the diaphragm: Normal.

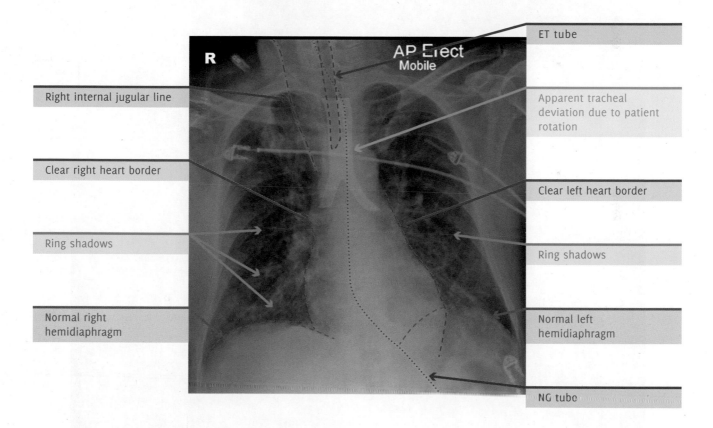

Labels on image: R · AP Erect Mobile · ET tube · Apparent tracheal deviation due to patient rotation · Right internal jugular line · Clear right heart border · Clear left heart border · Ring shadows · Ring shadows · Normal right hemidiaphragm · Normal left hemidiaphragm · NG tube

SUMMARY, INVESTIGATIONS AND MANAGEMENT

This X-ray demonstrates a correctly sited ET tube, NG tube and right internal jugular line. Background changes are in keeping with bronchiectasis.

The right internal jugular line is safe to use.

Previous imaging should be reviewed to determine if the bronchiectasis is new or progressive. A chest CT could better assess the bronchiectasis if considered necessary.

A 67-year-old male presents to ED with a productive cough, on a background of 2 weeks of nausea and vomiting. He has a history of dysphagia following a previous stroke. He is a nonsmoker. On examination, he has oxygen saturations of 85% in air, has an HR of 100 bpm and is febrile with a temperature of 39.5°C. There is dullness to percussion and coarse crackles in the right upper and mid zones. A chest X-ray is performed to assess for possible pneumonia or collapse.

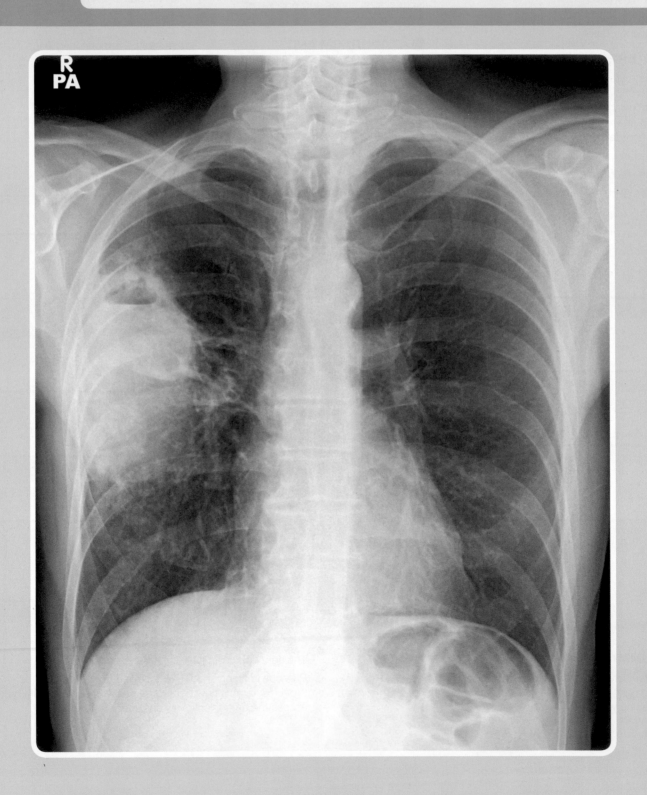

TECHNICAL INFORMATION

Patient ID: Anonymous
Projection: PA
Penetration: Adequate – vertebral bodies just visible behind heart
Inspiration: Adequate – eight anterior ribs visible
Rotation: The patient is slightly rotated to the left

● AIRWAY

The trachea is central after factoring in patient rotation.

● BREATHING

There is dense airspace opacification peripherally in the right upper and mid zones consistent with consolidation. An air-fluid level is visible superiorly in this region, suggesting a fluid collection.

The lungs are otherwise clear. The lungs are not hyperinflated.

The pleural spaces are clear.

Normal pulmonary vascularity.

● CIRCULATION AND MEDIASTINUM

The heart is not enlarged.

The heart borders are clear.

The aorta appears normal.

The mediastinum is central, not widened, with clear borders.

Normal size, shape and position of both hila.

● DIAPHRAGM AND DELICATES

Normal position and appearance of the hemidiaphragms.

No pneumoperitoneum.

The imaged skeleton is intact with no fractures or destructive bony lesions visible.

The visible soft tissues are unremarkable.

● EXTRAS AND REVIEW AREAS

No vascular lines, tubes or surgical clips.
Lung apices: Normal.
Hila: Normal.
Behind heart: Normal.
Costophrenic angles: Normal.
Below the diaphragm: Normal.

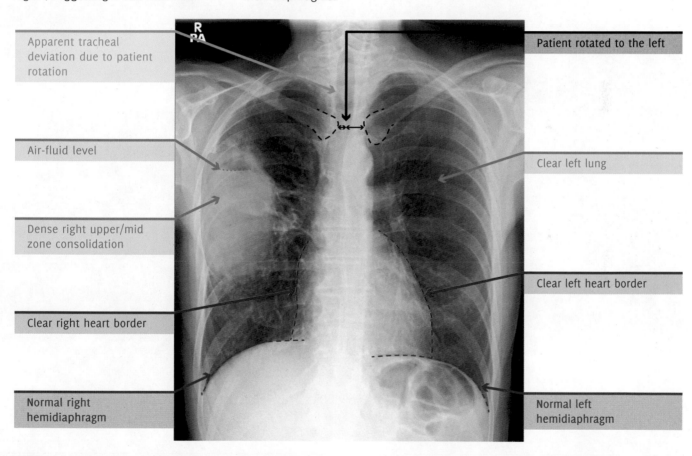

Apparent tracheal deviation due to patient rotation

Patient rotated to the left

Air-fluid level

Clear left lung

Dense right upper/mid zone consolidation

Clear left heart border

Clear right heart border

Normal right hemidiaphragm

Normal left hemidiaphragm

SUMMARY, INVESTIGATIONS AND MANAGEMENT

This X-ray demonstrates consolidation in the right upper and mid zone consistent with pneumonia. The air-fluid level is most likely in keeping with an abscess. Infection of a preexisting cavity is a possibility but is less likely.

The appearance is probably the result of aspiration pneumonia given the location of the pneumonia combined with the presence of an abscess and the clinical history of dysphagia. TB is in the differential diagnosis.

The patient should be barrier nursed. Initial blood tests may include FBC, U&Es, LFTs, bone profile, CRP and blood cultures. Sputum cultures and TB testing should also be performed.

The patient should be kept nil by mouth until a swallow assessment is performed. Broad-spectrum intravenous antibiotics should be started, with consideration of cover for tuberculosis and discussion with microbiology. A follow-up chest X-ray should be performed to ensure resolution of the pneumonia and abscess. If there is persisting abnormality a contrast-enhanced CT of the chest would be appropriate.

A 70-year-old female presents to ED acutely breathless after a mechanical fall. She has no significant past medical history. She is a nonsmoker. On examination, she has oxygen saturations of 88% in air, HR 95 bpm and BP 90/50 mmHg. There is increased resonance in the right hemithorax and reduced air entry. A chest X-ray is requested to assess for a possible pneumothorax.

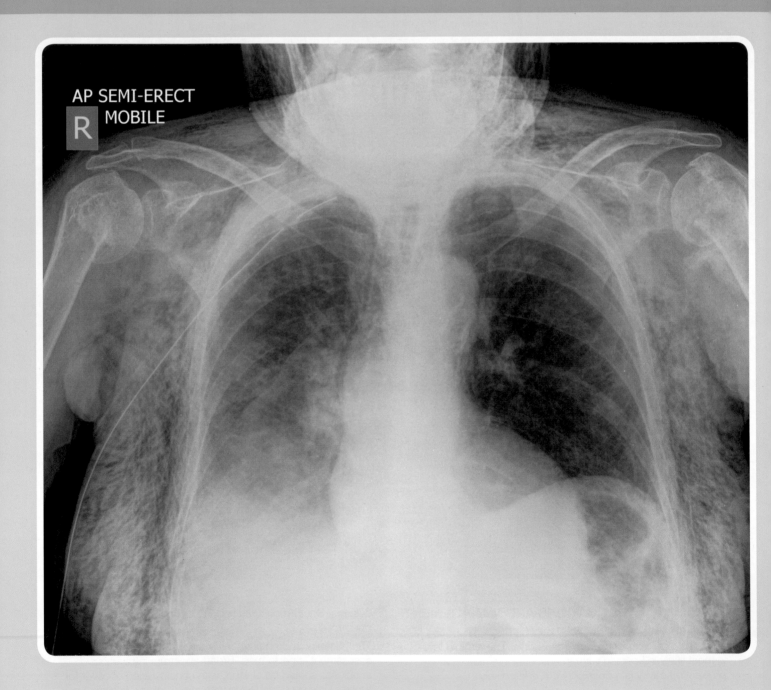

AP SEMI-ERECT
R MOBILE

TECHNICAL INFORMATION

Patient ID: Anonymous
Projection: AP semierect mobile
Penetration: Adequate– vertebral bodies just visible behind heart
Inspiration: Limited – five anterior ribs visible
Rotation: The patient is slightly rotated to the right

● AIRWAY

The trachea is central after factoring in patient rotation.

● BREATHING

A lung edge is visible in the right hemithorax, beyond which no lung markings are seen, consistent with a pneumothorax. There is increased opacification medially in the right lower zone, which may reflect contusions or be the result from the partially collapsed lung. The left lung is clear and is not hyperexpanded.

The right costophrenic angle is difficult to see and this may represent a small pleural effusion (most likely blood). The left pleural spaces are clear.

Normal pulmonary vascularity.

● CIRCULATION AND MEDIASTINUM

The heart does not appear enlarged, although its size cannot be accurately assessed on an AP X-ray.

The heart borders are clear.

The aorta appears normal.

There is a thin lucency along the right side of the mediastinum suggestive of pneumomediastinum. The mediastinum is central, not widened, with clear borders.

The hila are difficult to identify.

● DIAPHRAGM AND DELICATES

Normal appearance and position of left hemidiaphragm. The right hemidiaphragm is obscured. This may be due to a basal effusion/haemothorax or as a result of basal lung consolidation secondary to lung contusions.

No pneumoperitoneum.

There are right-sided rib fractures – it is difficult to accurately count the ribs but they appear to involve the right 4th, 6th and 7th ribs. Comminuted fracture of the left humeral head. Fracture of the right humeral neck.

There are extensive lucencies projected over the chest, axillae and neck, consistent with surgical emphysema.

● EXTRAS AND REVIEW AREAS

Right-sided chest drain in situ, with the tip projected over the right lung apex. No vascular lines or surgical clips.
Lung apices: Right-sided pneumothorax. Left apex is clear.
Hila: Difficult to assess.
Behind heart: Increased right retrocardiac opacification.
Costophrenic angles: Blunted right costophrenic angle. Normal on left.
Below the diaphragm: Normal.

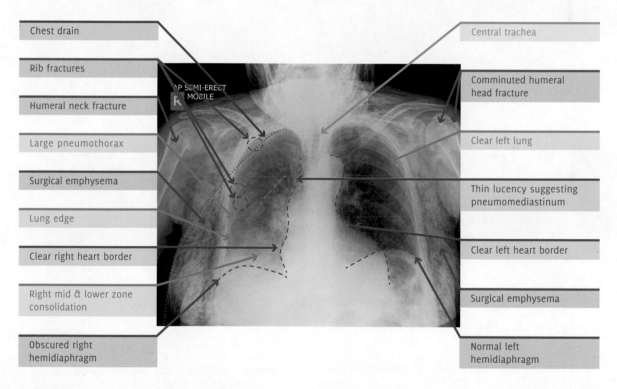

Chest drain

Rib fractures

Humeral neck fracture

Large pneumothorax

Surgical emphysema

Lung edge

Clear right heart border

Right mid & lower zone consolidation

Obscured right hemidiaphragm

Central trachea

Comminuted humeral head fracture

Clear left lung

Thin lucency suggesting pneumomediastinum

Clear left heart border

Surgical emphysema

Normal left hemidiaphragm

AP SEMI-ERECT MOBILE
R

SUMMARY, INVESTIGATIONS AND MANAGEMENT

This X-ray demonstrates a traumatic right-sided pneumothorax with extensive subcutaneous emphysema secondary to right posterior rib fractures. Consolidation in the right lower lobe is consistent with lung contusions. There is a probable small right-sided haemothorax and small-volume pneumomediastinum. Additionally there are fractures of the left humeral head and right humeral neck.

The patient needs to be assessed and resuscitated using the ATLS algorithm. The intercostal chest drain will need to be clinically reviewed and, if not adequately functioning, an alternative chest drain may need to be inserted.

Imaging with contrast-enhanced CT will provide more accurate assessment of the thoracic injuries. Other parts of the body (head, cervical spine, abdomen or pelvis) can also be imaged with CT depending on the clinical assessment. X-rays of both shoulders and any other possible fracture sites should be performed as part of the secondary survey, once the patient is stable.

A 75-year-old male presents to ED with confusion. There is no significant past medical history. He is a nonsmoker. On examination, he has oxygen saturations of 91% in air and is febrile with a temperature of 38.2°C. Lungs are resonant throughout, with good bilateral air entry. A chest X-ray is requested to assess for possible pneumonia.

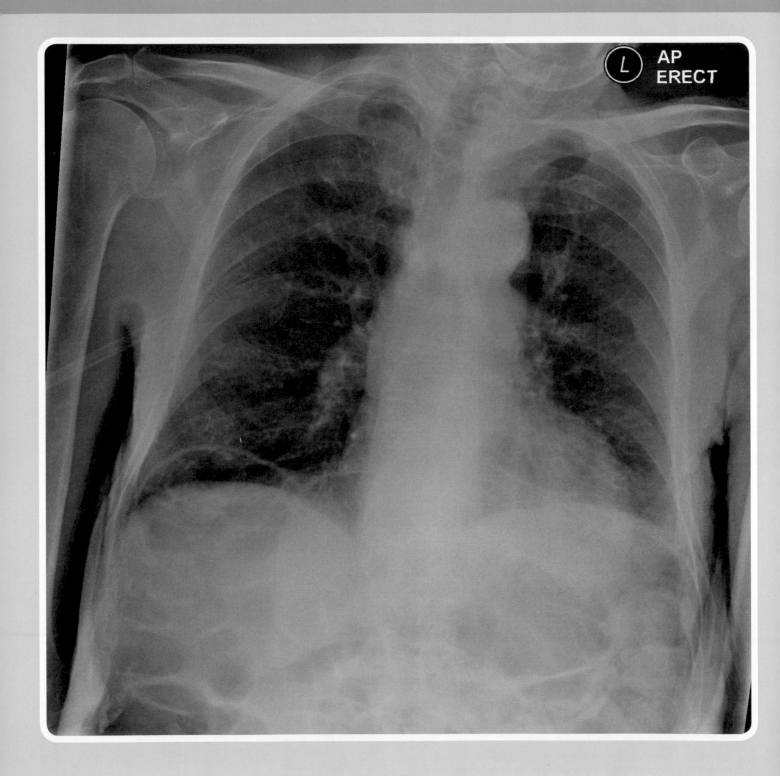

TECHNICAL INFORMATION

Patient ID: Anonymous
Projection: AP erect
Penetration: Adequate – vertebral bodies just visible behind heart
Inspiration: Adequate – six anterior ribs visible
Rotation: The patient is rotated to the right

● AIRWAY

The trachea is central after factoring in patient rotation.

● BREATHING

There is minor increased airspace opacification at the left base, which is in keeping with consolidation.

The lungs are otherwise clear. They are not hyperinflated.

The pleural spaces are clear.

Normal pulmonary vascularity.

● CIRCULATION AND MEDIASTINUM

The heart does not appear enlarged, although its size cannot be accurately assessed on an AP X-ray.

The heart borders are clear.

There is mild unfolding of the thoracic aorta.

The mediastinum is central, not widened, with clear borders.

Normal size, shape and position of both hila.

● DIAPHRAGM AND DELICATES

Normal appearance and position of both hemidiaphragms. There is increased lucency below the right hemidiaphragm. On closer inspection some bowel markings are visible at this site and there is a loop of large bowel in this region. No clear evidence of pneumoperitoneum.

There is an old left 6th rib fracture. The imaged skeleton is otherwise intact with no acute fractures or destructive bony lesions visible.

The visible soft tissues are unremarkable.

● EXTRAS AND REVIEW AREAS

There is oxygen tubing projected across the chest. No vascular lines or surgical clips.
Lung apices: Normal.
Hila: Normal.
Behind heart: Normal.
Costophrenic angles: Increased airspace opacification at the left costophrenic angle.
Below the diaphragm: Lucency beneath right hemidiaphragm.

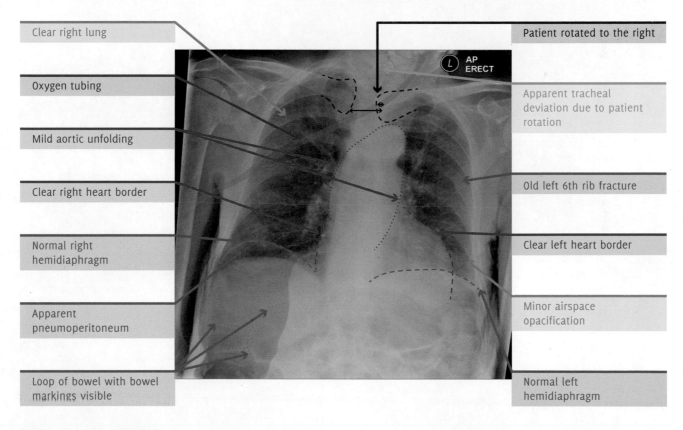

Clear right lung

Oxygen tubing

Mild aortic unfolding

Clear right heart border

Normal right hemidiaphragm

Apparent pneumoperitoneum

Loop of bowel with bowel markings visible

Patient rotated to the right

Apparent tracheal deviation due to patient rotation

Old left 6th rib fracture

Clear left heart border

Minor airspace opacification

Normal left hemidiaphragm

SUMMARY, INVESTIGATIONS AND MANAGEMENT

This X-ray demonstrates left lower zone consolidation, consistent with pneumonia.

The lucency beneath the right hemidiaphragm is likely to represent a loop of colon interposed between the liver and diaphragm as bowel markings are visible (Chilaiditi's sign).

The patient requires supplementary oxygen. Initial blood tests may include FBC, U&Es, LFTs, bone profile, CRP, ESR and TFTs. Sputum, urine and blood cultures may also be sent. He should be treated with appropriate antibiotics for community-acquired pneumonia and a follow-up chest X-ray performed to ensure resolution. The antibiotics may be oral or intravenous depending on the severity of pneumonia (CURB-65).

A review of any previous chest X-rays for similar appearances below the right hemidiaphragm would reassure that this is interposed bowel around the right hemidiaphragm rather than free gas. The patient's abdomen should be reexamined for any evidence of perforation, and if there is any clinical concern, a surgical opinion should be requested.

A 70-year-old male presents to ED with left-sided pleuritic chest pain and breathlessness following a 10-foot fall. There is no evidence of head injury, and no loss of consciousness. He has no significant past medical history. He is a nonsmoker. On examination, he has oxygen saturations of 92% in air and is haemodynamically stable. There is increased resonance in the left hemithorax, and reduced air entry. A chest X-ray is requested to assess for a possible pneumothorax.

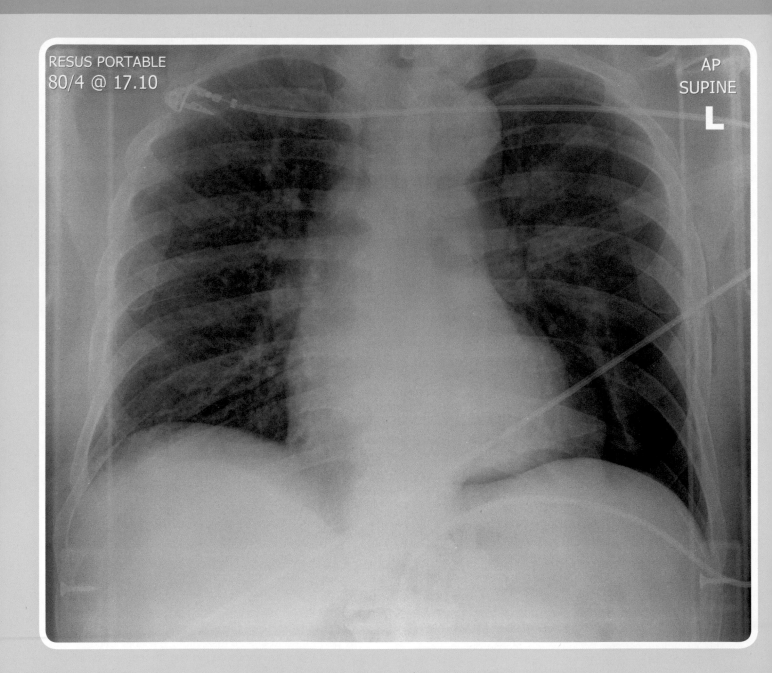

TECHNICAL INFORMATION

Patient ID: Anonymous
Projection: AP supine (portable)
Penetration: Adequate – vertebral bodies just visible behind heart
Inspiration: Adequate – six anterior ribs visible
Rotation: Not rotated

AIRWAY

The trachea is deviated slightly to the right.

BREATHING

A lung edge is visible in the left hemithorax, beyond which no lung markings are seen. There is also a deep left costophrenic angle with a sharply demarcated left heart border. All these features are consistent with a moderate/large left-sided pneumothorax.

The right lung is clear and is not hyperexpanded.

The right pleural spaces are clear and there is normal pulmonary vascularity.

CIRCULATION AND MEDIASTINUM

The heart does not appear enlarged, although its size cannot be accurately assessed on an AP X-ray.

There is a sharply demarcated left heart border secondary to the left-sided pneumothorax. The heart borders are clear.

The aorta appears normal.

The mediastinum is central with clear borders. Its size cannot be accurately assessed given the projection although it does not appear widened.

Normal size, shape and position of both hila.

DIAPHRAGM AND DELICATES

Normal appearance and position of the hemidiaphragms.

No pneumoperitoneum, although this is difficult to assess for on a supine film.

There are fractures of the left 5th and 6th ribs.

The visible soft tissues are unremarkable. Of note, there is no surgical emphysema.

EXTRAS AND REVIEW AREAS

ECG monitoring leads in situ. No vascular lines, tubes or surgical clips.

Two screws projected laterally over the lower part of the X-ray are presumably related to the spinal board the patient is lying on.

Lung apices: Left pneumothorax. Normal right apex.
Hila: Normal.
Behind heart: Normal.
Costophrenic angles: Left pneumothorax.
Below the diaphragm: Normal.

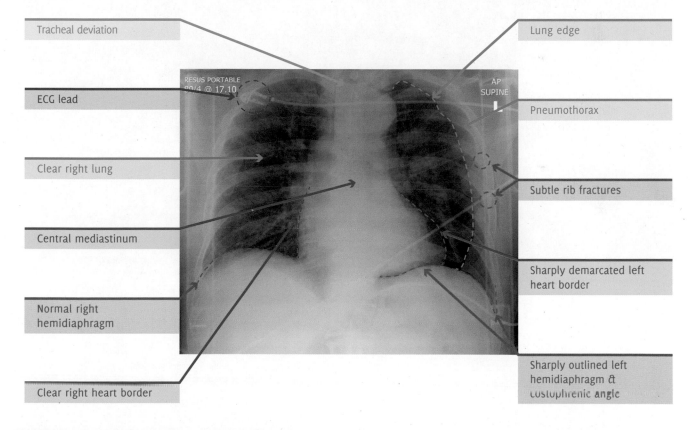

Tracheal deviation

ECG lead

Clear right lung

Central mediastinum

Normal right hemidiaphragm

Clear right heart border

RESUS PORTABLE
20/4 @ 17.10

AP SUPINE

Lung edge

Pneumothorax

Subtle rib fractures

Sharply demarcated left heart border

Sharply outlined left hemidiaphragm & costophrenic angle

SUMMARY, INVESTIGATIONS AND MANAGEMENT

This X-ray demonstrates a moderate/large left-sided pneumothorax associated with fractures of the left 5th and 6th ribs. The trachea is deviated slightly to the right. However, there is no lower mediastinal shift or flattening of the left hemidiaphragm. In addition, as the patient is haemodynamically stable, a tension pneumothorax is less likely.

The patient needs to be assessed and resuscitated using the ATLS algorithm. A left-sided intercostal chest drain will be required.

Imaging with contrast-enhanced CT will provide more accurate assessment of the thoracic injuries. Other parts of the body (head, cervical spine, abdomen or pelvis) can also be imaged with CT depending on the clinical assessment.

A 76-year-old female presents to ED with chest and shoulder discomfort following a mechanical fall. There is no significant past medical history. She is a nonsmoker. On examination, she has oxygen saturations of 100% in air and is afebrile. Her RR is 16 with an HR of 82 bpm. Lungs are resonant throughout, with good bilateral air entry. A chest X-ray is requested to assess for possible rib fractures or a pneumothorax.

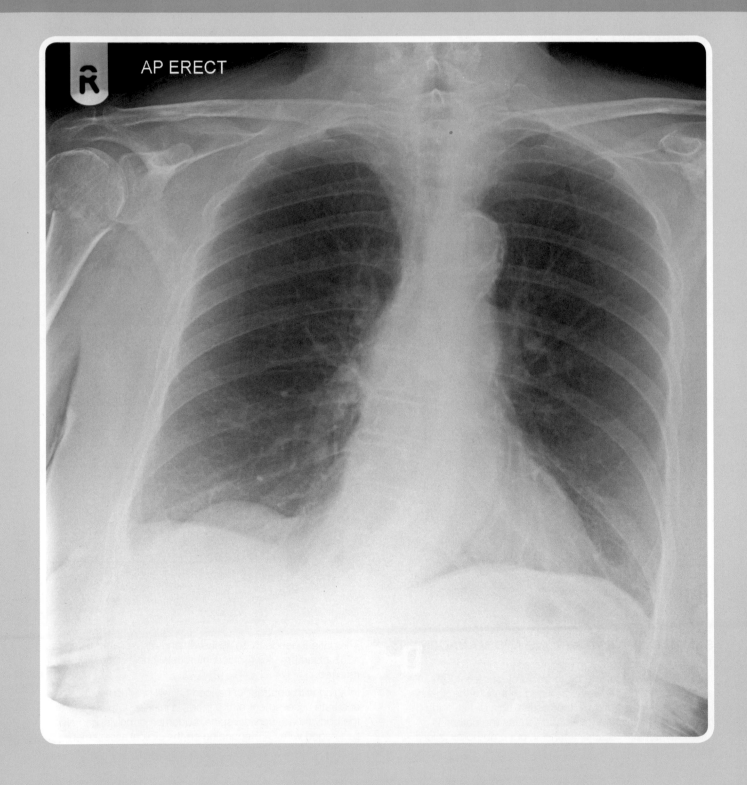

AP ERECT

TECHNICAL INFORMATION

Patient ID: Anonymous
Projection: AP erect
Penetration: Adequate – vertebral bodies just visible behind heart
Inspiration: Adequate – seven anterior ribs visible
Rotation: The patient is not rotated

● AIRWAY

The trachea is central.

● BREATHING

The lungs are clear.

The lungs are not hyperinflated.

The pleural spaces are clear.

Normal pulmonary vascularity.

● CIRCULATION AND MEDIASTINUM

The heart does not appear enlarged, although its size cannot be accurately assessed on an AP X-ray.

The heart borders are clear.

There is mild unfolding of the thoracic aorta.

The mediastinum is central, not widened, with clear borders.

Normal size, shape and position of both hila.

● DIAPHRAGM AND DELICATES

There is eventration of the right hemidiaphragm. Otherwise normal appearance and position of the hemidiaphragms.

No pneumoperitoneum.

There is a minimally displaced transverse fracture through the surgical neck of the right humerus. No other fractures or bony lesions.

The visible soft tissues are unremarkable.

● EXTRAS AND REVIEW AREAS

No vascular lines, tubes or surgical clips.
Lung apices: Normal.
Hila: Normal.
Behind heart: Normal.
Costophrenic angles: Normal.
Below the diaphragm: Normal.

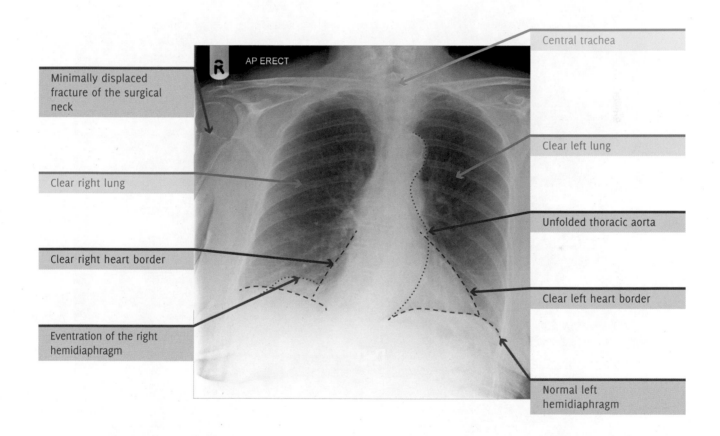

Minimally displaced fracture of the surgical neck

Clear right lung

Clear right heart border

Eventration of the right hemidiaphragm

Central trachea

Clear left lung

Unfolded thoracic aorta

Clear left heart border

Normal left hemidiaphragm

AP ERECT

SUMMARY, INVESTIGATIONS AND MANAGEMENT

This X-ray demonstrates a right-sided humeral neck fracture. No pneumothorax or rib fracture.

Dedicated X-rays of the right upper limb should be obtained. The patient should be referred to orthopaedics for further management, which will probably involve a sling and a follow-up X-ray.

An 80-year-old female presents to ED feeling unwell, with pyrexia and a productive cough. There is no significant past medical history. She is a nonsmoker. On examination, she has oxygen saturations of 93% in air and is febrile with a temperature of 38.2°C. There is dullness to percussion, reduced air entry and crackles in the left mid zone. A chest X-ray is requested to assess for possible pneumonia.

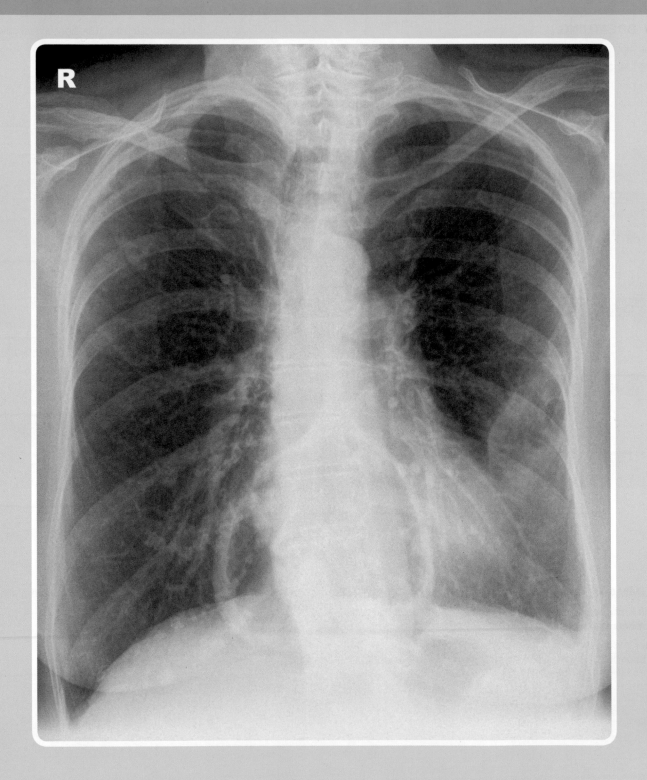

TECHNICAL INFORMATION

Patient ID: Anonymous
Projection: PA
Penetration: Adequate – vertebral bodies just visible behind heart
Inspiration: Adequate – six anterior ribs visible
Rotation: The patient is slightly rotated to the right

● AIRWAY

The trachea is central after factoring in patient rotation.

● BREATHING

There is left lower zone airspace opacification, with loss of clarity of the left heart border. The lungs are otherwise clear.

The lungs are not hyperinflated.

There is biapical pleural thickening and blunting of the left costophrenic angle in keeping with a small effusion.

Normal pulmonary vascularity.

● CIRCULATION AND MEDIASTINUM

The heart is not enlarged.

The left heart border is indistinct. The right heart border is clear.

There is a retrocardiac mass which has the density of gas.

The aorta appears normal.

The mediastinum is central, not widened, with clear borders.

Normal size, shape and position of both hila.

● DIAPHRAGM AND DELICATES

Normal appearance and position of the hemidiaphragms.

No pneumoperitoneum.

The imaged skeleton is intact with no fractures or destructive bony lesions visible.

The visible soft tissues are unremarkable.

● EXTRAS AND REVIEW AREAS

No vascular lines, tubes or surgical clips.
Lung apices: Biapical pleural thickening.
Hila: Normal.
Behind heart: Retrocardiac gas-filled opacity.
Costophrenic angles: Blunted left costophrenic angle.
Below the diaphragm: Normal.

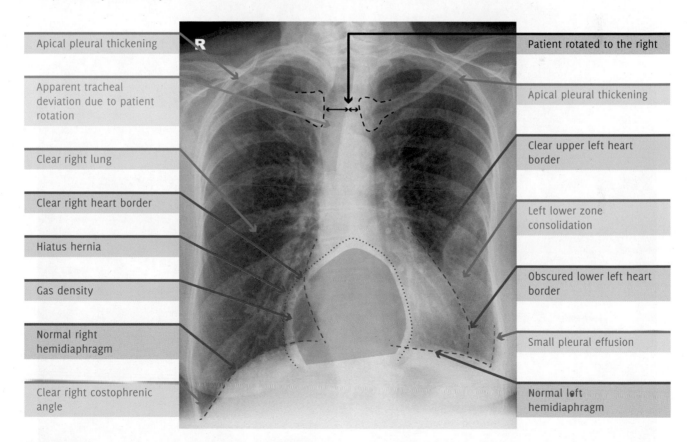

Left column labels (top to bottom): Apical pleural thickening; Apparent tracheal deviation due to patient rotation; Clear right lung; Clear right heart border; Hiatus hernia; Gas density; Normal right hemidiaphragm; Clear right costophrenic angle

Right column labels (top to bottom): Patient rotated to the right; Apical pleural thickening; Clear upper left heart border; Left lower zone consolidation; Obscured lower left heart border; Small pleural effusion; Normal left hemidiaphragm

SUMMARY, INVESTIGATIONS AND MANAGEMENT

This X-ray demonstrates left lower zone consolidation causing loss of clarity of the left heart border in keeping with a lingular pneumonia. There is a small effusion. The retrocardiac opacity is in keeping with an incidental hiatus hernia.

Initial blood tests may include FBC, U&Es, blood cultures and CRP. A sputum culture may also be taken.

The patient should be treated with appropriate antibiotics for community-acquired pneumonia and a follow-up chest X-ray performed to ensure resolution. The antibiotics may be oral or intravenous depending on the severity of pneumonia (CURB-65). The hiatus hernia and apical pleural thickening are incidental findings which do not require active management.

68

An 80-year-old male presents to ED with a 2-week history of a productive cough. There is no significant past medical history. He is a nonsmoker. On examination, he has oxygen saturations of 92% in air and is febrile with a temperature of 38°C. There is dullness to percussion and reduced air entry at the right lung base. A chest X-ray is requested to assess for possible pneumonia, effusion or collapse.

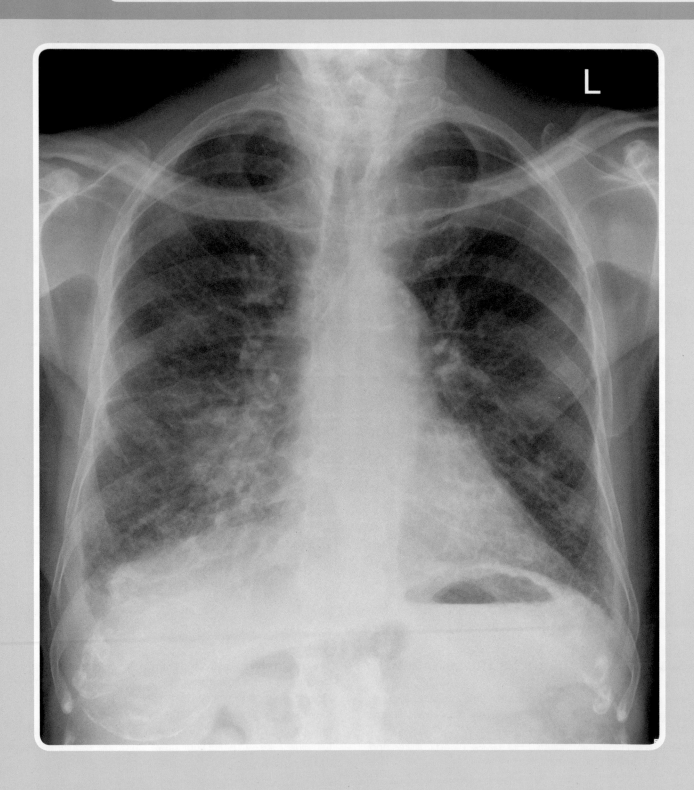

L

TECHNICAL INFORMATION

Patient ID: Anonymous

Projection: PA

Penetration: Adequate – vertebral bodies just visible behind heart

Inspiration: Adequate – seven anterior ribs visible

Rotation: The patient is slightly rotated to the left

● AIRWAY

The trachea is central after factoring in patient rotation.

● BREATHING

There is heterogeneous air-space opacification in the medial aspect of the right lower zone in keeping with consolidation. The rest of the lungs are clear. The lungs are not hyperinflated.

The right costophrenic angle is blunt, consistent with a small pleural effusion. There is minor blunting of the left costophrenic angle, which may represent pleural thickening or a small pleural effusion.

Normal pulmonary vascularity.

● CIRCULATION AND MEDIASTINUM

The heart is not enlarged.

The right heart border is indistinct. The left heart border is clear.

The mediastinum is central, not widened, with clear borders.

The aorta appears normal.

The right hilum is obscured by the consolidation. Normal size, shape and position of the left hilum.

● DIAPHRAGM AND DELICATES

Normal appearance and position of the left diaphragm. The right hemidiaphragm appears less distinct but is still visible.

No pneumoperitoneum.

The imaged skeleton is intact with no fracture or destructive bony lesion visible.

There is a well-defined, rounded, calcified lesion projected over the liver in the right upper quadrant. The soft tissues are otherwise unremarkable.

● EXTRAS AND REVIEW AREAS

No vascular lines, tubes or surgical clips.

Lung apices: Normal.

Hila: The right hilar region is not clear due to consolidation. The left hilum is normal.

Behind heart: Normal.

Costophrenic angles: Small right pleural effusion.

Below the diaphragm: There is a calcified mass projected over the liver.

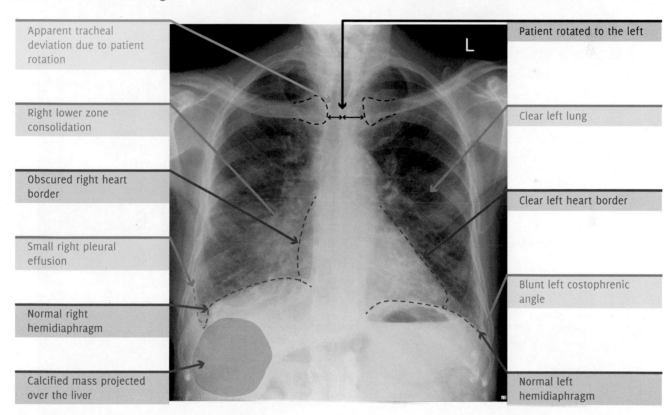

Apparent tracheal deviation due to patient rotation

Right lower zone consolidation

Obscured right heart border

Small right pleural effusion

Normal right hemidiaphragm

Calcified mass projected over the liver

Patient rotated to the left

Clear left lung

Clear left heart border

Blunt left costophrenic angle

Normal left hemidiaphragm

SUMMARY, INVESTIGATIONS AND MANAGEMENT

This X-ray demonstrates right lower zone consolidation, which given the clinical details is consistent with pneumonia. The right heart border is difficult to identify suggesting right middle lobe pneumonia. There is a large, peripherally calcified mass projected over the liver. This is typical for a hydatid (Echinococcal) cyst.

Initial blood tests may include FBC, U&Es, LFTs, bone profile, CRP and blood cultures. Sputum culture can also be checked. Appropriate antibiotics should be given to treat a community-acquired pneumonia, which may be oral or intravenous depending on the severity of pneumonia (CURB-65), with a follow-up chest X-ray to ensure resolution.

The calcification over the liver requires further evaluation, for example via ultrasound or CT scan. If it is a hydatid cyst, this may be managed surgically or medically (e.g. albendazole) and should be discussed with the infectious diseases team.

An 80-year-old male presents to ED with progressively worsening breathlessness. He used to work in the shipyards. He has a 60 pack-year smoking history. On examination, he has oxygen saturations of 92% in air and is febrile with a temperature of 38.2°C. His RR is 25 with an HR of 80 bpm. There are crackles and dullness to percussion at the right lung base. There is also finger clubbing. A chest X-ray is requested to assess for possible pneumonia or malignancy.

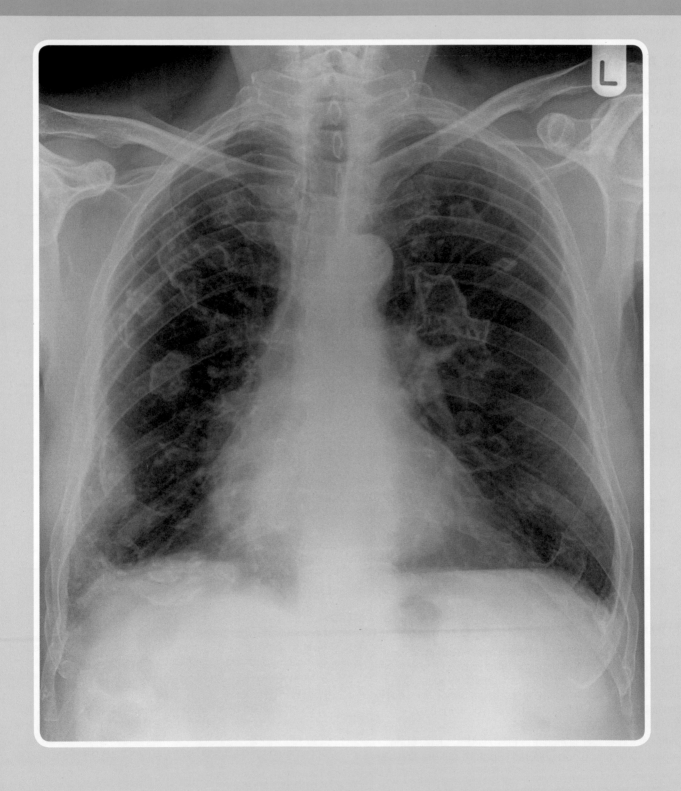

TECHNICAL INFORMATION

Patient ID: Anonymous
Projection: PA
Penetration: Adequate – vertebral bodies just visible behind heart
Inspiration: Adequate – eight anterior ribs visible
Rotation: The patient is mildly rotated to the right

● AIRWAY

The trachea is central after factoring in patient rotation.

● BREATHING

There is heterogeneous airspace opacification in the right lower zone in keeping with consolidation. The lungs are otherwise clear.

The lungs are not hyperinflated.

There are multiple irregular densities projected over the hemithoraces, consistent with calcified pleural plaques.

Normal pulmonary vascularity.

● CIRCULATION AND MEDIASTINUM

The heart is not enlarged.

The heart borders are clear. A left-sided epicardial fat pad is visible.

The aorta appears normal.

The mediastinum is central, not widened, with clear borders.

Normal size, shape and position of both hila.

● DIAPHRAGM AND DELICATES

There is calcification present overlying the right hemidiaphragm in keeping

with a pleural plaque. Otherwise normal appearance and position of the hemidiaphragms.

No pneumoperitoneum.

The imaged skeleton is intact with no fractures or destructive bony lesions visible.

The visible soft tissues are unremarkable.

● EXTRAS AND REVIEW AREAS

No vascular lines, tubes or surgical clips.
Lung apices: Normal.
Hila: Normal.
Behind heart: Normal.
Costophrenic angles: Consolidation at the right costophrenic angle.
Below the diaphragm: Normal.

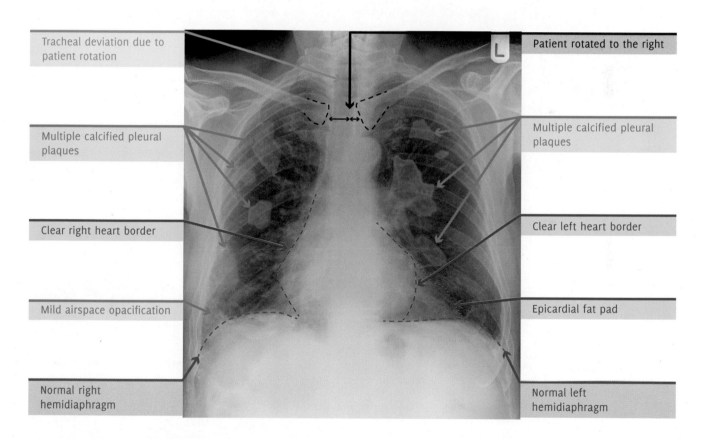

Tracheal deviation due to patient rotation

Multiple calcified pleural plaques

Clear right heart border

Mild airspace opacification

Normal right hemidiaphragm

Patient rotated to the right

Multiple calcified pleural plaques

Clear left heart border

Epicardial fat pad

Normal left hemidiaphragm

SUMMARY, INVESTIGATIONS AND MANAGEMENT

The X-ray demonstrates multiple irregularly shaped densities throughout both hemithoraces. These are consistent with calcified pleural plaques and indicate past asbestos exposure. Focal consolidation at the right costophrenic angle is in keeping with pneumonia.

Initial blood tests may include FBC, U&Es and CRP. Sputum and blood cultures may also be helpful. A follow-up chest

X-ray 4 to 6 weeks after appropriate antibiotics should be performed to ensure resolution of the pneumonia.

Previous imaging should be reviewed; if the pleural plaques are a new diagnosis the patient should be referred to respiratory for further assessment of asbestos-related lung disease.

ADVANCED CASES

A 58-year-old male is brought to ED after falling off a ladder. He has right-sided chest pain and breathlessness. He has no significant past medical history. He is a nonsmoker. On examination, he has oxygen saturations of 88% in air, his HR is 122 bpm and BP 108/68 mmHg. There is decreased air entry in the right hemithorax. A chest X-ray is requested to assess for a possible pneumothorax.

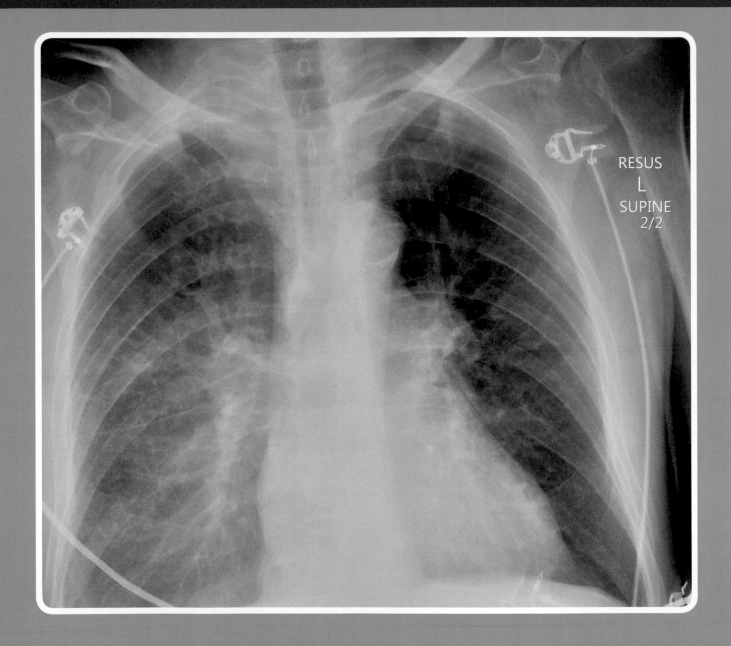

TECHNICAL INFORMATION

Patient ID: Anonymous
Projection: AP supine
Penetration: Adequate – vertebral bodies just visible behind heart
Inspiration: Adequate – six anterior ribs visible
Rotation: The patient is slightly rotated to the right

● AIRWAY

The trachea is central.

● BREATHING

The right lower zone and costophrenic angles have not been fully included on the X-ray.

There is hazy opacification in the right hemithorax compared with the left side. This is more marked in the lower and mid zones, and fades in the upper zone. Normal bronchovascular markings are clearly visible through the opacification and there are no air bronchograms.

The left lung is clear.

Normal pulmonary vascularity.

● CIRCULATION AND MEDIASTINUM

The heart size cannot be accurately assessed on an AP X-ray. The heart borders are clear.

The aorta appears normal.

The mediastinum is central, not widened, with clear borders.

Normal size, shape and position of both hila.

● DIAPHRAGM AND DELICATES

The right hemidiaphragm is not included on the X-ray. Normal appearance and position of the left hemidiaphragm.

It is not possible to accurately assess for pneumoperitoneum due to the limited X-ray coverage and supine positioning.

The imaged skeleton is intact with no fractures or destructive bony lesions visible.

● EXTRAS AND REVIEW AREAS

ECG monitoring leads in situ. No vascular lines, tubes or surgical clips.
Lung apices: Normal.
Hila: Normal.
Behind heart: Normal.
Costophrenic angles: Not included on the X-ray.
Below the diaphragm: Normal.

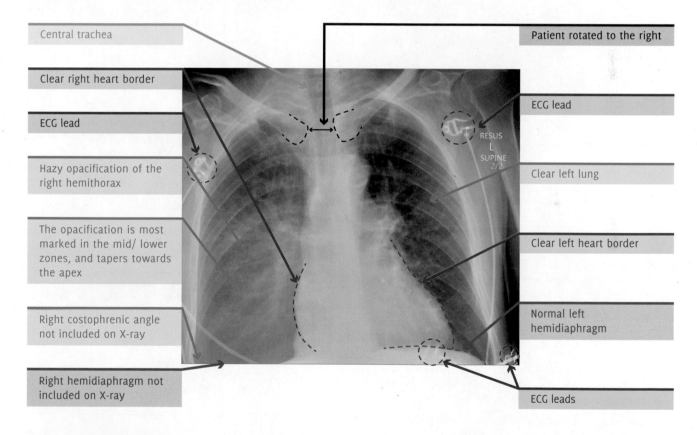

Central trachea

Clear right heart border

ECG lead

Hazy opacification of the right hemithorax

The opacification is most marked in the mid/ lower zones, and tapers towards the apex

Right costophrenic angle not included on X-ray

Right hemidiaphragm not included on X-ray

Patient rotated to the right

ECG lead

RESUS
L
SUPINE
2/2

Clear left lung

Clear left heart border

Normal left hemidiaphragm

ECG leads

SUMMARY, INVESTIGATIONS AND MANAGEMENT

This X-ray demonstrates hazy opacification in the right hemithorax. The presence of normal bronchovascular markings indicates the abnormality is outside the lung parenchyma. Given the supine projection, these findings are in keeping with fluid layering dependently in the posterior pleural space (i.e. a moderate right-sided pleural effusion). The opacification is most marked in the mid/lower zones as this is the most dependent part of the posterior pleural space in the supine position.

In the context of trauma, this effusion is likely to represent a haemothorax. There should be a high suspicion for underlying rib fractures even though none are visible on the X-ray. There is no evidence of pneumothorax, although this can be difficult to identify on a supine X-ray.

The patient needs to be assessed and resuscitated using the ATLS algorithm. Cardiothoracic surgery should be involved and a right-sided chest drain will be required.

Imaging with contrast-enhanced CT will provide more accurate assessment of the thorax. Other parts of the body (head, cervical spine, abdomen or pelvis) can also be imaged with CT depending on the clinical assessment.

A 28-year-old female presents to her GP feeling lethargic, breathless and with a dry cough. There is no significant past medical history. She is a nonsmoker. On examination, she has oxygen saturations of 100% in air and is afebrile. Her RR is 20 with an HR of 83 bpm. Lungs are resonant throughout, with good air entry bilaterally. She has enlarged lymph nodes in her neck. A chest X-ray is requested to assess for possible pneumonia, malignancy or an autoimmune disorder.

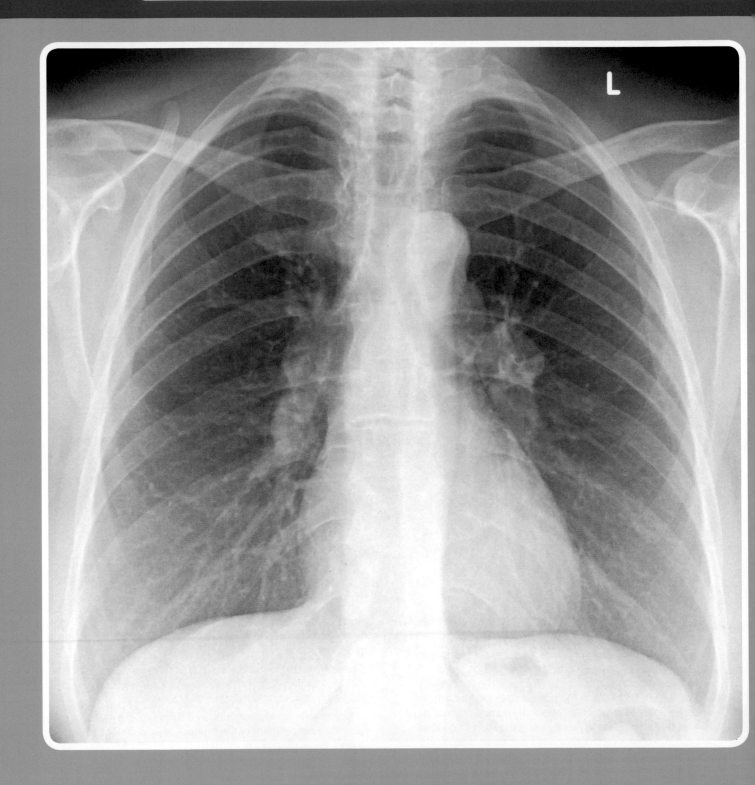

TECHNICAL INFORMATION

Patient ID: Anonymous
Projection: PA
Penetration: Adequate – vertebral bodies just visible behind heart
Inspiration: Adequate – seven anterior ribs visible
Rotation: The patient is not rotated

● AIRWAY

The trachea is central.

● BREATHING

The lungs are clear.

The lungs are not hyperinflated.

The pleural spaces are clear.

Normal pulmonary vascularity.

● CIRCULATION AND MEDIASTINUM

The heart is not enlarged.

The heart borders are clear.

The aorta appears normal.

There is a convex contour to the aortopulmonary window in keeping with lymph node enlargement. The mediastinum is otherwise normal. In particular there is no widening of the right paratracheal stripe.

Both hila have a lobulated convex appearance.

● DIAPHRAGM AND DELICATES

Normal appearance and position of the hemidiaphragms.

No pneumoperitoneum.

The imaged skeleton is intact with no fractures or destructive bony lesions visible.

The visible soft tissues are unremarkable.

● EXTRAS AND REVIEW AREAS

No vascular lines, tubes or surgical clips.
Lung apices: Normal.
Hila: Bilateral hilar and aortopulmonary window lymph nodes.
Behind heart: Normal.
Costophrenic angles: Normal.
Below the diaphragm: Normal.

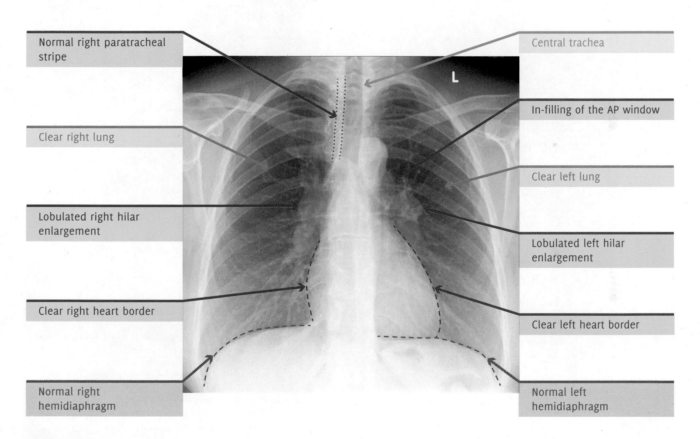

Normal right paratracheal stripe

Central trachea

Clear right lung

In-filling of the AP window

Clear left lung

Lobulated right hilar enlargement

Lobulated left hilar enlargement

Clear right heart border

Clear left heart border

Normal right hemidiaphragm

Normal left hemidiaphragm

SUMMARY, INVESTIGATIONS AND MANAGEMENT

This chest X-ray demonstrates symmetrical hilar lymph node enlargement, with further aortopulmonary window nodes. There is no widening of the right paratracheal stripe to indicate paratracheal lymph node enlargement, and the lung parenchyma appears normal. In the context of the history, the findings are consistent with sarcoidosis (Stage I). The symmetrical hilar appearance makes other causes of lymph node enlargement, such as lymphoma and TB, unlikely.

Initial blood tests may include FBC, U&Es, LFTs, bone profile, serum ACE levels, urinalysis and ECG. High-resolution CT of the chest can be performed if more detailed chest imaging is required. Corticosteroids may be prescribed.

A 34-year-old female presents to the respiratory outpatient clinic for follow-up after a double lung transplant. She has a background of cystic fibrosis, for which she had the surgery. She is a nonsmoker. On examination, she has oxygen saturations of 100% in air and is afebrile. Her RR is 16 with an HR of 73 bpm. Lungs are resonant throughout and there is good air entry bilaterally. A chest X-ray is requested as part of routine follow-up care to look for any possible transplant complications (e.g. fibrosis or infection).

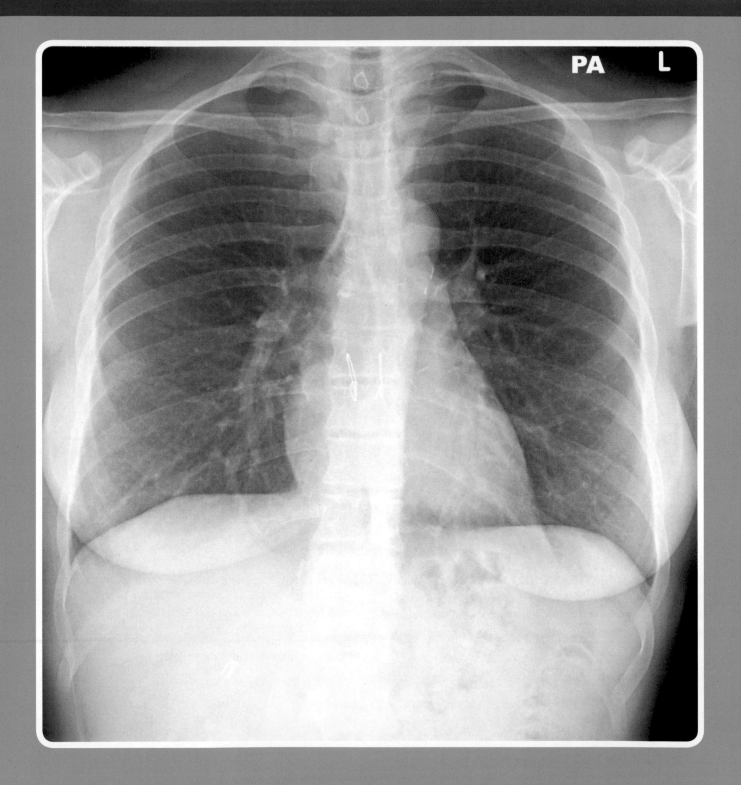

TECHNICAL INFORMATION

Patient ID: Anonymous
Projection: PA
Penetration: Adequate – vertebral bodies just visible behind heart
Inspiration: Adequate – eight anterior ribs visible
Rotation: The patient is not rotated

● AIRWAY

The trachea is central.

● BREATHING

The lungs are clear.

The lungs are not hyperinflated.

The pleural spaces are clear.

Normal pulmonary vascularity.

● CIRCULATION AND MEDIASTINUM

The heart is not enlarged.

The heart borders are clear.

The aorta appears normal.

The mediastinum is central, not widened, with clear borders.

Normal size, shape and position of both hila.

● DIAPHRAGM AND DELICATES

Normal appearance and position of the hemidiaphragms.

No pneumoperitoneum.

The imaged skeleton is intact with no fractures or destructive bony lesions visible.

The visible soft tissues are unremarkable.

● EXTRAS AND REVIEW AREAS

There are surgical clips projected bilaterally over the hilar regions. There are transverse sternotomy sutures projected over the lower mediastinum in the midline.

No vascular lines or tubes.
Lung apices: Normal.
Hila: Normal.
Behind heart: Normal.
Costophrenic angles: Normal.
Below the diaphragm: Normal.

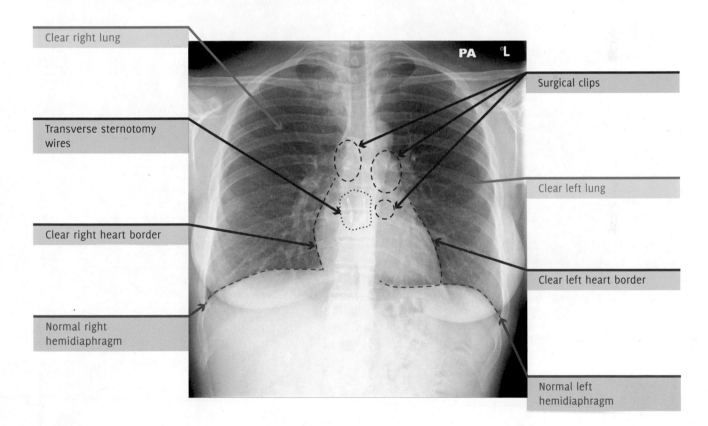

Clear right lung

Transverse sternotomy wires

Clear right heart border

Normal right hemidiaphragm

PA   L

Surgical clips

Clear left lung

Clear left heart border

Normal left hemidiaphragm

SUMMARY, INVESTIGATIONS AND MANAGEMENT

This X-ray demonstrates surgical clips and transverse sternotomy wires, consistent with a previous double lung transplant, presumably for end-stage cystic fibrosis. The lungs and pleural spaces are clear.

No specific additional management is required based on the X-ray. Routine posttransplant investigations should be obtained, including lung function testing, bronchoscopy and monitoring levels of any immunosuppressant therapy.

A 46-year-old male presents to ED with a feeling of general lethargy, malaise, pyrexia and flulike symptoms. There is no significant past medical history, and he is a nonsmoker. On examination, he has oxygen saturations of 89% in air and is febrile with a temperature of 38°C. Lungs are resonant throughout with good bilateral air entry. A chest X-ray is requested to assess for possible pneumonia.

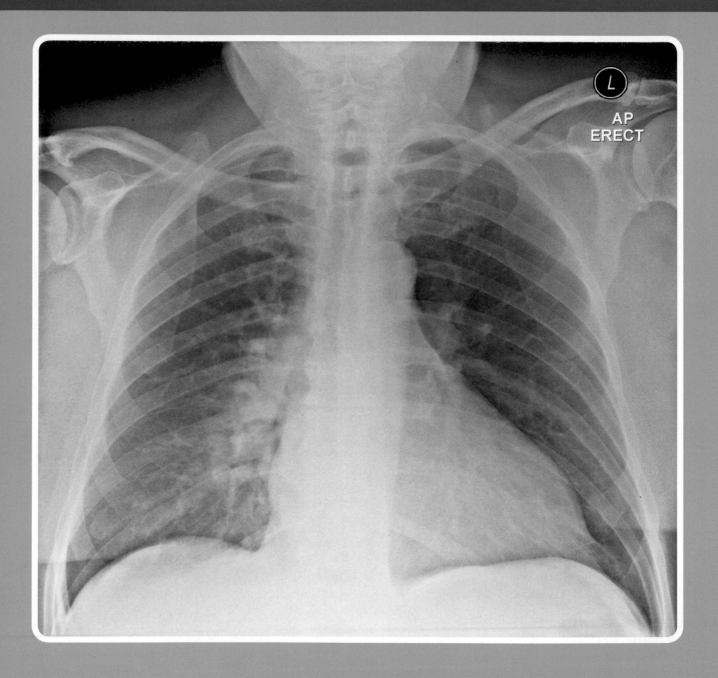

TECHNICAL INFORMATION

Patient ID: Anonymous
Projection: AP erect
Penetration: Adequate – vertebral bodies just visible behind heart
Inspiration: Adequate – seven anterior ribs visible
Rotation: Not rotated

● AIRWAY

The trachea is central.

● BREATHING

The lungs are clear, although the left costophrenic angle has not been fully included.

The lungs are not hyperinflated.

The pleural spaces are clear.

Normal pulmonary vascularity.

● CIRCULATION AND MEDIASTINUM

The heart is not enlarged.

The heart borders are clear.

The aorta appears normal.

The mediastinum is central, not widened, with clear borders.

The right hilum is enlarged and abnormally dense. Normal size, shape and position of the left hilum.

● DIAPHRAGM AND DELICATES

Normal appearance and position of the hemidiaphragms.

No pneumoperitoneum.

The imaged skeleton is intact with no fractures or destructive bony lesions visible.

The visible soft tissues are unremarkable.

● EXTRAS AND REVIEW AREAS

No vascular lines, tubes or surgical clips.
Lung apices: Normal.
Hila: Enlarged, dense right hilum. Normal left hilum.
Behind heart: Normal.
Costophrenic angles: Normal.
Below the diaphragm: Normal.

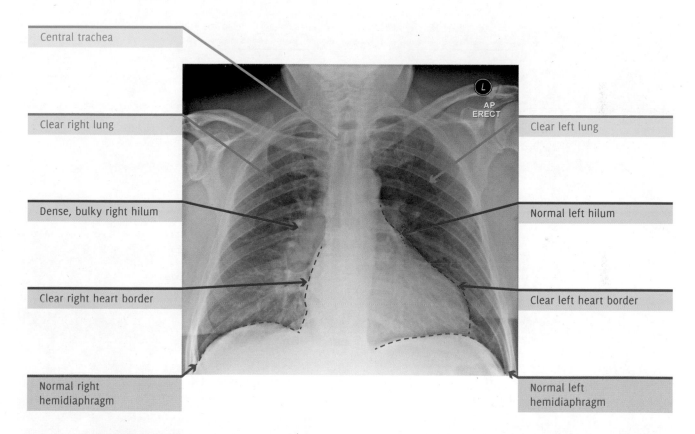

Central trachea

Clear right lung · Clear left lung

Dense, bulky right hilum · Normal left hilum

Clear right heart border · Clear left heart border

Normal right hemidiaphragm · Normal left hemidiaphragm

SUMMARY, INVESTIGATIONS AND MANAGEMENT

This X-ray demonstrates an enlarged, dense right hilum, likely due to hilar lymph node enlargement. The differential diagnosis includes infection, such as tuberculosis and histoplasmosis, lymphoma, sarcoidosis and metastatic disease.

The patient needs further clinical and radiological assessment to narrow the differential diagnosis. Initial blood tests may include FBC, U&Es, ESR, LFTs, bone profile, serum ACE and spirometry. Autoantibody screening, quantiferon (for TB) and other tests should be considered.

Any previous relevant imaging should be reviewed. A CT of the chest could be performed for further assessment. The abdomen and pelvis should also be imaged if malignant disease is considered likely. If lymphoma is considered, then the neck should also be included.

The patient should be referred to respiratory/oncology services for further management, which may include biopsy and MDT discussion.

A 55-year-old man is in the intensive care unit. He was found collapsed on the street the previous day and was brought to the ED via ambulance. He was haemodynamically unstable on arrival with diffuse crackles in his lungs. The first chest X-ray showed marked pulmonary oedema. He was commenced on a furosemide infusion, and an intraaortic balloon pump was inserted. A repeat chest X-ray is requested the next day to assess his response to treatment.

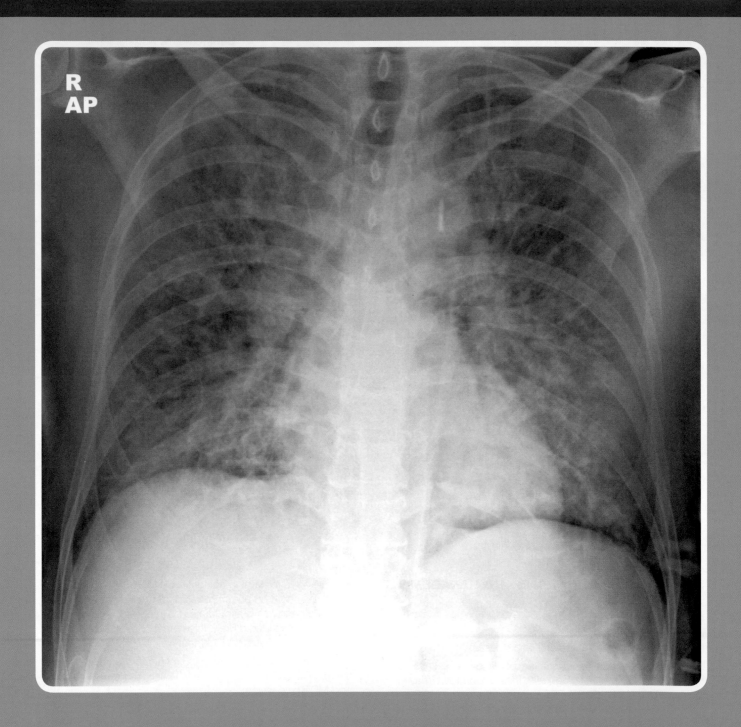

TECHNICAL INFORMATION

Patient ID: Anonymous
Projection: AP
Penetration: Adequate – vertebral bodies just visible behind heart
Inspiration: Adequate – six anterior ribs visible
Rotation: Not rotated

● AIRWAY

The trachea is central.

● BREATHING

There is generalized interstitial opacification with increased pulmonary vascularity seen within the upper lobes, in keeping with bilateral upper lobe venous blood diversion. There is bilateral airspace opacification in the perihilar regions.

The lungs are not hyperinflated.

The pleural spaces are clear.

● CIRCULATION AND MEDIASTINUM

The heart is not enlarged, even allowing for the magnification caused by the AP projection.

The heart borders are clear.

The aorta appears normal.

The mediastinum is central, not widened, with clear borders.

Both hila appear enlarged but they are in a normal position, with no increased density.

● DIAPHRAGM AND DELICATES

Normal appearance and position of the hemidiaphragms.

No pneumoperitoneum.

The imaged skeleton is intact with no fractures or destructive bony lesions visible.

The visible soft tissues are unremarkable.

● EXTRAS AND REVIEW AREAS

There is a radio-opacity projected over the arch of the aorta, in keeping with an intraaortic balloon pump. No vascular lines, tubes or surgical clips.
Lung apices: Increased vascularity within the apices of the lung indicating upper lobe blood diversion.
Hila: Increased alveolar opacification in the hilar region.
Behind heart: Normal.
Costophrenic angles: Normal.
Below the diaphragm: Normal.

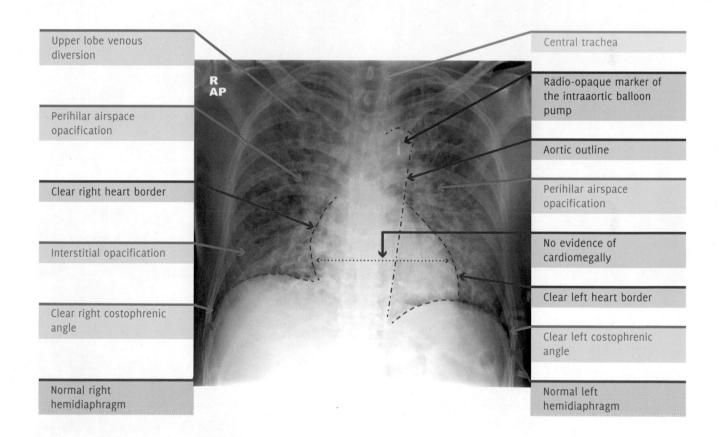

Upper lobe venous diversion

Perihilar airspace opacification

Clear right heart border

Interstitial opacification

Clear right costophrenic angle

Normal right hemidiaphragm

Central trachea

Radio-opaque marker of the intraaortic balloon pump

Aortic outline

Perihilar airspace opacification

No evidence of cardiomegally

Clear left heart border

Clear left costophrenic angle

Normal left hemidiaphragm

SUMMARY, INVESTIGATIONS AND MANAGEMENT

This X-ray demonstrates interstitial and alveolar opacification along with upper lobe venous diversion, in keeping with pulmonary oedema. There is an intraaortic balloon pump in situ, suggesting this is cardiogenic pulmonary oedema.

The chest X-ray should be compared with previous X-rays to assess for interval change. An ECHO (if not already performed) should be considered to assess left ventricular function. The patient's oxygenation and ventilation status can be monitored with serial arterial blood gases. Continue fluid monitoring/management and cardiovascular support in the ICU. Diuretic therapy may need to be optimized if the pulmonary oedema is worsening.

Serial chest X-rays should be performed to assess response to treatment.

A 78-year-old female presents to ED after a mechanical fall, which was preceded by light-headedness. She has severe right-sided chest pain. There is no significant past medical history. She is a nonsmoker. On examination, she has oxygen saturations of 92% in air and is afebrile. Her RR is 24 with an HR of 90 bpm. Lungs are resonant throughout, with good bilateral air entry. A chest X-ray is requested to assess for possible rib fractures or a pneumothorax.

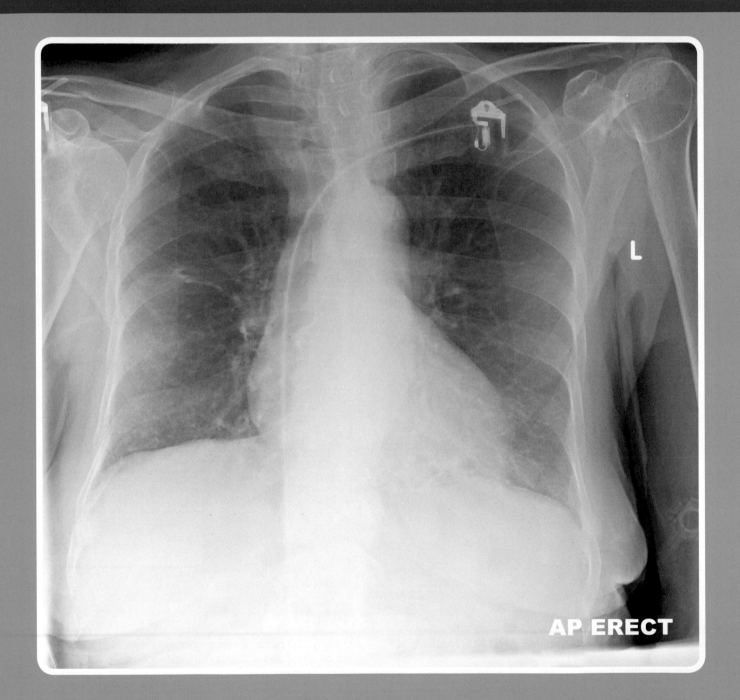

L

AP ERECT

TECHNICAL INFORMATION

Patient ID: Anonymous
Projection: AP erect
Penetration: Adequate – vertebral bodies just visible behind heart
Inspiration: Adequate – six anterior ribs visible
Rotation: The patient is rotated to the right

● AIRWAY

The trachea is central after factoring in patient rotation.

● BREATHING

The lungs are clear.

The lungs are not hyperinflated.

The pleural spaces are clear.

Normal pulmonary vascularity.

● CIRCULATION AND MEDIASTINUM

The heart is not enlarged, although its size cannot be accurately assessed on an AP X-ray.

The heart borders are clear.

There is mild unfolding of the thoracic aorta.

The mediastinum is central allowing for patient rotation, not widened and with clear borders.

Normal size, shape and position of both hila.

● DIAPHRAGM AND DELICATES

Normal appearance and position of the hemidiaphragms.

No pneumoperitoneum.

The partially imaged right humeral head is abnormally positioned, lying inferior to the coracoid process. This is suggestive of an anterior dislocation. The imaged skeleton is otherwise intact with no fractures or destructive bony lesions visible.

The visible soft tissues are unremarkable.

● EXTRAS AND REVIEW AREAS

ECG monitoring leads in situ. No vascular lines, tubes or surgical clips.
Lung apices: Normal.
Hila: Normal.
Behind heart: Normal.
Costophrenic angles: Normal.
Below the diaphragm: Normal.

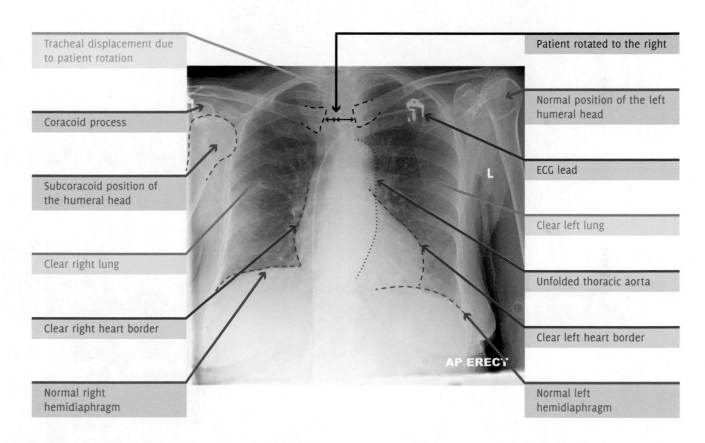

Tracheal displacement due to patient rotation

Coracoid process

Subcoracoid position of the humeral head

Clear right lung

Clear right heart border

Normal right hemidiaphragm

Patient rotated to the right

Normal position of the left humeral head

ECG lead

Clear left lung

Unfolded thoracic aorta

Clear left heart border

Normal left hemidiaphragm

L

AP ERECT

SUMMARY, INVESTIGATIONS AND MANAGEMENT

The X-ray demonstrates a likely anterior dislocation of the right shoulder. The lungs are clear and there is no rib fracture or pneumothorax visible.

The patient's right shoulder should be assessed, in particular looking for distal neurovascular compromise. Dedicated

X-rays of the right shoulder are required to confirm the dislocation. It should be reduced, with a postreduction X-ray to confirm the reduction was successful.

The episode of light-headedness needs to be assessed. Initial blood tests may include FBC, U&Es, glucose, bone profile and CRP. An ECG would also be helpful.

A 16-year-old female presents to her GP with a chest wall deformity. There is no significant past medical history. She is a nonsmoker. On examination, she has oxygen saturations of 100% in air and is afebrile. Her RR is 17 with an HR of 70 bpm. Lungs are resonant throughout, with good bilateral air entry. A chest X-ray is requested to assess for any bony abnormalities.

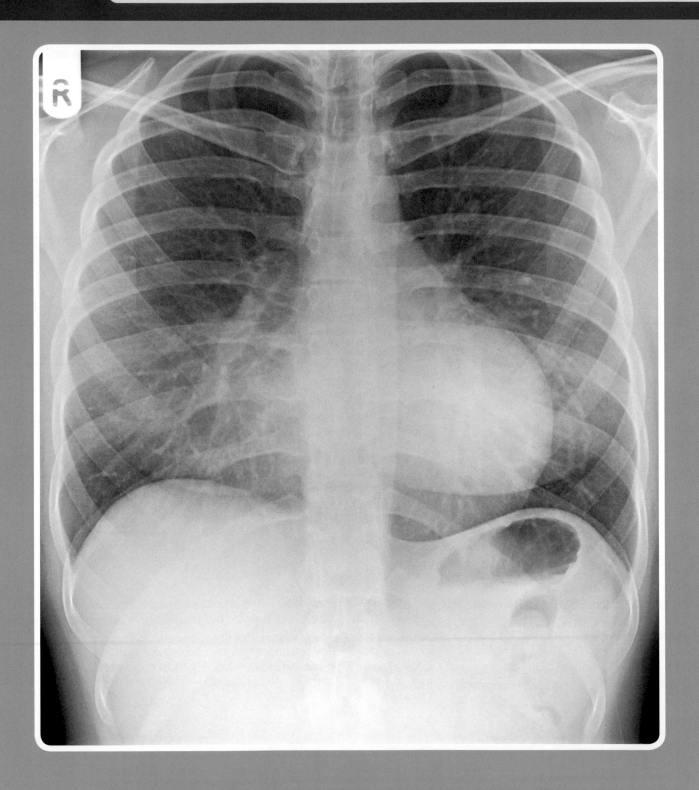

TECHNICAL INFORMATION

Patient ID: Anonymous
Projection: PA
Penetration: Adequate – vertebral bodies just visible behind heart
Inspiration: Adequate – eight anterior ribs visible
Rotation: Not rotated

● AIRWAY

The trachea is central.

● BREATHING

There is heterogeneous air-space opacification medially in the right lower zone. The lungs are otherwise clear.

The lungs are not hyperinflated.

The pleural spaces are clear.

Normal pulmonary vascularity.

● CIRCULATION AND MEDIASTINUM

The heart is not enlarged.

The right heart border is difficult to identify as it is projected over the vertebral column and appears indistinct. The left heart border is clear.

The mediastinum is central, not widened, with clear borders.

Normal size, shape and position of both hila.

● DIAPHRAGM AND DELICATES

Normal appearance and position of the hemidiaphragms.

No pneumoperitoneum.

The ribs are abnormally orientated – their posterior aspects are horizontally orientated while anteriorly they are nearly vertical. No fractures or other bony changes.

The visible soft tissues are unremarkable.

● EXTRAS AND REVIEW AREAS

No vascular lines, tubes or surgical clips.
Lung apices: Normal.
Hila: Normal.
Behind heart: Obscured right heart border.
Costophrenic angles: Normal.
Below the diaphragm: Normal.

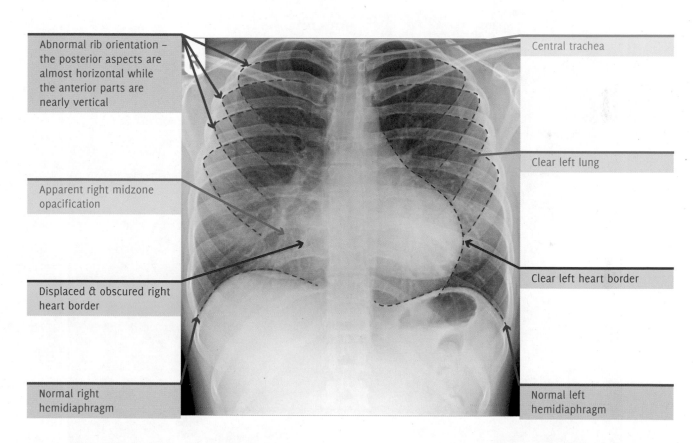

Abnormal rib orientation – the posterior aspects are almost horizontal while the anterior parts are nearly vertical

Apparent right midzone opacification

Displaced & obscured right heart border

Normal right hemidiaphragm

Central trachea

Clear left lung

Clear left heart border

Normal left hemidiaphragm

SUMMARY, INVESTIGATIONS AND MANAGEMENT

This X-ray demonstrates an indistinct right heart border with adjacent opacification. This may represent right middle lobe consolidation or collapse. However, in combination with the abnormal rib orientation and clinical history of chest wall deformity, the appearances are consistent with pectus excavatum.

Further management will depend on the effects of the chest wall deformity. No further assessment or treatment may be required. Pulmonary function tests and an ECHO can be performed to assess any pulmonary and/or cardiovascular compromise. The patient should be referred to cardiothoracics if surgery is contemplated. A CT of the chest may be required to assess the underlying anatomy presurgery.

A 40-year-old male presents to ED with recurrent episodes of haemoptysis. He has a history of IV drug use in the past and has a 20 pack-year smoking history. On examination, he has oxygen saturations of 90% in air and is afebrile. His RR is 20 with an HR of 80 bpm. There are crackles and wheeze in the upper zones of both the lungs. A chest X-ray is requested to assess for possible pneumonia, tuberculosis, malignancy or COPD.

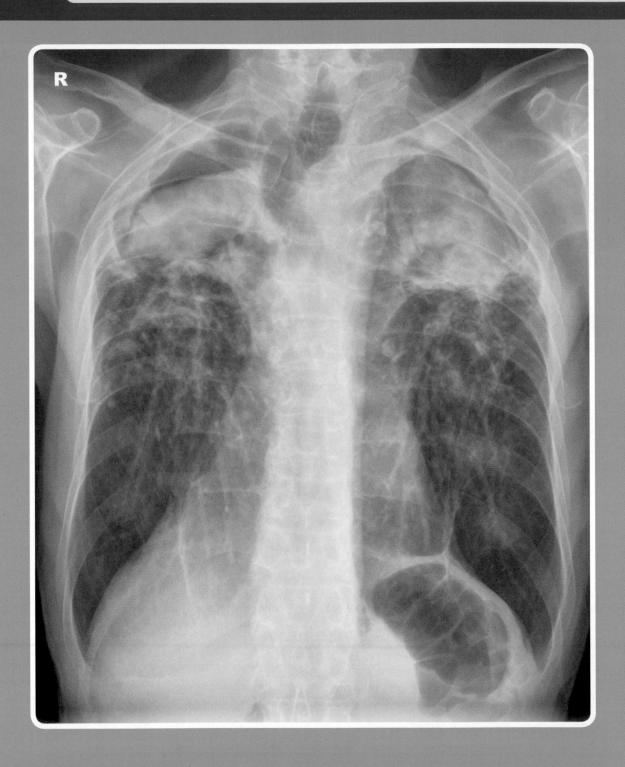

TECHNICAL INFORMATION

Patient ID: Anonymous
Projection: PA
Penetration: Adequate – vertebral bodies just visible behind heart
Inspiration: Adequate – seven anterior ribs visible
Rotation: The patient is not rotated

● AIRWAY

The upper trachea is central. The mid trachea is deviated to the right in keeping with right upper zone volume loss.

● BREATHING

There are bilateral upper and mid zone abnormalities with coarsened bronchovascular lung markings. There is increased lucency at the apices, in keeping with cavitation. In addition, there are rounded/ovoid soft tissue density masses in both apices.

These are outlined by thin crescents of air. There is pleural thickening at both apices. The lower zones are unremarkable.

The lungs are not hyperinflated.

● CIRCULATION AND MEDIASTINUM

The heart is not enlarged.

The heart borders are clear.

The aorta is difficult to identify.

The mediastinum is central and not widened. Its upper borders are difficult to identify.

Both hila are markedly elevated indicating bilateral upper zone volume loss.

● DIAPHRAGM AND DELICATES

The medial aspect of the right hemidiaphragm is obscured by an

epicardial fat pad. Normal appearance and position of the left hemidiaphragm.

No pneumoperitoneum.

The imaged skeleton is intact with no fractures or destructive bony lesions visible. In particular there are no bony changes associated with previous radiotherapy.

The visible soft tissues are unremarkable.

● EXTRAS AND REVIEW AREAS

No vascular lines, tubes or surgical clips.
Lung apices: Bilateral apical cavities with soft tissues masses.
Hila: Bilateral elevation of the hila.
Behind heart: Normal.
Costophrenic angles: Normal.
Below the diaphragm: Normal.

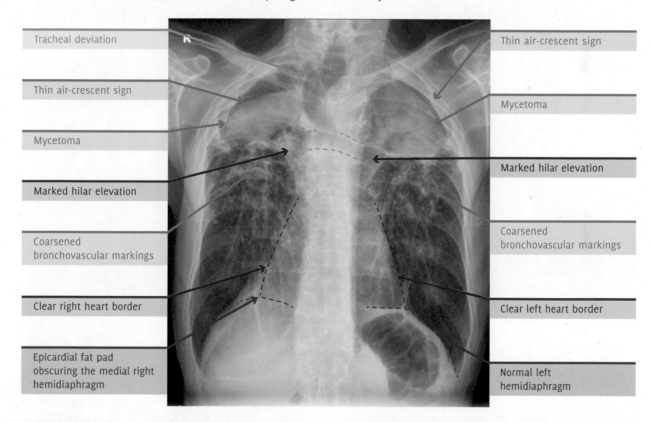

Left labels (top to bottom):
- Tracheal deviation
- Thin air-crescent sign
- Mycetoma
- Marked hilar elevation
- Coarsened bronchovascular markings
- Clear right heart border
- Epicardial fat pad obscuring the medial right hemidiaphragm

Right labels (top to bottom):
- Thin air-crescent sign
- Mycetoma
- Marked hilar elevation
- Coarsened bronchovascular markings
- Clear left heart border
- Normal left hemidiaphragm

SUMMARY, INVESTIGATIONS AND MANAGEMENT

This X-ray demonstrates bilateral upper zone fibrosis with large apical cavities. There are also bilateral apical soft tissues masses with air crescent signs, in keeping with mycetomas.

The differential diagnosis for upper lobe fibrosis includes old TB, pneumoconiosis, ankylosing spondylitis, previous radiotherapy and sarcoidosis. Given the patient's background and the large cavities, TB is the most likely cause.

Supplementary oxygen should be given. Initial blood tests may include FBC, U&Es and CRP. Sputum cultures should be obtained. An arterial blood gas may also be helpful.

Appropriate antibiotic/antifungal therapy should be considered following discussion with respiratory and microbiology, bearing in mind that old TB does not require active treatment.

Comparison with previous imaging would be useful to assess for progression of changes. An HRCT of the chest would provide more detailed assessment if required. Input from the respiratory team would be helpful to guide further management.

A 57-year-old male presents to ED with right-sided pleuritic chest pain and fever. He has a background of oesophageal cancer treated with an oesophagectomy. Three weeks ago he underwent radiofrequency ablation of a liver metastasis. He is a nonsmoker. On examination, he has oxygen saturations of 90% in air and is febrile with a temperature of 39.5°C. His RR is 35 with an HR of 100 bpm. There is reduced air entry in the right lower zone, with dullness to percussion. A chest X-ray is requested to assess for possible pneumonia, collapse or pleural effusion.

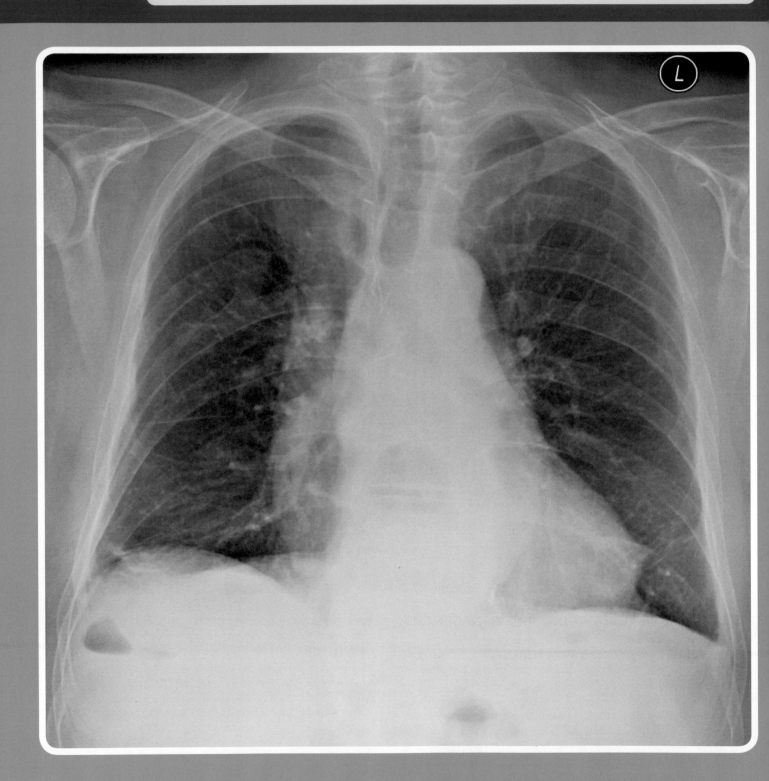

TECHNICAL INFORMATION

Patient ID: Anonymous
Projection: PA
Penetration: Adequate – vertebral bodies just visible behind heart
Inspiration: Adequate – six anterior ribs visible
Rotation: The patient is rotated to the right

● AIRWAY

The trachea is central after factoring in patient rotation.

● BREATHING

There is minor atelectasis in the right lower zone. The lungs are otherwise clear.

The lungs are not hyperinflated.

The pleural spaces are clear.

Normal pulmonary vascularity.

● CIRCULATION AND MEDIASTINUM

The heart appears enlarged, although assessment of the size is difficult due to patient rotation.

The heart borders are clear.

The mediastinum is central, not widened and with clear borders. There is an air-fluid level projected over the lower mediastinum.

Normal size, shape and position of both hila.

● DIAPHRAGM AND DELICATES

Normal appearance and position of the hemidiaphragms.

No pneumoperitoneum.

There is partial resection of the posterior aspect of the right 6th rib. The imaged skeleton is otherwise intact with no fractures or destructive bony lesions visible.

There is a lucent area projected over the liver in the right upper quadrant. The visible soft tissues are otherwise unremarkable.

● EXTRAS AND REVIEW AREAS

There are surgical clips projected over the upper and mid mediastinum. No vascular lines or tubes.
Lung apices: Normal.
Hila: Normal.
Behind heart: Air-fluid level and surgical clips.
Costophrenic angles: Normal.
Below the diaphragm: Lucent area projected over the liver.

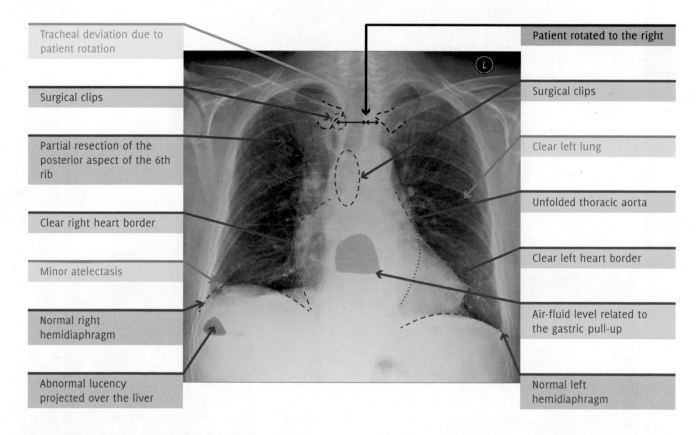

Left column labels:
- Tracheal deviation due to patient rotation
- Surgical clips
- Partial resection of the posterior aspect of the 6th rib
- Clear right heart border
- Minor atelectasis
- Normal right hemidiaphragm
- Abnormal lucency projected over the liver

Right column labels:
- Patient rotated to the right
- Surgical clips
- Clear left lung
- Unfolded thoracic aorta
- Clear left heart border
- Air-fluid level related to the gastric pull-up
- Normal left hemidiaphragm

SUMMARY, INVESTIGATIONS AND MANAGEMENT

The X-ray demonstrates evidence of a previous oesophagectomy with gastric pull up (there is partial resection of the right 6th rib, surgical clips and a mediastinal air-fluid level). The lucent area projected over the liver is in keeping with gas. This may represent an abscess given the clinical history and previous radiofrequency ablation, or alternatively it could be bowel gas.

Initial blood tests may include FBC, U&Es, LFTs, CRP and blood cultures.

Previous imaging and notes should be reviewed to assess the site of the previous radiofrequency ablation. Further imaging in the form of contrast-enhanced CT of the abdomen would be useful for assessing the liver.

If an abscess is confirmed, treatment would include appropriate antibiotics and percutaneous drainage under ultrasound guidance.

A 19-year-old male presents to ED with increasing wheeze and breathlessness. He is a known asthmatic. He is a nonsmoker. On examination, he has oxygen saturations of 85% in air and is afebrile. His RR is 30 with an HR of 80 bpm. There are scattered wheezes throughout the lungs with reduced air entry. A chest X-ray is requested to assess for possible pneumonia or a pneumothorax.

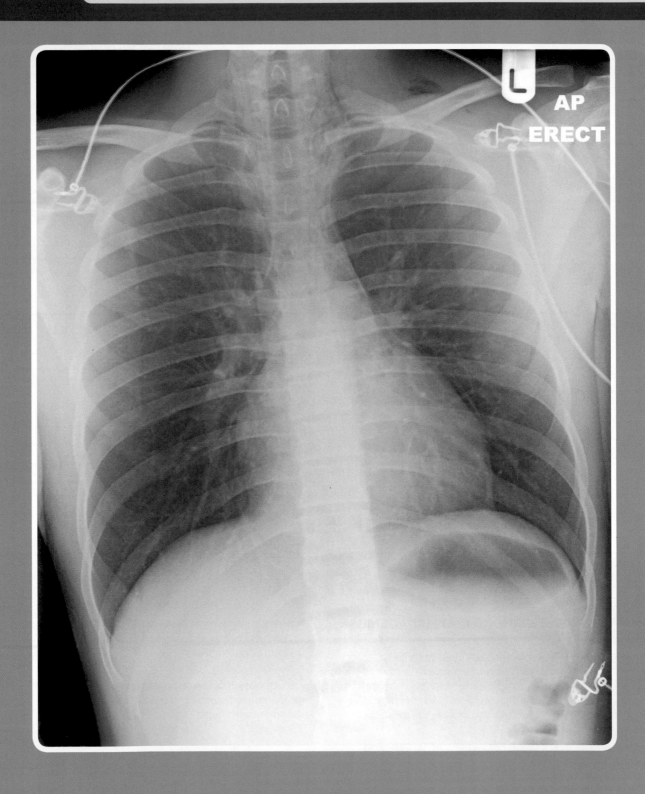

TECHNICAL INFORMATION

Patient ID: Anonymous
Projection: AP erect
Penetration: Adequate – vertebral bodies just visible behind heart
Inspiration: Adequate – eight anterior ribs visible
Rotation: The patient is not rotated

● AIRWAY

The trachea is central.

● BREATHING

The lungs are clear.

The lungs are not hyperinflated.

The pleural spaces are clear.

Normal pulmonary vascularity.

● CIRCULATION AND MEDIASTINUM

The heart does not appear enlarged, although its size cannot be accurately assessed on an AP X-ray.

The heart borders are clear.

The aorta appears normal.

The mediastinum is central and not widened. There are bilateral linear and curvilinear lucencies outlining the mediastinal contours, extending into the soft tissues of the neck and down towards the heart.

Normal size, shape and position of both hila.

● DIAPHRAGM AND DELICATES

Normal appearance and position of the hemidiaphragms.

No pneumoperitoneum.

The imaged skeleton is intact with no fractures or destructive bony lesions visible.

There is a small volume of surgical emphysema in the left supraclavicular fossa. The visible soft tissues are otherwise unremarkable.

● EXTRAS AND REVIEW AREAS

ECG monitoring leads in situ. No vascular lines, tubes or surgical clips.
Lung apices: Normal.
Hila: Normal.
Behind heart: Normal.
Costophrenic angles: Normal.
Below the diaphragm: Normal.

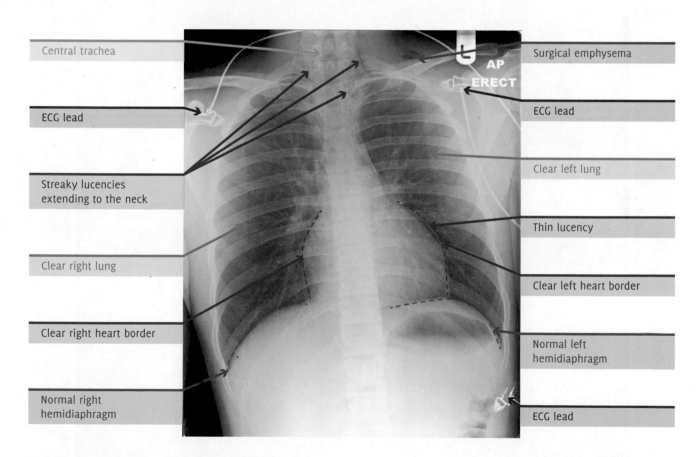

Central trachea

ECG lead

Streaky lucencies extending to the neck

Clear right lung

Clear right heart border

Normal right hemidiaphragm

Surgical emphysema

AP ERECT

ECG lead

Clear left lung

Thin lucency

Clear left heart border

Normal left hemidiaphragm

ECG lead

SUMMARY, INVESTIGATIONS AND MANAGEMENT

This X-ray demonstrates curvilinear lucencies outlining the cardiomediastinal contours associated with surgical emphysema. In the context of asthma, this is likely to reflect a pneumomediastinum. No evidence of pneumothorax or pleural effusion.

Supplementary oxygen should be given alongside nebulized bronchodilators and oral corticosteroids. Initial blood tests may include FBC, U&Es, CRP and an arterial blood gas. A peak flow may also be helpful. Pneumomediastinum in this context can usually be managed conservatively.

A 22-year-old male presents to his GP with progressive exertional breathlessness. He has lost some weight over the last few weeks and feels lethargic. There is no significant past medical history, and he is a nonsmoker. On examination, he has oxygen saturations of 100% in air and is afebrile. There is dullness to percussion and reduced air entry in the left lower zone. A chest X-ray is requested to assess for possible pneumonia, effusion or collapse.

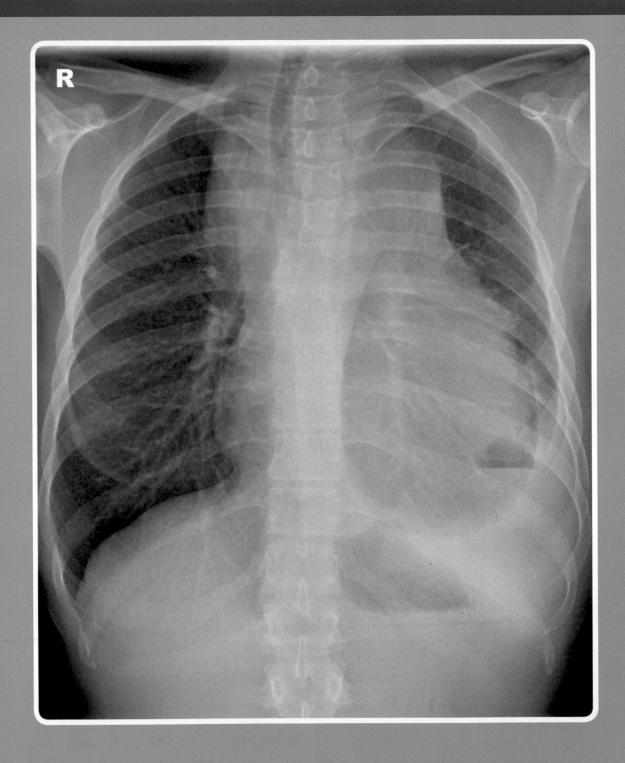

TECHNICAL INFORMATION

Patient ID: Anonymous
Projection: PA
Penetration: Adequate – vertebral bodies just visible behind heart
Inspiration: Adequate – eight anterior ribs visible
Rotation: Not rotated

● AIRWAY

The trachea is deviated to the right.

● BREATHING

There is opacification at the left costophrenic angle, in keeping with a pleural abnormality (either effusion or mass). The lungs are otherwise clear.

The lungs are not hyperinflated.

Normal pulmonary vascularity.

● CIRCULATION AND MEDIASTINUM

There is marked widening of the superior mediastinum, including the right paratracheal stripe, in keeping with a mediastinal mass.

The left paravertebral line and aortic knuckle/thoracic aorta are preserved and the left hilar structures can be seen through this mass (hilum overlay sign), indicating that the mass is not in the posterior or middle mediastinum, respectively.

The left heart border is obscured by the mediastinal mass. It is therefore difficult to assess the heart size. The right heart border is preserved.

The aorta appears normal.

Normal size, shape and position of both hila.

● DIAPHRAGM AND DELICATES

The left hemidiaphragm is largely obscured but appears elevated. Normal position and appearance of the right hemidiaphragm.

No pneumoperitoneum.

The imaged skeleton is intact with no fractures or destructive bony lesions visible.

The soft tissues are unremarkable.

● EXTRAS AND REVIEW AREAS

No vascular lines, tubes or surgical clips.
Lung apices: Mediastinal soft tissue mass encroaches into the left apex.
Hila: Normal (left hilum overlay sign).
Behind heart: Normal.
Costophrenic angles: Left-sided pleural effusion.
Below the diaphragm: Normal.

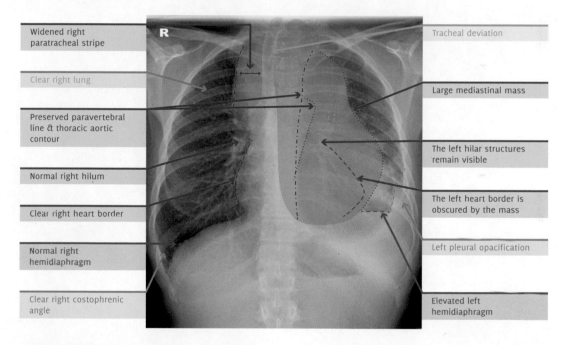

Widened right paratracheal stripe

Clear right lung

Preserved paravertebral line & thoracic aortic contour

Normal right hilum

Clear right heart border

Normal right hemidiaphragm

Clear right costophrenic angle

R

Tracheal deviation

Large mediastinal mass

The left hilar structures remain visible

The left heart border is obscured by the mass

Left pleural opacification

Elevated left hemidiaphragm

SUMMARY, INVESTIGATIONS AND MANAGEMENT

This X-ray demonstrates a large mediastinal mass. The loss of the left heart border, combined with preserved hila and thoracic aorta, indicates this is an anterior mediastinal mass. There is an additional left-sided pleural abnormality, which may represent a pleural effusion or pleural metastatic disease. Possible elevation of the left hemidiaphragm may relate to damage to the left phrenic nerve.

The differentials of an anterior mediastinal mass include lymphoma, thyroid malignancy, thymoma (although usually in older patients) and teratoma.

The patient needs urgent referral to oncology. A full examination to assess for lymph node enlargement should be undertaken. Initial blood tests may include FBC, U&Es, LFTs, bone profile and TFTs.

Further imaging in the form of contrast-enhanced CT of the chest should be performed. If lymphoma is suspected, then the neck, abdomen and pelvis should also be included in the CT. An ultrasound examination could assess the pleural abnormality and may permit tissue sampling; otherwise, a CT-guided anterior mediastinal mass biopsy may be required for a histological diagnosis.

The patient should be referred to respiratory/oncology services for further management, which may include biopsy and MDT discussion. Treatment, which may include surgery, radiotherapy, chemotherapy or palliative treatment, will depend on the outcome of the MDT discussion, investigations and the patient's wishes.

A 30-year-old female is referred for a chest X-ray by her GP. She has persistent shortness of breath. There is no significant past medical history. She is a nonsmoker. On examination, she is apyrexial, with oxygen saturations of 95% in air. There is dullness on percussion and inspiratory crackles in the right upper zone. A chest X-ray is requested to look for possible pneumonia or collapse.

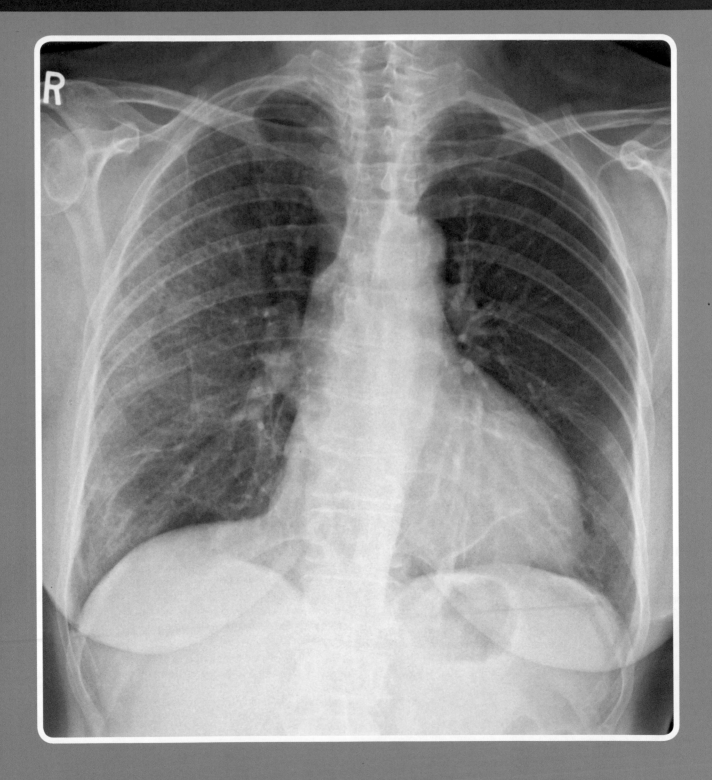

TECHNICAL INFORMATION

Patient ID: Anonymous
Projection: PA
Penetration: Adequate – vertebral bodies just visible behind heart
Inspiration: Adequate – six anterior ribs visible
Rotation: The patient is rotated to the right

● AIRWAY

The trachea is central after factoring in patient rotation.

● BREATHING

There is peripheral ground-glass opacification in the right upper and mid zones. Minor atelectasis is present in the left lower zone. The lungs are otherwise clear.

The lungs are not hyperinflated.

The pleural spaces are clear.

Normal pulmonary vascularity.

● CIRCULATION AND MEDIASTINUM

The heart is not enlarged.

The heart borders are clear.

The aorta appears normal.

The mediastinum is central, not widened, with clear borders.

Normal size, shape and position of both hila.

● DIAPHRAGM AND DELICATES

Normal appearance and position of the hemidiaphragms.

No pneumoperitoneum.

The imaged skeleton is intact with no fractures or destructive bony lesions visible.

The visible soft tissues are unremarkable.

● EXTRAS AND REVIEW AREAS

No vascular lines, tubes or surgical clips.
Lung apices: Normal.
Hila: Normal.
Behind heart: Normal.
Costophrenic angles: Normal.
Below the diaphragm: Normal.

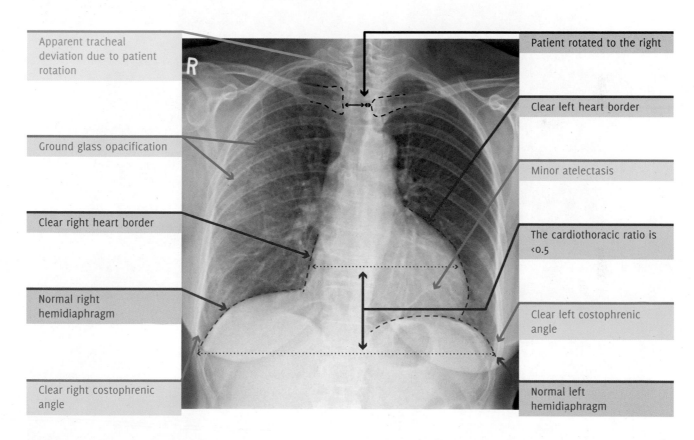

Apparent tracheal deviation due to patient rotation

Ground glass opacification

Clear right heart border

Normal right hemidiaphragm

Clear right costophrenic angle

Patient rotated to the right

Clear left heart border

Minor atelectasis

The cardiothoracic ratio is <0.5

Clear left costophrenic angle

Normal left hemidiaphragm

SUMMARY, INVESTIGATIONS AND MANAGEMENT

This X-ray demonstrates peripheral ground-glass opacification in the right upper and mid zones. The differential diagnosis is wide and includes infection (especially viral infection), eosinophilic pneumonia, interstitial pneumonias, hypersensitivity pneumonitis and pulmonary oedema.

Initial blood tests may include FBC, U&Es and CRP. An ECG and arterial blood gas may also be helpful. Any previous imaging should be reviewed to assess whether this is a new or longstanding abnormality. Appropriate antibiotics should be considered. Referral to the respiratory team may be helpful.

A 32-year-old male presents to the ED with worsening shortness of breath. There is no significant past medical history and he is a nonsmoker. On examination, he has oxygen saturations of 99% in air and is afebrile. There is dullness to percussion and crackles with reduced air entry in the left lower zone. A chest X-ray is requested to assess for possible pneumonia, collapse or effusion.

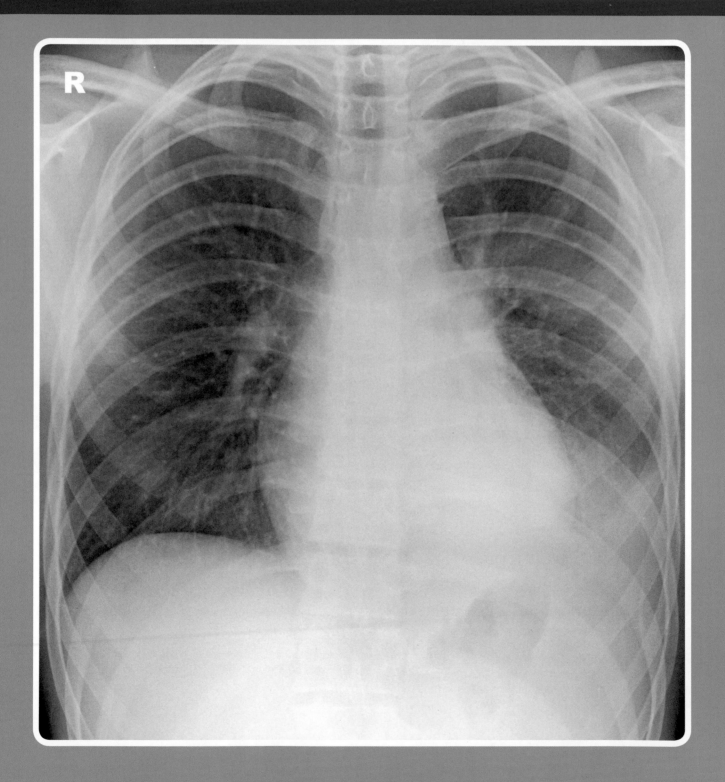

TECHNICAL INFORMATION

Patient ID: Anonymous
Projection: PA
Penetration: Adequate – vertebral bodies just visible behind heart
Inspiration: Adequate – seven anterior ribs visible
Rotation: Not rotated

● AIRWAY

The trachea is central.

● BREATHING

There is heterogeneous airspace opacification in the left lower zone including the left retrocardiac position. Some air bronchograms are visible in this region, consistent with consolidation. The right lung is clear. The lungs are not hyperinflated.

There is blunting of the left costophrenic angle, in keeping with a pleural effusion. There is also opacification in the left mid/upper zone. This has a very sharp curvilinear inferior margin and probably represents fluid encysted in the oblique fissure. The right-sided pleural spaces are clear.

Normal pulmonary vascularity.

● CIRCULATION AND MEDIASTINUM

The heart is not enlarged.

The heart borders are clear.

The aorta appears normal.

The mediastinum is central, not widened, with clear borders.

Normal size, shape and position of both hila.

● DIAPHRAGM AND DELICATES

The left hemidiaphragm is obscured. Normal position and appearance of the right hemidiaphragm.

No pneumoperitoneum.

The imaged skeleton is intact with no fractures or destructive bony lesions visible.

The visible soft tissues are unremarkable.

● EXTRAS AND REVIEW AREAS

No vascular lines, tubes or surgical clips.
Lung apices: Normal.
Hila: Normal.
Behind heart: Left retrocardiac consolidation.
Costophrenic angles: Blunting of the left.
Below the diaphragm: Normal.

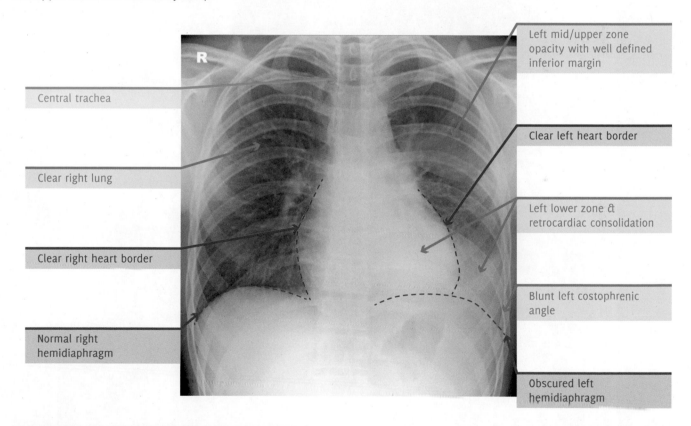

Central trachea

Clear right lung

Clear right heart border

Normal right hemidiaphragm

Left mid/upper zone opacity with well defined inferior margin

Clear left heart border

Left lower zone & retrocardiac consolidation

Blunt left costophrenic angle

Obscured left hemidiaphragm

SUMMARY, INVESTIGATIONS AND MANAGEMENT

This X-ray demonstrates left lower zone consolidation, obscuring the left hemidiaphragm but with the left heart border preserved. The appearances are consistent with left lower lobe pneumonia. A left-sided pleural effusion is present. The opacity in the left mid/upper zone has a very sharp curvilinear inferior margin and most likely represents fluid encysted in the oblique fissure (pseudotumour).

Initial blood tests may include FBC, U&Es, CRP and blood cultures. A sputum culture may also be obtained.

The patient should be treated with appropriate antibiotics for community-acquired pneumonia and a follow-up chest X-ray performed in 4 to 6 weeks to ensure resolution. The antibiotics may be oral or intravenous depending on the severity of pneumonia (CURB-65). No specific additional action is required for the pseudotumour.

Ultrasound could be used to further assess the volume of the pleural effusion, particularly if a diagnostic pleural aspiration is being considered.

A 35-year-old male presents to ED with worsening shortness of breath and a fever. He is an IV drug user. He has a 10 pack-year smoking history. On examination, he has oxygen saturations of 89% in air and is febrile with a temperature of 39°C. Lungs are resonant with good bilateral air entry and occasional crackles throughout. A systolic murmur is audible. A chest X-ray is requested to assess for possible pneumonia or pulmonary oedema.

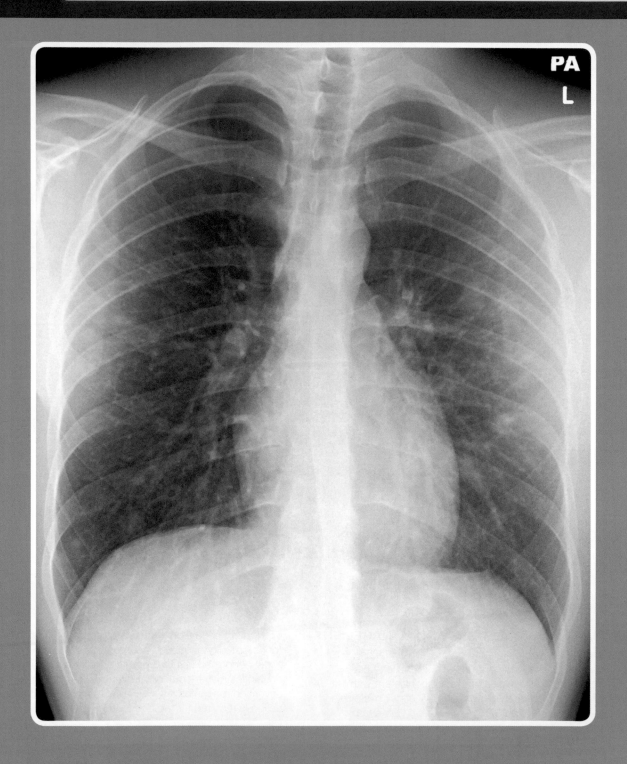

TECHNICAL INFORMATION

Patient ID: Anonymous
Projection: PA
Penetration: Adequate – vertebral bodies just visible behind heart
Inspiration: Adequate – eight anterior ribs visible
Rotation: Not rotated

● AIRWAY

The trachea is central.

● BREATHING

There are multiple ill-defined nodules seen throughout both lungs. They are all less than 1 cm in size. There is no cavitation or visible calcification and no consolidation.

The lungs are not hyperinflated.

The pleural spaces are clear.

Normal pulmonary vascularity.

● CIRCULATION AND MEDIASTINUM

The heart is not enlarged.

The heart borders are clear.

The aorta appears normal.

The mediastinum is central, not widened, with clear borders.

Normal size, shape and position of both hila.

● DIAPHRAGM AND DELICATES

Normal appearance and position of the hemidiaphragms.

No pneumoperitoneum.

The imaged skeleton is intact with no fractures or destructive bony lesions visible.

The visible soft tissues are unremarkable.

● EXTRAS AND REVIEW AREAS

No vascular lines, tubes or surgical clips.
Lung apices: Normal.
Hila: Normal.
Behind heart: At least one nodule is projected over the right side of the cardiac silhouette.
Costophrenic angles: Normal.
Below the diaphragm: Normal.

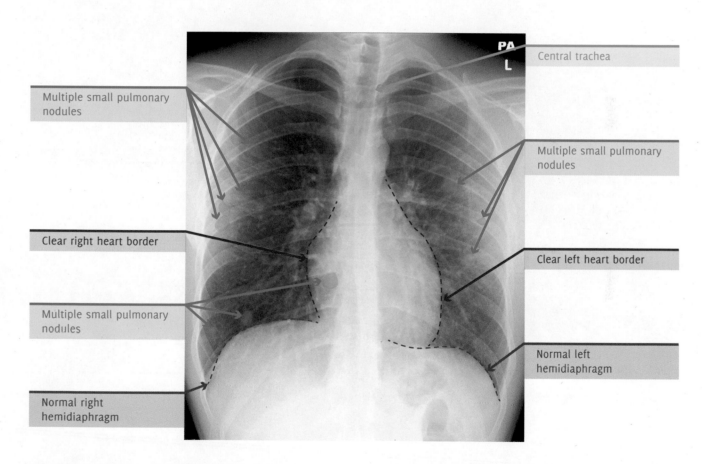

Multiple small pulmonary nodules

Central trachea

Multiple small pulmonary nodules

Clear right heart border

Clear left heart border

Multiple small pulmonary nodules

Normal left hemidiaphragm

Normal right hemidiaphragm

SUMMARY, INVESTIGATIONS AND MANAGEMENT

This X-ray demonstrates multiple ill-defined lung nodules (5–10 mm). There is a wide differential for these appearances but in combination with the clinical history, septic emboli and other forms of infection, such as fungal or TB, are highest on the list. Other differentials include metastases, autoimmune conditions, such as granulomatosis with polyangiitis, vascular malformations and sarcoidosis.

Supplementary oxygen should be given. Initial blood tests may include FBC, U&Es, CRP, ESR, LFTs, bone profile and three sets of blood cultures. A sputum culture and urine culture may also be helpful. After blood cultures are taken, appropriate antibiotics should be commenced.

An ECHO to assess the murmur and look for evidence of vegetations should be done. A contrast-enhanced CT would provide a better assessment of the pulmonary nodules.

A 40-year-old male presents to ED with shortness of breath. There is no significant past medical history. He is a nonsmoker. On examination, he has oxygen saturations of 100% in air and is afebrile. His RR is 20 with an HR of 80 bpm. Lungs are resonant throughout, with good bilateral air entry. A chest X-ray is requested to assess for possible pneumonia or a pneumothorax.

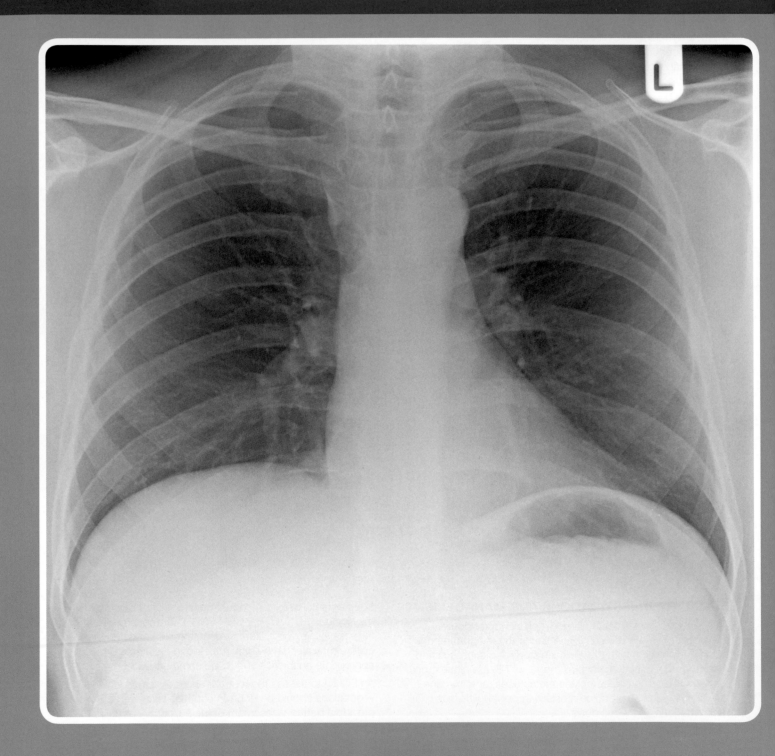

TECHNICAL INFORMATION

Patient ID: Anonymous
Projection: PA
Penetration: Adequate – vertebral bodies just visible behind heart
Inspiration: Adequate – six anterior ribs visible
Rotation: The patient is not rotated

● AIRWAY

The trachea is central.

● BREATHING

There is a thin curvilinear line (convex relative to the mediastinum) crossing the apex of the right lung. The lungs are otherwise clear.

The lungs are not hyperinflated.

The pleural spaces are clear.

Normal pulmonary vascularity.

● CIRCULATION AND MEDIASTINUM

The heart is not enlarged.

The heart borders are clear.

The aorta appears normal.

The mediastinum is central, not widened, with clear borders.

Normal size, shape and position of both hila.

● DIAPHRAGM AND DELICATES

Normal appearance and position of the hemidiaphragms.

No pneumoperitoneum.

The imaged skeleton is intact with no fractures or destructive bony lesions visible.

The visible soft tissues are unremarkable.

● EXTRAS AND REVIEW AREAS

No vascular lines, tubes or surgical clips.
Lung apices: Fine curvilinear line in the right apex.
Hila: Normal.
Behind heart: Normal.
Costophrenic angles: Normal.
Below the diaphragm: Normal.

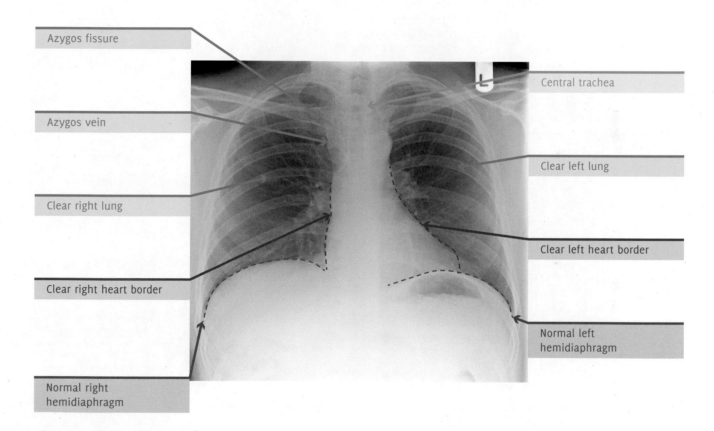

SUMMARY, INVESTIGATIONS AND MANAGEMENT

This X-ray demonstrates a fine curvilinear opacity in the right apex, which is in keeping with an azygos fissure and azygos lobe. This is a normal variant and requires no further investigation. No cause for breathlessness demonstrated.

Further investigations are therefore required to account for the clinical presentation. Initial blood tests may include FBC, U&Es, CRP and D-Dimer. A blood gas may be helpful. If there is a strong suspicion of a PE, a CTPA would be indicated.

A 43-year-old female presents to ED with left-sided chest pain. She has recently returned from New Zealand. She is a nonsmoker. On examination, she has oxygen saturations of 98% in air and is afebrile. Lungs are resonant throughout with good bilateral air entry. She is tender over the left side of her chest. A chest X-ray is requested to assess for possible pneumonia, pneumothorax or PE.

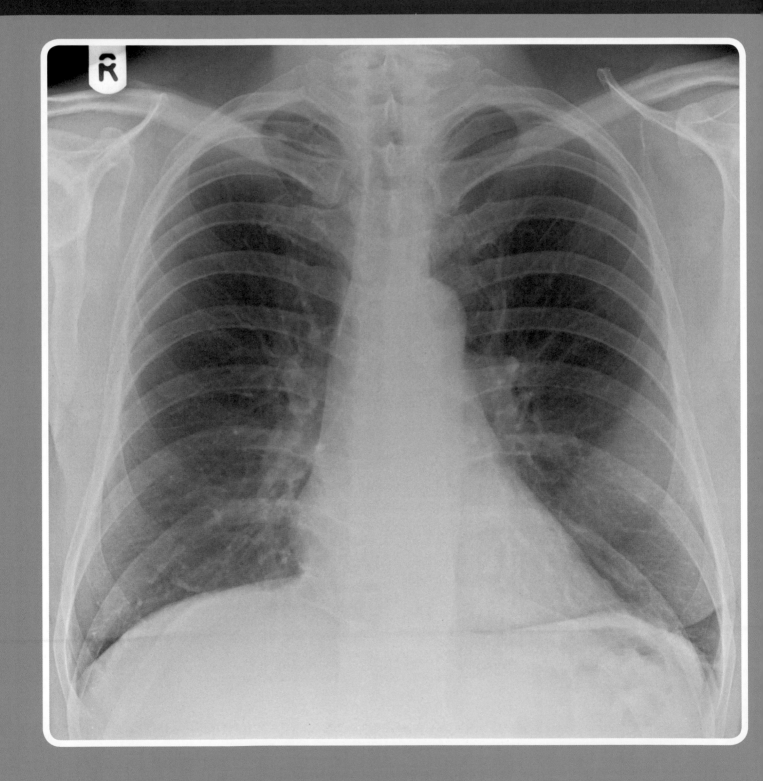

TECHNICAL INFORMATION

Patient ID: Anonymous
Projection: PA
Penetration: Adequate – vertebral bodies just visible behind heart
Inspiration: Adequate – seven anterior ribs visible
Rotation: The patient is slightly rotated to the right

● AIRWAY

The trachea is central after factoring in patient rotation.

● BREATHING

There is an ill-defined left lower zone opacification in the region of the left 5th rib. The remainder of the lungs are clear.

The lungs are not hyperinflated.

The pleural spaces are clear.

Normal pulmonary vascularity.

● CIRCULATION AND MEDIASTINUM

The heart is not enlarged.

The heart borders are clear.

The aorta appears normal.

The mediastinum is central, not widened, with clear borders.

Normal size, shape and position of both hila.

● DIAPHRAGM AND DELICATES

Normal appearance and position of the diaphragm.

No pneumoperitoneum.

There is destruction of the anterior aspect of the right 5th rib. No other destructive bony lesions or bony changes are visible.

The visible soft tissues are unremarkable.

● EXTRAS AND REVIEW AREAS

No vascular lines, tubes or surgical clips.
Lung apices: Normal.
Hila: Normal.
Behind heart: Normal.
Costophrenic angles: Normal.
Below the diaphragm: Normal.

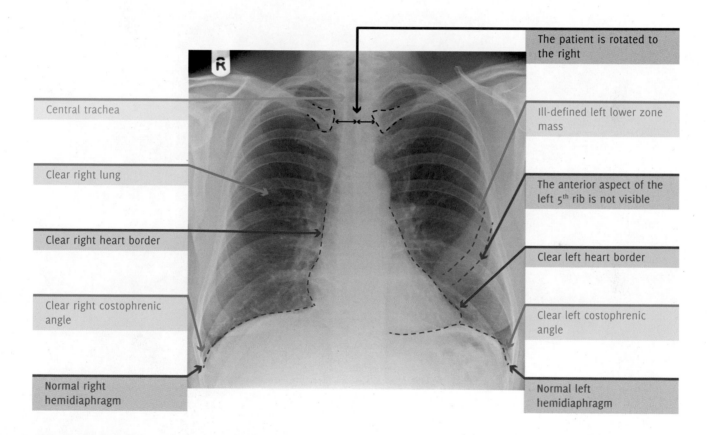

The patient is rotated to the right

Central trachea

Ill-defined left lower zone mass

Clear right lung

The anterior aspect of the left 5th rib is not visible

Clear right heart border

Clear left heart border

Clear right costophrenic angle

Clear left costophrenic angle

Normal right hemidiaphragm

Normal left hemidiaphragm

SUMMARY, INVESTIGATIONS AND MANAGEMENT

The X-ray demonstrates an ill-defined left lower zone mass associated with rib destruction. The differentials include a lung tumour with localized rib invasion, a pleural mass with rib destruction or a primary rib lesion (e.g. myeloma, plasmacytoma, metastasis or sarcoma).

Initial blood tests may include FBC, U&Es, LFTs, bone profile and a myeloma screen.

A staging CT chest, abdomen and pelvis with IV contrast should be performed.

Depending on the underlying aetiology, the patient should be referred to respiratory, oncology or haematology services for further management, which may include biopsy and MDT discussion. Treatment, which may include surgery, radiotherapy, chemotherapy or palliative treatment, will depend on the outcome of the MDT discussion, investigations and the patient's wishes.

A 50-year-old male presents to his GP with worsening right shoulder/chest pain. He has a 50 pack-year smoking history. On examination, he has oxygen saturations of 100% in air and is afebrile. His RR is 17 with an HR of 75 bpm. Lungs are resonant throughout, with good bilateral air entry. A chest X-ray is requested to assess for a possible apical lung tumour.

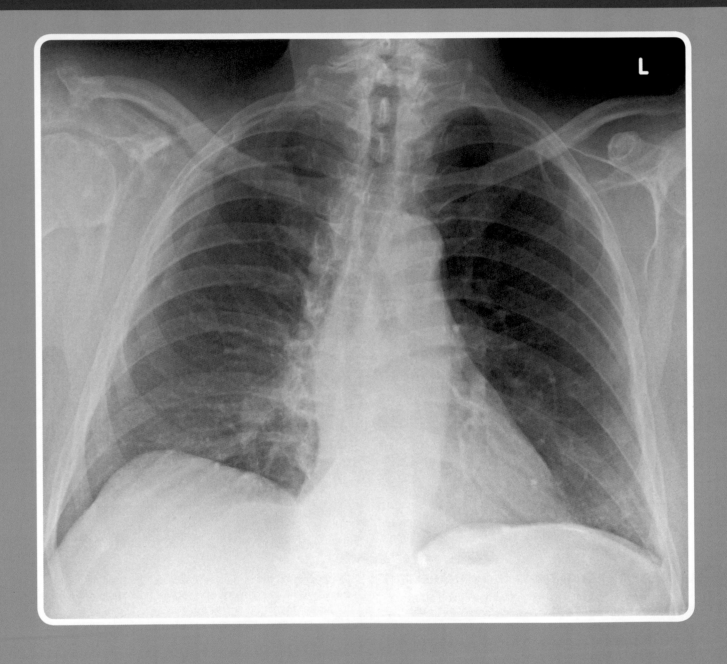

TECHNICAL INFORMATION

Patient ID: Anonymous
Projection: PA
Penetration: Adequate – vertebral bodies just visible behind heart
Inspiration: Adequate – six anterior ribs visible
Rotation: The patient is slightly rotated to the left

● AIRWAY

The trachea is central.

● BREATHING

The lungs are clear.

The lungs are not hyperinflated.

The pleural spaces are clear, apart from minor blunting of the left costophrenic angle.

Normal pulmonary vascularity.

● CIRCULATION AND MEDIASTINUM

The heart is not enlarged.

The heart borders are clear.

The aorta appears normal.

The mediastinum is central, not widened, with clear borders.

Normal size, shape and position of both hila.

● DIAPHRAGM AND DELICATES

Mild blunting of the left costophrenic angle, which may represent pleural thickening or a small effusion. Otherwise normal appearance and position of the hemidiaphragms.

No pneumoperitoneum.

The right scapula has a permeative destructive appearance in the region of the coracoid and acromion. The right proximal humerus and right clavicle appear normal. There are no other destructive bone lesions.

The visible soft tissues are unremarkable.

● EXTRAS AND REVIEW AREAS

No vascular lines, tubes or surgical clips.
Lung apices: Normal.
Hila: Normal.
Behind heart: Normal.
Costophrenic angles: Mild blunting of the left costophrenic angle.
Below the diaphragm: Normal.

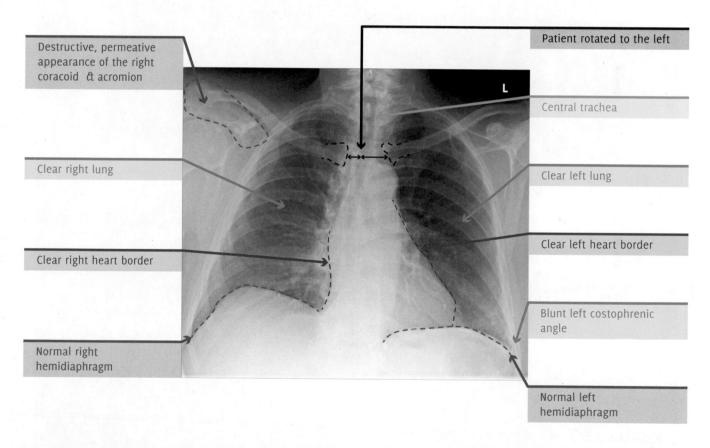

Destructive, permeative appearance of the right coracoid & acromion

Clear right lung

Clear right heart border

Normal right hemidiaphragm

Patient rotated to the left

L

Central trachea

Clear left lung

Clear left heart border

Blunt left costophrenic angle

Normal left hemidiaphragm

SUMMARY, INVESTIGATIONS AND MANAGEMENT

This X-ray demonstrates a subtle bony destruction of the right scapula which is likely accounting for the patient's symptoms. The differential for this aggressive lesion includes malignancy (primary tumours, e.g. sarcoma, plasmacytoma or metastatic disease) and infection. Metastatic disease is most likely in a patient of this age.

Dedicated X-rays of the right shoulder should be performed. Initial blood tests may include FBC, U&Es, CRP, ESR, LFTs and bone profile.

A contrast-enhanced CT of the chest, abdomen and pelvis to look for malignancy should be performed. If required, the scapula lesion could be imaged in more detail with MRI. The patient should be referred to oncology if malignancy is confirmed.

A 58-year-old male presents to ED with left-sided pleuritic chest pain. He had a left hemicolectomy for bowel cancer 6 days previously. He is a nonsmoker. On examination, he has oxygen saturations of 90% in air and is febrile. His RR is 23 with an HR of 90 bpm. Lungs are resonant throughout, with good bilateral air entry. A chest X-ray is requested to assess for a possible pneumonia or PE.

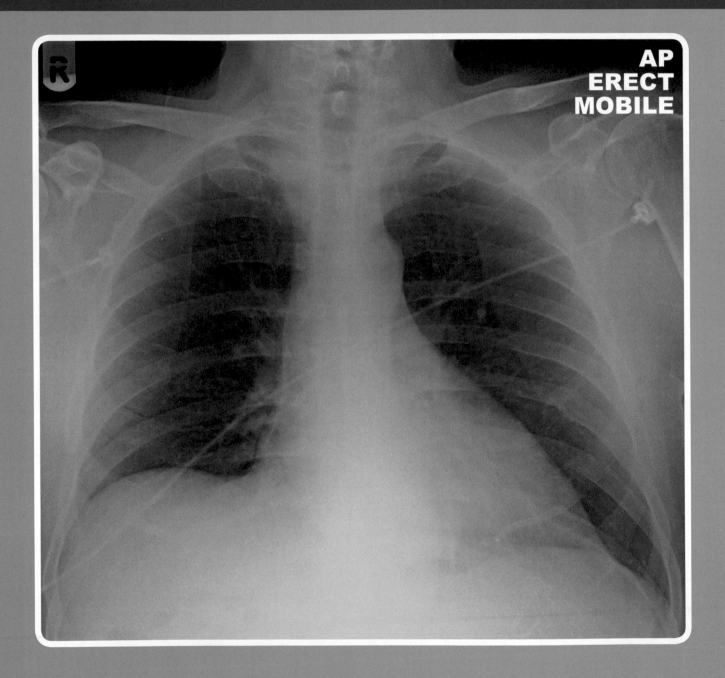

R

AP
ERECT
MOBILE

TECHNICAL INFORMATION

Patient ID: Anonymous
Projection: Mobile AP erect
Penetration: Adequate – vertebral bodies just visible behind heart
Inspiration: Adequate – six anterior ribs visible
Rotation: The patient is not rotated

● AIRWAY

The trachea is central.

● BREATHING

The lungs are clear.

The lungs are not hyperinflated.

The pleural spaces are clear.

Normal pulmonary vascularity.

● CIRCULATION AND MEDIASTINUM

The heart size cannot be accurately assessed on an AP X-ray. The heart borders are clear.

The aorta appears normal.

The mediastinum is central, not widened and with clear borders.

Normal size, shape and position of both hila.

● DIAPHRAGM AND DELICATES

Normal appearance and position of the hemidiaphragms.

No pneumoperitoneum.

The imaged skeleton is intact with no fractures or destructive bony lesions visible.

The visible soft tissues are unremarkable.

● EXTRAS AND REVIEW AREAS

ECG monitoring leads in situ.

There is a subtle curvilinear radio-opacity beneath the left hemidiaphragm, in the left upper quadrant. Its appearance is in keeping with a surgical swab.

No vascular lines, tubes or surgical clips.
Lung apices: Normal.
Hila: Normal.
Behind heart: Normal.
Costophrenic angles: Normal.
Below the diaphragm: Probable surgical swap in the left upper quadrant.

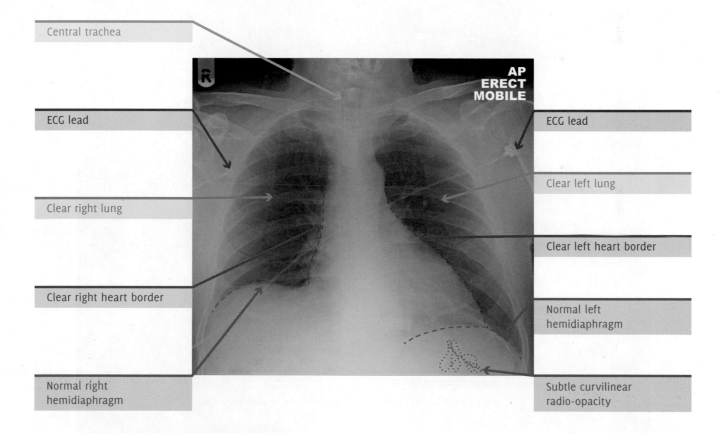

Central trachea

ECG lead

Clear right lung

Clear right heart border

Normal right hemidiaphragm

AP ERECT MOBILE

ECG lead

Clear left lung

Clear left heart border

Normal left hemidiaphragm

Subtle curvilinear radio-opacity

SUMMARY, INVESTIGATIONS AND MANAGEMENT

This X-ray demonstrates a foreign body in the left upper quadrant. Its appearance is consistent with a retained surgical swab, which is probably accounting for the patient's deterioration. The lungs are clear.

The patient should be discussed urgently with the surgical team regarding the possibility of a retained swab from the recent hemicolectomy. He needs to be assessed to ensure the swab is not on his skin/clothing. Initial blood tests may include FBC, U&Es, CRP, blood cultures and crossmatch. If further imaging is needed, a CT of the abdomen with IV contrast could be performed. Surgical exploration and removal of the swab is likely to be required.

A 60-year-old female presents to her GP for a health insurance medical. She has a 50 pack-year smoking history. On examination, she has oxygen saturations of 99% in air and is afebrile. Her RR is 16 with an HR of 72 bpm. Lungs are resonant throughout, with good bilateral air entry. A chest X-ray is requested as part of the health insurance assessment.

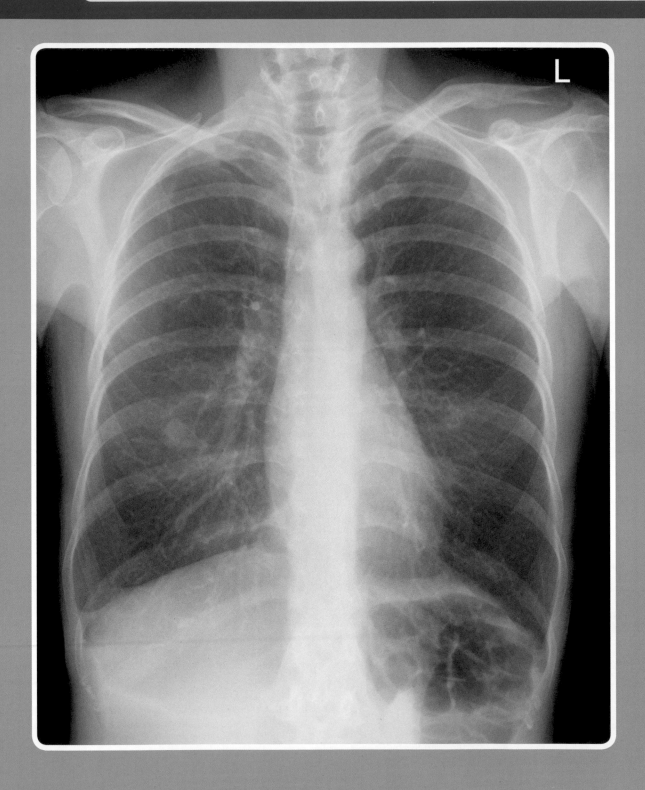

TECHNICAL INFORMATION

Patient ID: Anonymous
Projection: PA
Penetration: Adequate – vertebral bodies just visible behind heart
Inspiration: Adequate – eight anterior ribs visible
Rotation: Not rotated

● AIRWAY

The trachea is central.

● BREATHING

There are two small, well-defined circular densities within the right and left mid zones, projected over the anterior aspects of the 5th ribs. The lungs are otherwise clear.

The lungs appear hyperexpanded with flattening of the diaphragms, in keeping with COPD.

There is pleural thickening at the lung apices and costophrenic angles.

Normal pulmonary vascularity.

● CIRCULATION AND MEDIASTINUM

The heart is not enlarged.

The heart borders are clear.

The aorta appears normal.

The mediastinum is central, not widened, with clear borders.

Normal size, shape and position of both hila.

● DIAPHRAGM AND DELICATES

The hemidiaphragms are flattened. There is minor blunting of the costophrenic angles in keeping with pleural thickening.

No pneumoperitoneum.

There is an old, healed left clavicular fracture. The imaged skeleton is otherwise intact with no destructive bony lesions visible.

The visible soft tissues are unremarkable.

● EXTRAS AND REVIEW AREAS

No vascular lines, tubes or surgical clips.
Lung apices: Biapical pleural thickening.
Hila: Normal.
Behind heart: Normal.
Costophrenic angles: Pleural thickening bilaterally.
Below the diaphragm: Normal.

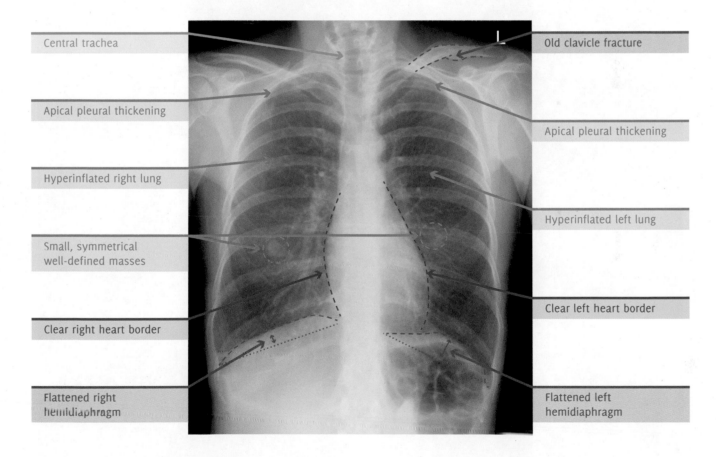

Central trachea — Old clavicle fracture

Apical pleural thickening — Apical pleural thickening

Hyperinflated right lung — Hyperinflated left lung

Small, symmetrical well-defined masses

Clear right heart border — Clear left heart border

Flattened right hemidiaphragm — Flattened left hemidiaphragm

SUMMARY, INVESTIGATIONS AND MANAGEMENT

This X-ray demonstrates hyperinflated lungs, in keeping with COPD. The two well-defined, symmetrical circular densities in the mid zones are likely to represent nipple shadows. The remainder of the X-ray is unremarkable.

No specific action is required. If there is clinical uncertainty, a repeat chest X-ray with nipple markers should be performed for clarification.

A 60-year-old male presents to ED with severe left-sided pleuritic chest pain. He has a 50 pack-year smoking history. On examination, he has oxygen saturations of 100% in air and is afebrile. Lungs are resonant throughout and there is good bilateral air entry. He is focally tender over the left upper chest wall. A chest X-ray is requested to assess for possible pneumonia or a pneumothorax.

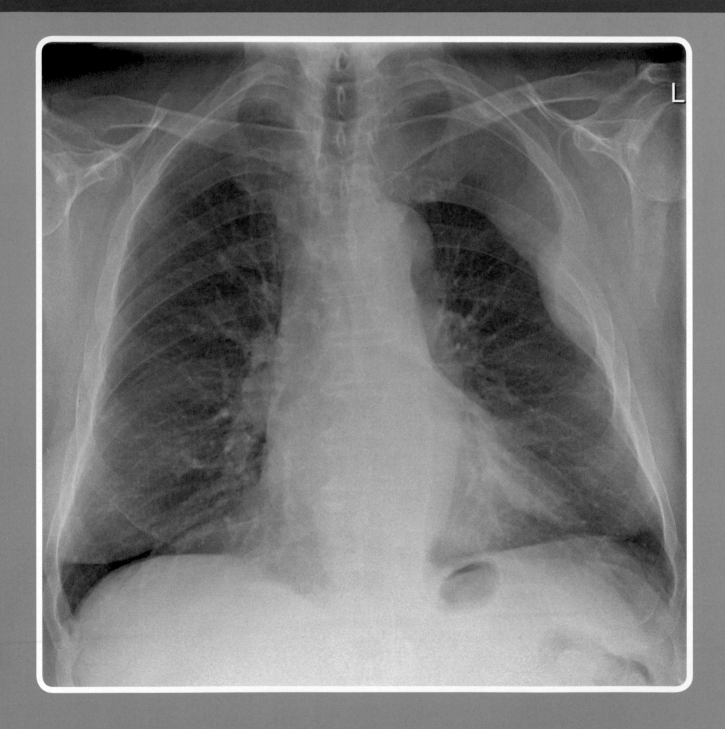

L

TECHNICAL INFORMATION

Patient ID: Anonymous
Projection: PA
Penetration: Adequate – vertebral bodies just visible behind heart
Inspiration: Adequate – seven anterior ribs visible
Rotation: Not rotated

● AIRWAY

The trachea is central.

● BREATHING

There is homogeneous peripheral opacification in the left upper and mid zones. Some lung markings can be seen through this. Inferiorly, the opacity makes an obtuse angle with the chest wall, suggesting it is within the pleural space or chest wall rather than lung parenchyma. The lateral margin of the lesion is difficult to identify.

The right lung is clear.

The lungs are not hyperinflated.

The right-sided pleural space is clear.

Normal pulmonary vascularity.

● CIRCULATION AND MEDIASTINUM

The heart is not enlarged.

The heart borders are clear. There is an epicardial fat pad at the right cardiophrenic angle.

There is mild unfolding of the thoracic aorta.

The mediastinum is central, not widened, with clear borders.

Normal size, shape and position of both hila.

● DIAPHRAGM AND DELICATES

Normal appearance and position of the hemidiaphragms.

No pneumoperitoneum.

The posterolateral aspect of the left 4th rib is not visible. The imaged skeleton is otherwise intact with no fractures or other destructive bony lesions visible.

The soft tissues are unremarkable.

● EXTRAS AND REVIEW AREAS

No vascular lines, tubes or surgical clips.
Lung apices: Increased soft tissue opacification within the left apex.
Hila: Normal.
Behind heart: Normal.
Costophrenic angles: Normal.
Below the diaphragm: Normal.

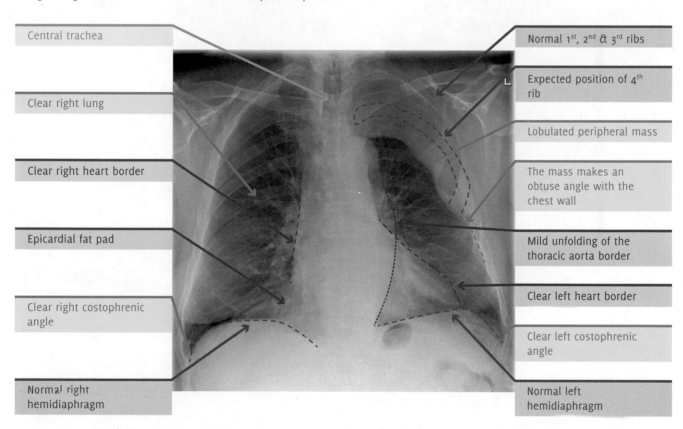

Central trachea	Normal 1st, 2nd & 3rd ribs
Clear right lung	Expected position of 4th rib
Clear right heart border	Lobulated peripheral mass
	The mass makes an obtuse angle with the chest wall
Epicardial fat pad	Mild unfolding of the thoracic aorta border
	Clear left heart border
Clear right costophrenic angle	
	Clear left costophrenic angle
Normal right hemidiaphragm	Normal left hemidiaphragm

SUMMARY, INVESTIGATIONS AND MANAGEMENT

This X-ray demonstrates a peripheral lobulated abnormality in the left upper and mid hemithorax with destruction of the underlying left 4th rib. The abnormal lesion makes an obtuse angle with the chest wall. The findings are suggestive of an aggressive pleural or extrapleural mass. The differentials include pleural-based tumours (e.g. mesothelioma, adenocarcinoma metastases or invasive thymoma) and chest wall masses (rib metastasis, plasmacytoma or sarcoma).

Initial blood tests may include FBC, U&Es, LFTs and bone profile.

Previous imaging should be reviewed to ascertain if this is a new abnormality. A contrast-enhanced CT of the chest would provide more information on the mass.

The patient should be referred to respiratory/oncology services for further management, which may include biopsy and MDT discussion. Treatment, which may include surgery, radiotherapy, chemotherapy or palliative treatment, will depend on the outcome of the MDT discussion, investigations and the patient's wishes.

A 67-year-old female presents to her GP with chest pain on inspiration. She previously had surgery for breast cancer 10 years ago. She is a nonsmoker. On examination, she has oxygen saturations of 100% in air and is afebrile. Her RR is 16 with an HR of 75 bpm. There is some localized tenderness over the ribs bilaterally. A chest X-ray is requested to assess for a pneumothorax or rib fracture.

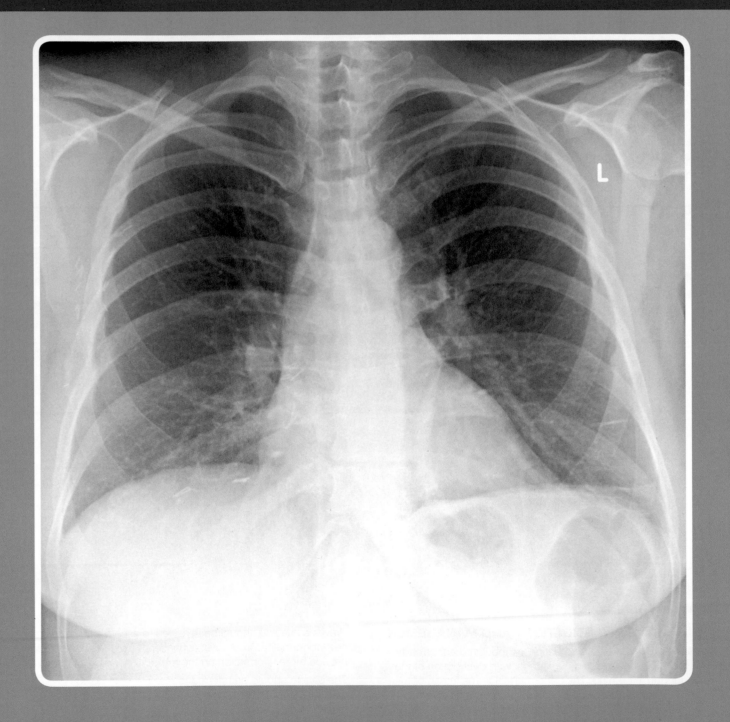

TECHNICAL INFORMATION

Patient ID: Anonymous
Projection: PA
Penetration: Adequate – vertebral bodies just visible behind heart
Inspiration: Adequate – six anterior ribs visible
Rotation: The patient is slightly rotated to the right

● AIRWAY

The trachea is central after factoring in patient rotation.

● BREATHING

There is minor linear atelectasis in the left lower zone. The lungs are otherwise clear.

The lungs are not hyperinflated.

The pleural spaces are clear.

Normal pulmonary vascularity.

● CIRCULATION AND MEDIASTINUM

The heart is not enlarged.

The heart borders are clear.

The aorta appears normal.

The mediastinum is central, not widened, with clear borders.

Normal size, shape and position of both hila.

● DIAPHRAGM AND DELICATES

Normal appearance and position of the hemidiaphragms.

No pneumoperitoneum.

There is a subtle expansile lucent lesion within the lateral aspect of the left 5th rib. A further lesion is present in the right 6th rib. The right 3rd and left 6th ribs also have abnormal areas.

The visible soft tissues are unremarkable.

● EXTRAS AND REVIEW AREAS

There are multiple surgical clips within the right axilla and overlying the right breast, in keeping with previous breast surgery with axillary node clearance.
Lung apices: Normal.
Hila: Normal.

Behind heart: Normal.
Costophrenic angles: Minor left atelectasis.
Below the diaphragm: Normal.

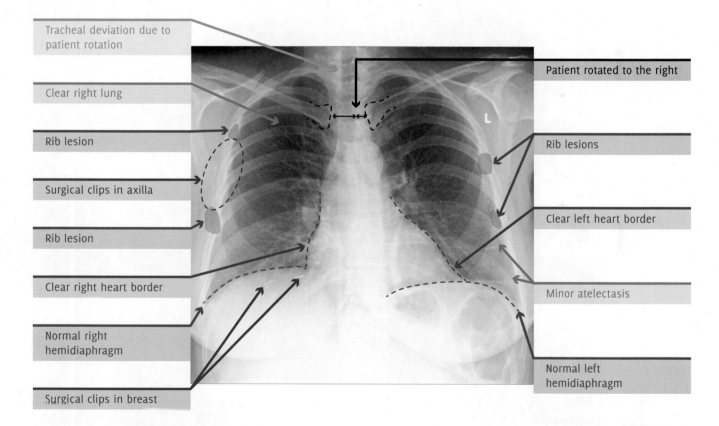

Tracheal deviation due to patient rotation

Clear right lung

Rib lesion

Surgical clips in axilla

Rib lesion

Clear right heart border

Normal right hemidiaphragm

Surgical clips in breast

Patient rotated to the right

Rib lesions

Clear left heart border

Minor atelectasis

Normal left hemidiaphragm

SUMMARY, INVESTIGATIONS AND MANAGEMENT

This X-ray demonstrates bilateral rib lesions. In the context of previous breast and axillary surgery for breast cancer, these rib lesions are highly suspicious for metastatic deposits.

This patient needs restaging with contrast-enhanced CT of the chest, abdomen and pelvis and referred to oncology for further management.

A 68-year-old female presents to her GP with unintentional weight loss. She has a 50 pack-year smoking history. On examination, she has oxygen saturations of 100% in air and is afebrile. Lungs are resonant throughout with good bilateral air entry. There is a left-sided Horner syndrome. A chest X-ray is requested to assess for possible malignancy.

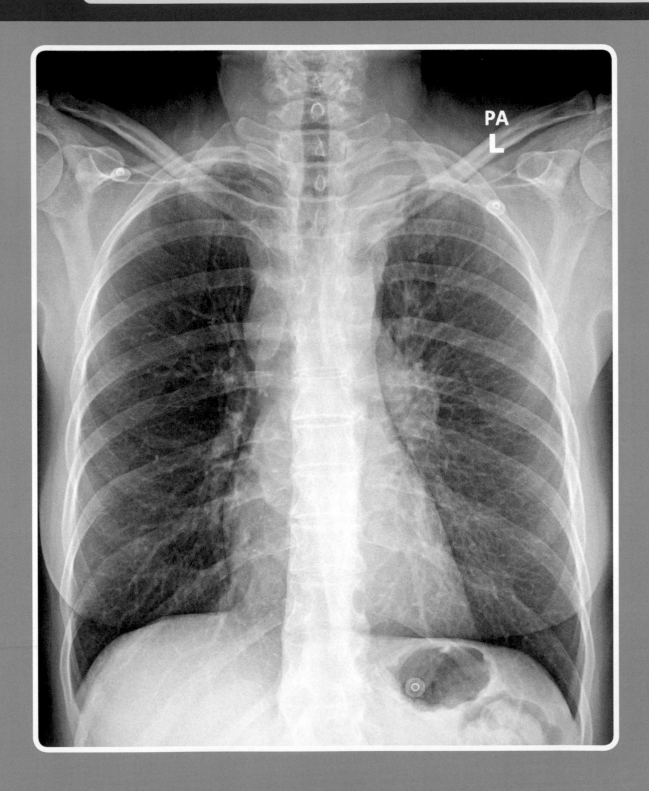

TECHNICAL INFORMATION

Patient ID: Anonymous
Projection: PA
Penetration: Adequate – vertebral bodies just visible behind heart
Inspiration: Adequate – eight anterior ribs visible
Rotation: Not rotated

● AIRWAY

The trachea is central.

● BREATHING

There is asymmetry of the lung apices with increased density in the left apex. A subtle lace-like opacification in the left lung is present, in keeping with interstitial opacification.

The right lung is clear.

The lungs are not hyperinflated. There is coarsening of the bronchovascular markings, in keeping with COPD.

The pleural spaces are clear.

● CIRCULATION AND MEDIASTINUM

The heart is not enlarged.

The heart borders are clear. There is a well-defined lobulated mass projected over the right side of the cardiac silhouette, which is separate to the right hilum.

The aorta appears normal.

There is widening of the right paratracheal stripe. The mediastinum has clear borders.

Normal size, shape and position of right hila. The left hilum is enlarged and dense, consistent with lymph node enlargement.

● DIAPHRAGM AND DELICATES

Normal appearance and position of the hemidiaphragms.

No pneumoperitoneum.

The imaged skeleton is intact with no fractures or destructive bony lesions visible. In particular, the left 1st and 2nd ribs appear intact.

The visible soft tissues are unremarkable.

● EXTRAS AND REVIEW AREAS

ECG electrodes in situ.

No vascular lines, tubes or surgical clips.
Lung apices: Left apical mass.
Hila: Enlarged, dense left hilum.
Behind heart: Right retrocardiac mass.
Costophrenic angles: Normal.
Below the diaphragm: Normal.

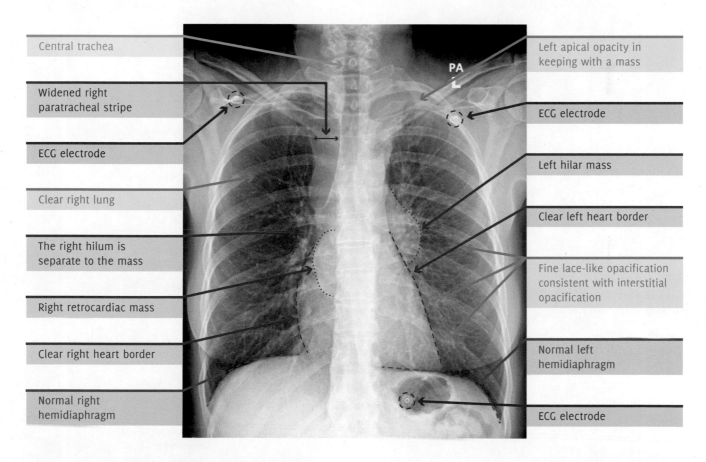

Central trachea

Widened right paratracheal stripe

ECG electrode

Clear right lung

The right hilum is separate to the mass

Right retrocardiac mass

Clear right heart border

Normal right hemidiaphragm

Left apical opacity in keeping with a mass

ECG electrode

Left hilar mass

Clear left heart border

Fine lace-like opacification consistent with interstitial opacification

Normal left hemidiaphragm

ECG electrode

SUMMARY, INVESTIGATIONS AND MANAGEMENT

The X-ray demonstrates a left apical mass, which is likely accounting for the Horner syndrome. There is evidence of mediastinal lymph node enlargement (widened right paratracheal stripe, dense left hilum and right retrocardiac mass). The interstitial opacification in the left lung probably represents malignant spread via the lymphatics (lymphangitis carcinomatosis).

Initial blood tests may include FBC, U&Es, LFTs and bone profile.

A staging CT chest and abdomen with IV contrast should be performed.

The patient should be referred to respiratory/oncology services for further management, which may include biopsy and MDT discussion. Treatment, which may include surgery, radiotherapy, chemotherapy or palliative treatment, will depend on the outcome of the MDT discussion, investigations and the patient's wishes.

A 70-year-old female presented to her GP with a 3-week history of a cough. She described recent weight loss and 'constantly feeling tired'. She has a 45 pack-year smoking history. On examination, she has oxygen saturations of 98% in air and is afebrile. Lungs are resonant throughout, with good air entry bilaterally. There is a dry cough and cachexia. The GP requests a chest X-ray to assess for possible malignancy.

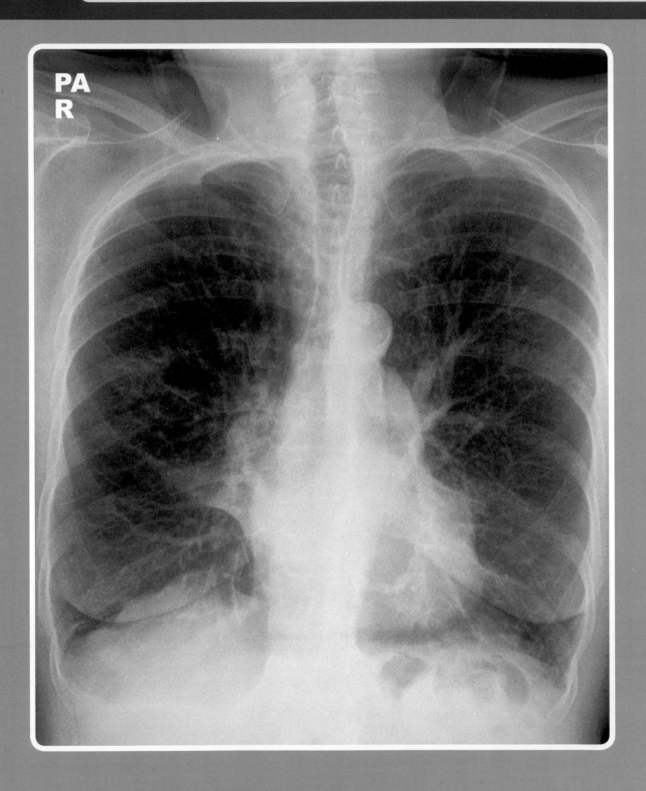

PA R
R

TECHNICAL INFORMATION

Patient ID: Anonymous
Projection: PA
Penetration: Adequate – vertebral bodies just visible behind heart
Inspiration: Adequate – eight anterior ribs visible
Rotation: Not rotated

● AIRWAY

The trachea is central.

● BREATHING

The lungs are hyperinflated with coarsening of the lung markings.

There is increased density in the medial aspect of the right lower zone. The horizontal fissure cannot be identified. Additionally, there is a 2-cm opacity in the right mid zone projected over the posterior intercostal space of the 7th and 8th ribs.

The left lung is clear.

The pleural spaces are clear.

Normal pulmonary vascularity.

● CIRCULATION AND MEDIASTINUM

The heart is not enlarged.

The right heart border is indistinct. The left heart border is clear.

The aorta appears normal.

The mediastinum is central.

The right hilum is bulky with a convex margin and increased density. Normal size, shape and position of the left hilum.

● DIAPHRAGM AND DELICATES

The medial aspect of the right hemidiaphragm is slightly elevated. The left hemidiaphragm is flattened, but in a normal position.

No pneumoperitoneum.

The imaged skeleton is intact with no fractures or destructive bony lesions visible.

The visible soft tissues are unremarkable.

● EXTRAS AND REVIEW AREAS

No vascular lines, tubes or surgical clips.
Lung apices: Normal.
Hila: Right hilum is bulky, with a convex margin and increased density.
Behind heart: Normal.
Costophrenic angles: Normal.
Below the diaphragm: Normal.

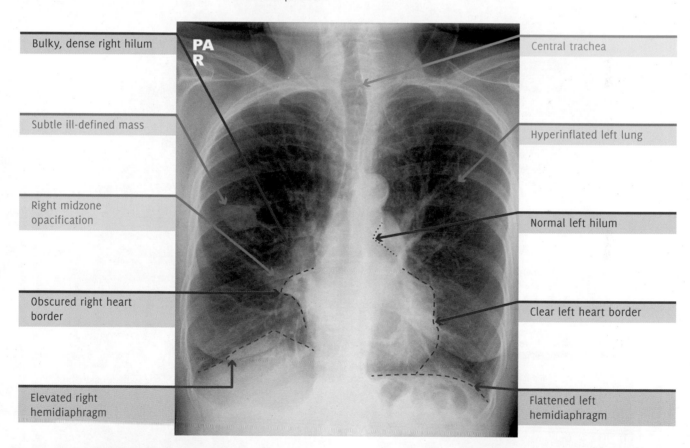

Bulky, dense right hilum

Subtle ill-defined mass

Right midzone opacification

Obscured right heart border

Elevated right hemidiaphragm

PA R

Central trachea

Hyperinflated left lung

Normal left hilum

Clear left heart border

Flattened left hemidiaphragm

SUMMARY, INVESTIGATIONS AND MANAGEMENT

This X-ray demonstrates a right middle lobe collapse (opacification obscuring the right heart border and mild elevation of the right hemidiaphragm). Additionally, the right hilum is abnormal and there is an ill-defined opacity in the right mid zone.

The lungs are hyperinflated with coarsening of the markings, in keeping with COPD.

The most likely diagnosis is underlying malignancy. Mucus plugging or a foreign body could also cause collapse but is less likely, given the lung mass and abnormal right hilum. Initial

blood tests may include FBC, U&Es, LFTs, bone profile, CRP, ESR and TFTs.

The patient should be urgently referred to respiratory/oncology services for further management. This will include an urgent outpatient CT chest with IV contrast performed to assess for an underlying tumour. A CT of the abdomen will usually also be acquired at the same time to enable lung cancer staging.

Further treatment may include surgery, radiotherapy, chemotherapy or palliative treatment, depending on the outcome of the MDT discussion and the patient's wishes.

A 71-year-old male presents to his GP with a chronic cough and right shoulder pain. He has a 40 pack-year smoking history. On examination, he has oxygen saturations of 96% in air and is afebrile. Lungs are resonant throughout with good bilateral air entry and occasional wheeze. There is a full range of movement in the shoulder, but some weakness in the right hand. A chest X-ray is requested to assess for possible malignancy.

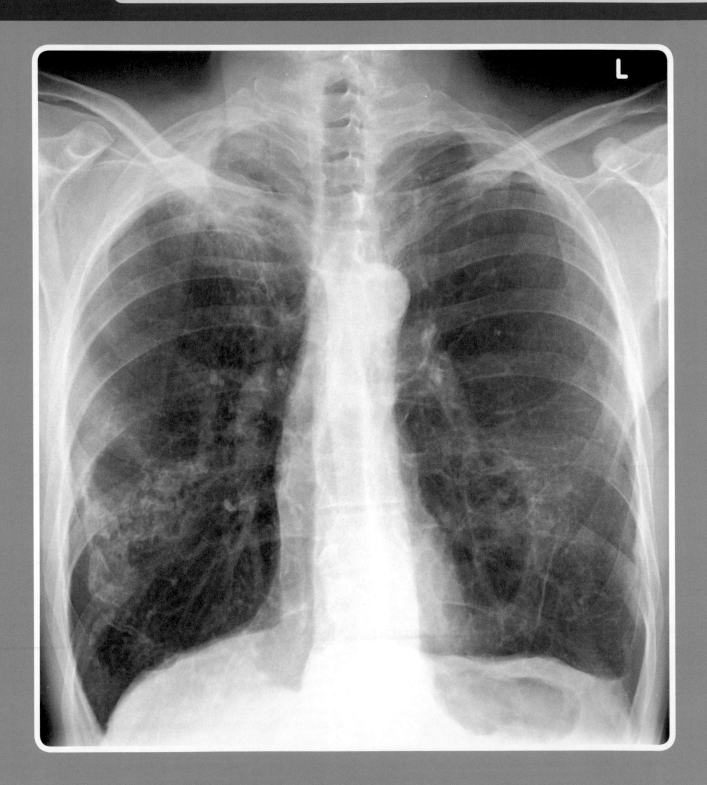

TECHNICAL INFORMATION

Patient ID: Anonymous
Projection: PA
Penetration: Adequate – vertebral bodies just visible behind heart
Inspiration: Adequate – seven anterior ribs visible
Rotation: The patient is slightly rotated to the right

● AIRWAY

The trachea is central after factoring in patient rotation.

● BREATHING

The lung apices are asymmetrical with right apical opacification. There are bilateral calcified pleural plaques, in keeping with previous asbestos exposure.

The lungs are hyperinflated in keeping with COPD, but otherwise clear.

The pleural spaces are clear, apart from the pleural plaques.

Normal pulmonary vascularity.

● CIRCULATION AND MEDIASTINUM

The heart is not enlarged.

The heart borders are clear.

The aorta appears normal.

The mediastinum is central, not widened, with clear borders.

Normal size, shape and position of both hila.

● DIAPHRAGM AND DELICATES

Both hemidiaphragms are flattened but clear.

No pneumoperitoneum.

The posterolateral aspect of the right 3rd rib is not visible, in keeping

with localized destruction. No other destructive bone lesions or other bony changes.

The soft tissues are unremarkable.

● EXTRAS AND REVIEW AREAS

No vascular lines, tubes or surgical clips.
Lung apices: There is a right apical mass with associated destruction of the right 3rd rib.
Hila: Normal.
Behind heart: Normal.
Costophrenic angles: Normal.
Below the diaphragm: Normal.

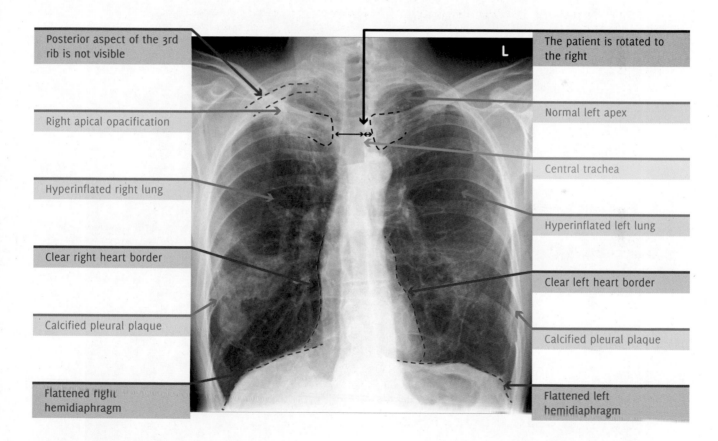

Posterior aspect of the 3rd rib is not visible

Right apical opacification

Hyperinflated right lung

Clear right heart border

Calcified pleural plaque

Flattened right hemidiaphragm

The patient is rotated to the right

Normal left apex

Central trachea

Hyperinflated left lung

Clear left heart border

Calcified pleural plaque

Flattened left hemidiaphragm

SUMMARY, INVESTIGATIONS AND MANAGEMENT

This X-ray demonstrates a right apical mass with associated destruction of the right 3rd rib. There are background changes of COPD and previous asbestos exposure. The findings are in keeping with a primary lung (Pancoast) tumour with direct involvement of the adjacent rib. Given the previous asbestos exposure, mesothelioma is one of the differentials.

Initial blood tests may include FBC, U&Es, LFTs and bone profile.

A staging CT chest and abdomen with IV contrast should be performed.

The patient should be referred to respiratory/oncology services for further management, which may include biopsy and MDT discussion. Treatment, which may include surgery, radiotherapy, chemotherapy or palliative treatment, will depend on the outcome of the MDT discussion, investigations and the patient's wishes.

A 75-year-old male presents to ED feeling unwell with a productive cough. He was diagnosed with pneumonia 2 weeks earlier, but has not been taking his antibiotics. He is a nonsmoker. On examination, he has oxygen saturations of 90% in air and is febrile, with a temperature of 38.2°C. There are crackles, reduced air entry and dullness to percussion in the right mid and lower zones. A chest X-ray is requested to assess for possible collapse, consolidation or effusion.

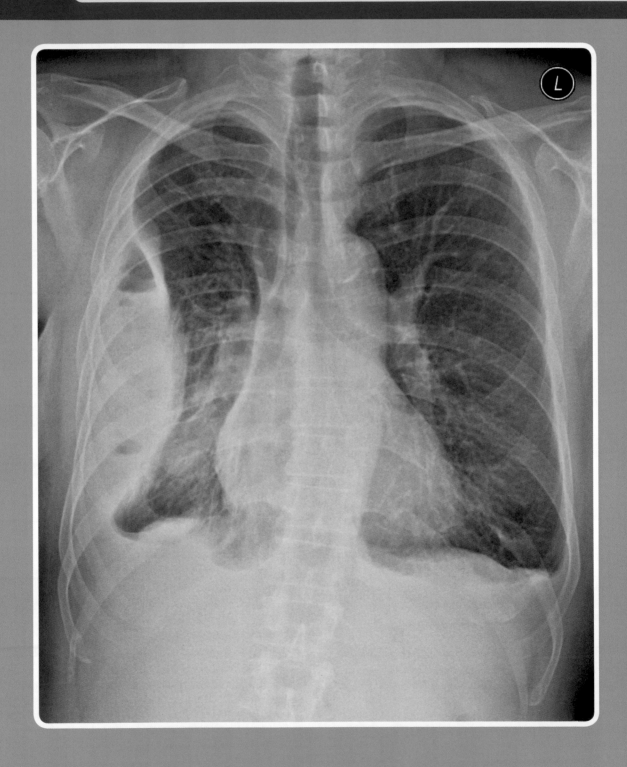

TECHNICAL INFORMATION

Patient ID: Anonymous
Projection: PA
Penetration: Adequate – vertebral bodies just visible behind heart
Inspiration: Adequate – nine anterior ribs visible
Rotation: The patient is slightly rotated to the right

● AIRWAY

The trachea is central after factoring patient rotation.

● BREATHING

Heterogeneous opacification is present in the right mid and lower zones. There is a loculated right-sided pleural collection tracking up to the right apex. It contains several pockets of gas and an air-fluid level superiorly. The adjacent pleura appears thickened.

The left lung is clear. The lungs are not hyperinflated.

A small left pleural effusion is present.

Normal pulmonary vascularity.

● CIRCULATION AND MEDIASTINUM

The heart is not enlarged.

The heart borders are clear.

The mediastinum is central, not widened, with clear borders.

Normal size, shape and position of both hila.

● DIAPHRAGM AND DELICATES

The right hemidiaphragm is indistinct. Normal appearance and position of the left hemidiaphragm.

No pneumoperitoneum.

The imaged skeleton is intact with no fractures or destructive bony lesions visible.

The visible soft tissues are unremarkable.

● EXTRAS AND REVIEW AREAS

No vascular lines, tubes or surgical clips.
Lung apices: Normal.
Hila: Normal.
Behind heart: Increased right retrocardiac opacification.
Costophrenic angles: Blunt costophrenic angles bilaterally.
Below the diaphragm: Normal.

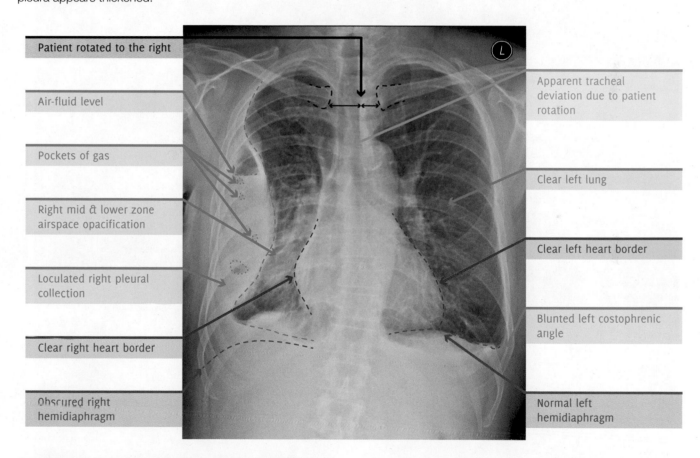

Labels (left): Patient rotated to the right · Air-fluid level · Pockets of gas · Right mid & lower zone airspace opacification · Loculated right pleural collection · Clear right heart border · Obscured right hemidiaphragm

Labels (right): Apparent tracheal deviation due to patient rotation · Clear left lung · Clear left heart border · Blunted left costophrenic angle · Normal left hemidiaphragm

SUMMARY, INVESTIGATIONS AND MANAGEMENT

The X-ray demonstrates a right-sided loculated pleural effusion with pleural thickening and an air-fluid level. There is associated heterogeneous opacification in the right mid and lower zones. The findings are consistent with an empyema and adjacent pneumonia. A small left pleural effusion is present.

Supplementary oxygen needs to be given.

Initial blood tests may include a FBC, U&Es, LFTs, CRP, coagulation and blood cultures. Sputum cultures should also be obtained.

The patient should be discussed with respiratory and/or infectious diseases.

A chest CT with IV contrast would delineate the right-sided abnormalities more clearly. Additionally, it could exclude associated lung abscesses. Ultrasound-guided drainage of the right pleural collection should be performed, and the patient should be started on appropriate intravenous antibiotics. Interval imaging to ensure resolution will be required.

A 79-year-old female presents to ED with worsening shortness of breath. She has a background of mitral regurgitation. She is a nonsmoker. On examination, she has oxygen saturations of 94% in air and is afebrile. Her RR is 22 with an HR of 90 bpm. There are scattered crackles in both the lung bases, in addition to bibasal dullness to percussion. A chest X-ray is requested to assess for possible pulmonary oedema.

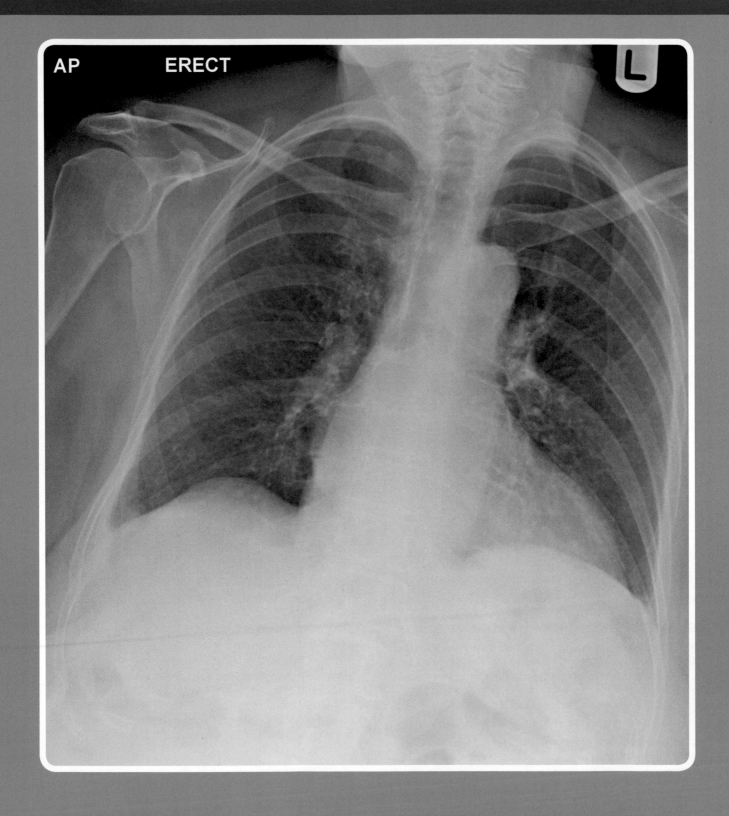

AP   ERECT   L

TECHNICAL INFORMATION

Patient ID: Anonymous
Projection: AP erect
Penetration: Adequate – vertebral bodies just visible behind heart
Inspiration: Adequate – six anterior ribs visible
Rotation: The patient is not rotated

● AIRWAY

The trachea is central.

● BREATHING

The lungs are clear.

The lungs are not hyperinflated.

There is minor blunting of the costophrenic angles. The pleural spaces are otherwise clear.

Normal pulmonary vascularity.

● CIRCULATION AND MEDIASTINUM

The cardiac size cannot be accurately assessed on this AP X-ray.

There is a double right heart border. The left heart border is clear.

The aorta appears normal.

The mediastinum is central, not widened with clear borders. The carina is splayed.

Normal size, shape and position of both hila.

● DIAPHRAGM AND DELICATES

Minor blunting of the costophrenic angles which may represent pleural thickening or small effusions. Otherwise normal appearance and position of the hemidiaphragms.

No pneumoperitoneum.

The imaged skeleton is intact with no fractures or destructive bony lesions visible.

The visible soft tissues are unremarkable.

● EXTRAS AND REVIEW AREAS

No vascular lines, tubes or surgical clips.
Lung apices: Normal.
Hila: Normal.
Behind heart: Double right heart border and splayed carina.
Costophrenic angles: Minor blunting.
Below the diaphragm: Normal.

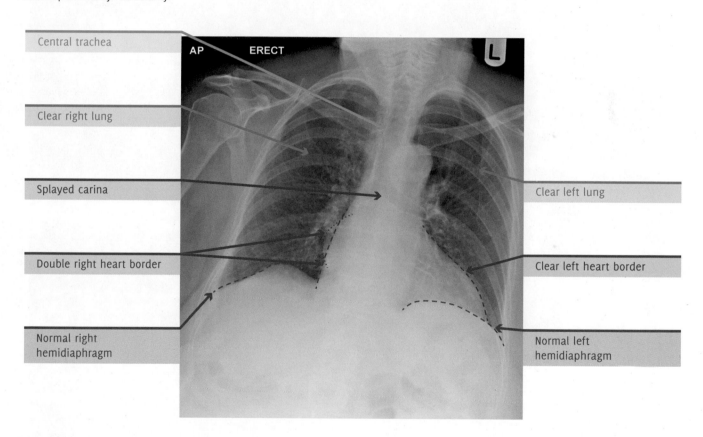

Central trachea

Clear right lung

Splayed carina

Double right heart border

Normal right hemidiaphragm

AP   ERECT   L

Clear left lung

Clear left heart border

Normal left hemidiaphragm

SUMMARY, INVESTIGATIONS AND MANAGEMENT

This X-ray demonstrates a double right heart border associated with splayed carina, consistent with left atrial enlargement – this is compatible with the known history of mitral regurgitation. There is minor blunting of the costophrenic angles which may represent small effusions or pleural thickening. There is no evidence of pulmonary oedema.

Initial blood tests may include FBC, U&Es and CRP. Previous X-rays should be reviewed to assess whether the findings are new or longstanding. An ECG should be performed. An ECHO would allow assessment of the cardiac function and the degree of any regurgitation. Depending on the results, medical (diuretic) or surgical management may be needed for the valve disease.

A 79-year-old male presents to ED with chest pain, a cough and fever. He has previously had a CABG. He is a nonsmoker. On examination, he has oxygen saturations of 99% in air and is febrile with a temperature of 39.5°C. His RR is 22 with an HR of 95 bpm. Lungs are resonant throughout, with good bilateral air entry. A chest X-ray is requested to assess for possible pneumonia.

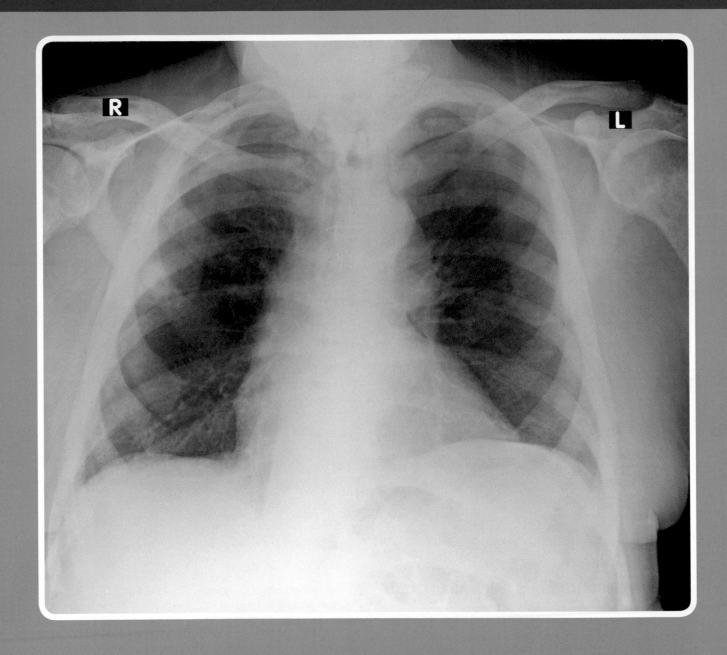

TECHNICAL INFORMATION

Patient ID: Anonymous
Projection: PA
Penetration: Slightly underpenetrated – vertebral bodies not clearly visible behind the heart
Inspiration: Adequate – six anterior ribs visible
Rotation: The patient is rotated to the right

● AIRWAY

The trachea is central after factoring in patient rotation.

● BREATHING

The lungs are clear.

The lungs are not hyperinflated.

The pleural spaces are clear.

Normal pulmonary vascularity.

● CIRCULATION AND MEDIASTINUM

The heart is not enlarged.

The heart borders are clear.

There is unfolding of the thoracic aorta.

The mediastinum is central, not widened, with clear borders.

Normal size, shape and position of both hila.

● DIAPHRAGM AND DELICATES

Normal appearance and position of the hemidiaphragms.

No pneumoperitoneum.

The bones have an abnormal texture, appearing diffusely sclerotic. The imaged skeleton is otherwise intact with no fracture or destructive bony lesion visible.

The visible soft tissues are unremarkable.

● EXTRAS AND REVIEW AREAS

Sternotomy wires in situ.
Lung apices: Normal.
Hila: Normal.
Behind heart: Normal.
Costophrenic angles: Normal.
Below the diaphragm: Normal.

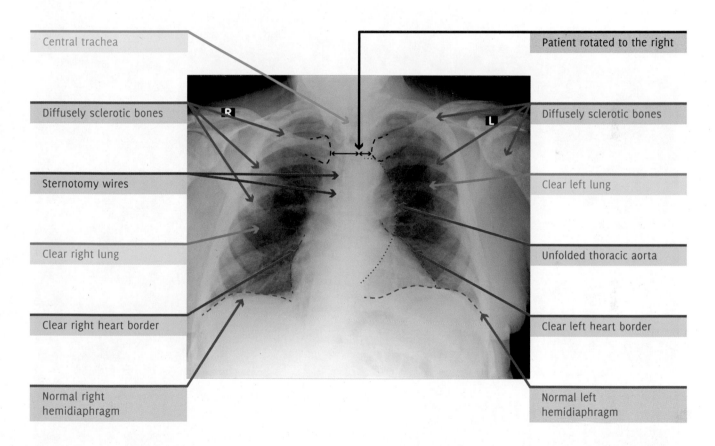

Central trachea

Patient rotated to the right

Diffusely sclerotic bones

Diffusely sclerotic bones

Sternotomy wires

Clear left lung

Clear right lung

Unfolded thoracic aorta

Clear right heart border

Clear left heart border

Normal right hemidiaphragm

Normal left hemidiaphragm

SUMMARY, INVESTIGATIONS AND MANAGEMENT

The X-ray demonstrates diffusely sclerotic bones. In a male patient of this age, the most likely cause is sclerotic metastases from prostate cancer.

Previous imaging and medical notes should be reviewed to assess whether the patient is known to have an underlying malignancy, especially prostate cancer. Initial blood tests may include FBC, U&Es, PSA, LFTs and a bone profile. A digital rectal examination of the prostate should be performed. The patient should be discussed with urology and oncology for further management.

An 18-year-old female presents to ED with acute shortness of breath and pleuritic chest pain. She has known sickle cell disease, with multiple recent hospital admissions. She is a nonsmoker. On examination, she has oxygen saturations of 94% in air and is febrile with a temperature of 39°C. Her RR is 20 with an HR of 80 bpm. There are scattered crackles throughout the lungs. A chest X-ray is requested to assess for possible pneumonia, pneumothorax or an acute chest syndrome.

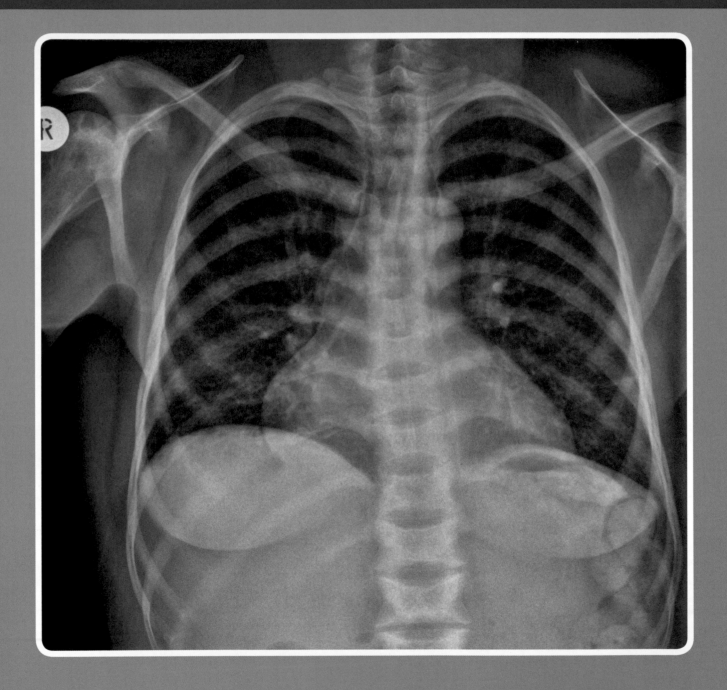

TECHNICAL INFORMATION

Patient ID: Anonymous
Projection: PA
Penetration: Overpenetrated – vertebral bodies clearly visible behind heart
Inspiration: Adequate – six anterior ribs visible
Rotation: The patient is not rotated

● AIRWAY

The trachea is central.

● BREATHING

There is minor linear atelectasis in the left mid zone. The lungs are otherwise clear.

The lungs are not hyperinflated.

The pleural spaces are clear.

Normal pulmonary vascularity.

● CIRCULATION AND MEDIASTINUM

The cardiothoracic ratio is 0.6, consistent with cardiomegaly. The heart borders are clear.

The aorta appears normal.

The mediastinum is central, not widened with clear borders.

Normal size, shape and position of both hila.

● DIAPHRAGM AND DELICATES

Normal appearance and position of the hemidiaphragms. No pneumoperitoneum.

There are mixed sclerotic/lucent changes seen within the right humeral head. The ribs have a mottled bony texture. There are biconcave vertebral endplate changes resulting in 'H'-shaped vertebrae.

The visible soft tissues are unremarkable.

● EXTRAS AND REVIEW AREAS

No vascular lines, tubes or surgical clips.
Lung apices: Normal.
Hila: Normal.
Behind heart: Normal.
Costophrenic angles: Normal.
Below the diaphragm: Normal.

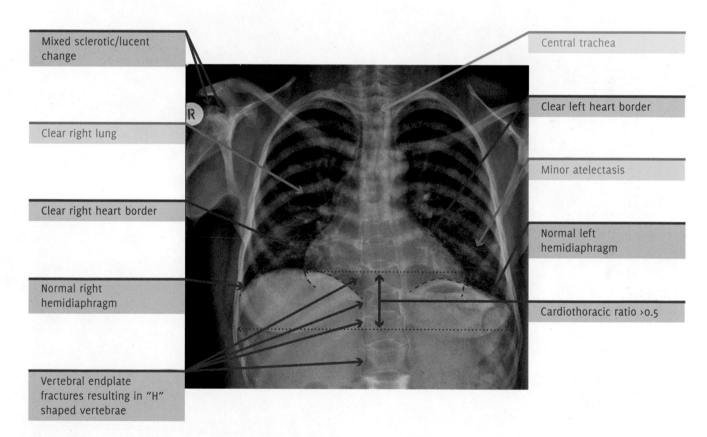

Mixed sclerotic/lucent change

Clear right lung

Clear right heart border

Normal right hemidiaphragm

Vertebral endplate fractures resulting in "H" shaped vertebrae

Central trachea

Clear left heart border

Minor atelectasis

Normal left hemidiaphragm

Cardiothoracic ratio >0.5

SUMMARY, INVESTIGATIONS AND MANAGEMENT

This X-ray demonstrates multiple chronic features of sickle cell anaemia. The 'H'-shaped vertebrae are the result of endplate infarcts, while the changes in the right humeral head reflect avascular necrosis from a previous sickle cell crisis. The cardiomegaly is presumably related to severe anaemia. There is no consolidation, effusion or pneumothorax.

A clinical concern remains for a sickle cell acute chest syndrome. Initial blood tests may include FBC, U&Es, LFTs and CRP.

Analgesia and appropriate antibiotics should be administered. Depending on the haemoglobin, a transfusion may be required.

An 80-year-old male presents to ED with increasing shortness of breath. He has a background of two previous MIs. He has a 50 pack-year smoking history. On examination, he has oxygen saturations of 92% in air and is afebrile. His RR is 20 with an HR of 90 bpm. There are scattered crackles at the lung bases, with dullness to percussion. A chest X-ray is requested to assess for possible pulmonary oedema, collapse or pneumonia.

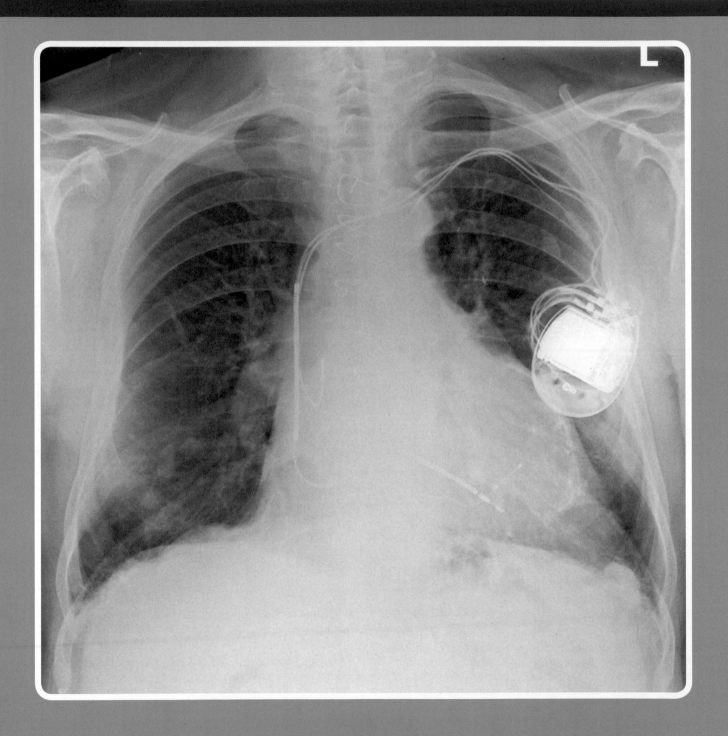

TECHNICAL INFORMATION

Patient ID: Anonymous
Projection: PA
Penetration: Underpenetrated – vertebral bodies not visible behind heart
Inspiration: Adequate – seven anterior ribs visible
Rotation: The patient is slightly rotated to the left

● AIRWAY

The trachea is central after factoring in patient rotation.

● BREATHING

The lungs are clear, apart from prominent end-on vessels seen in the right lower zone.

The lungs are not hyperinflated.

There is minor blunting of the costophrenic angles, which may represent small effusions or pleural thickening.

● CIRCULATION AND MEDIASTINUM

The cardiothoracic ratio is 0.56 in keeping with cardiomegaly. There is a curvilinear calcification projected peripherally over the left side of the cardiac silhouette.

The aorta appears normal.

The heart borders are clear.

The mediastinum is central, not widened, with clear borders.

The left hilum is difficult to see due to the enlarged cardiac silhouette. The right hilum is bulky, which is likely due to vascular prominence.

● DIAPHRAGM AND DELICATES

There is mild blunting of the costophrenic angles bilaterally, which may represent pleural thickening or small effusions. Otherwise normal appearance and position of the hemidiaphragms.

No pneumoperitoneum.

The imaged skeleton is intact with no fractures or destructive bony lesions visible.

The visible soft tissues are unremarkable.

● EXTRAS AND REVIEW AREAS

Triple-chamber pacemaker in situ, with the tips of the leads appropriately projected over the right atrium, right ventricle and left ventricle. Midline sternotomy sutures and coronary artery bypass graft clips.
Lung apices: Normal.
Hila: Bulky right hilum due to vessels. The left is obscured.
Behind heart: Calcified area projected over the left ventricle.
Costophrenic angles: Minor bilateral blunting.
Below the diaphragm: Normal.

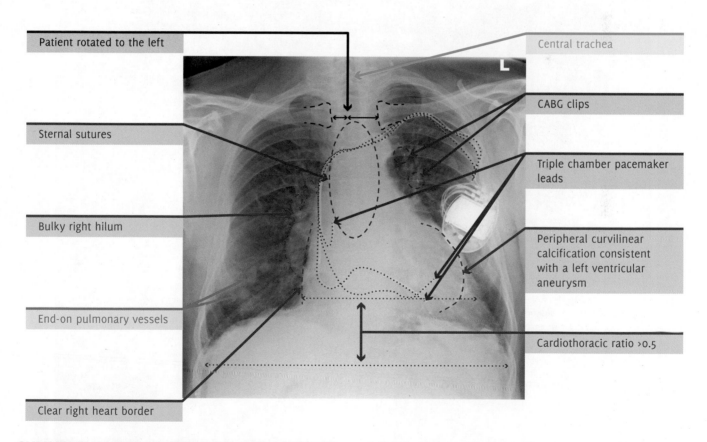

Patient rotated to the left

Central trachea

L

CABG clips

Sternal sutures

Triple chamber pacemaker leads

Bulky right hilum

Peripheral curvilinear calcification consistent with a left ventricular aneurysm

End-on pulmonary vessels

Cardiothoracic ratio >0.5

Clear right heart border

SUMMARY, INVESTIGATIONS AND MANAGEMENT

This X-ray demonstrates cardiomegaly with probable shallow pleural effusions in keeping with a degree of heart failure. The triple-chamber pacemaker is consistent with a history of congestive heart failure. There is no pulmonary oedema visible.

The calcified area projected over the left ventricle is consistent with a calcified left ventricular aneurysm secondary to previous myocardial infarcts.

Initial blood tests may include FBC, U&Es and CRP.

An ECG should be performed. An ECHO would allow assessment of the cardiac function and pacemaker testing may be appropriate. Previous X-rays should be reviewed to assess whether the costophrenic angle blunting is new (i.e. effusion) or longstanding (i.e. likely pleural thickening). Heart failure medication should be reviewed and optimized where possible.

An 85-year-old female presents to ED with increasing confusion, pyrexia and a productive cough. There is no significant past medical history. She is a nonsmoker. On examination, she has oxygen saturations of 93% in air and is febrile with a temperature of 38°C. There is dullness to percussion, reduced air entry and crackles in the right upper zone. A chest X-ray is requested to assess for possible pneumonia.

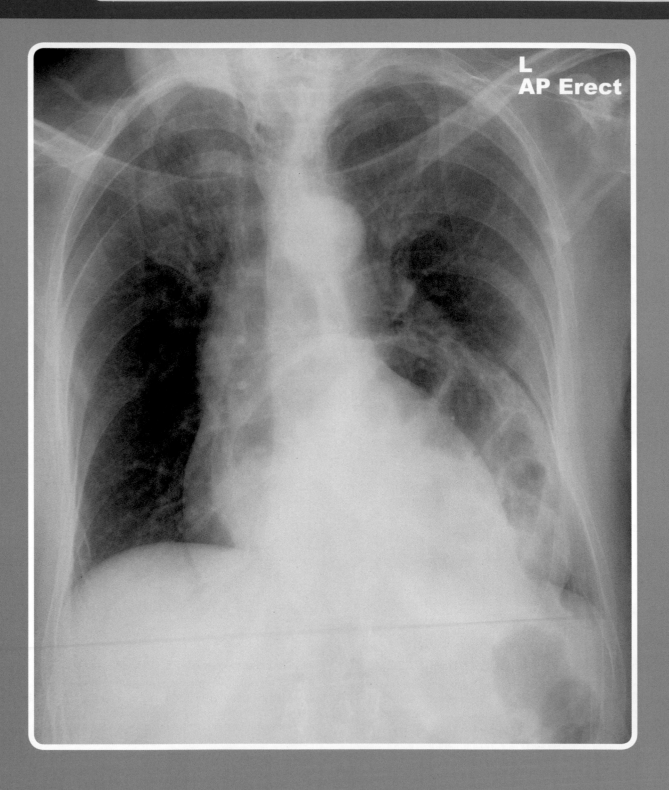

TECHNICAL INFORMATION

Patient ID: Anonymous
Projection: AP erect
Penetration: Adequate – vertebral bodies just visible behind heart
Inspiration: Inadequate – five anterior ribs visible
Rotation: The patient is rotated to the right

● AIRWAY

The trachea is projected to the right of the midline, which may be related to patient rotation and/or right upper lobe volume loss.

● BREATHING

There is increased airspace opacification in the right upper lobe. It has a sharp concave inferior margin, which is in keeping with an elevated horizontal fissure. There is a large mass projected over the left lower zone, retrocardiac area and lower mediastinum. The lungs are otherwise clear.

The lungs are not hyperinflated.

The pleural spaces are clear.

Normal pulmonary vascularity.

● CIRCULATION AND MEDIASTINUM

The heart does not appear enlarged, although its size cannot be accurately assessed on an AP X-ray.

The heart borders are clear.

The aorta appears normal.

There is a large mass projected over the heart/lower mediastinum. It contains gas and haustral folds within it, and is splaying the carina.

The mediastinum is displaced to the right, which is likely related to patient rotation and possibly volume loss in the right hemithorax. It has clear borders.

Normal size and shape of both hila. The left hilum appears elevated relative to the right. No hilar mass.

● DIAPHRAGM AND DELICATES

The medial aspect of the left hemidiaphragm is obscured. Normal appearance and position of the right hemidiaphragm.

No pneumoperitoneum.

The imaged skeleton is intact with no fractures or destructive bony lesions visible.

The visible soft tissues are unremarkable.

● EXTRAS AND REVIEW AREAS

No vascular lines, tubes or surgical clips.
Lung apices: Airspace opacification in the right apex.
Hila: Elevated left hilum.
Behind heart: Retrocardiac mass with areas of gas lucency. Splayed carina.
Costophrenic angles: Normal.
Below the diaphragm: Normal.

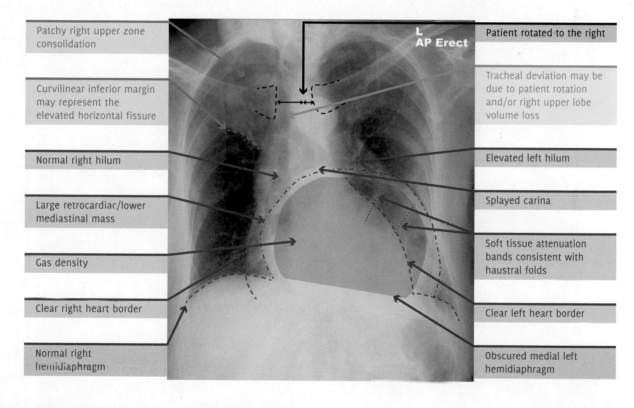

Patchy right upper zone consolidation

Curvilinear inferior margin may represent the elevated horizontal fissure

Normal right hilum

Large retrocardiac/lower mediastinal mass

Gas density

Clear right heart border

Normal right hemidiaphragm

L
AP Erect

Patient rotated to the right

Tracheal deviation may be due to patient rotation and/or right upper lobe volume loss

Elevated left hilum

Splayed carina

Soft tissue attenuation bands consistent with haustral folds

Clear left heart border

Obscured medial left hemidiaphragm

SUMMARY, INVESTIGATIONS AND MANAGEMENT

This X-ray demonstrates consolidation in the right upper lobe, in keeping with pneumonia. Additionally, there is the suggestion of right-sided volume loss, which may indicate partial collapse, although the patient rotation makes this difficult to confirm. The large mass projected over the lower mediastinum and left lower zone contains haustral folds and is consistent with a large hiatus hernia containing colon. The hernia is displacing the carina and left hilum.

Initial blood tests may include FBC, U&Es, blood cultures and CRP. A sputum culture may also be taken. The patient should be treated with appropriate antibiotics for community-acquired pneumonia and a follow-up chest X-ray performed to ensure resolution. The antibiotics may be oral or intravenous depending on the severity of pneumonia (CURB-65).

Review by surgeons may be useful to assess future management of large bowel containing hiatus hernia, although this is likely an incidental finding.

An 85-year-old male presents to his GP with shortness of breath, haemoptysis and weight loss. He has a 50 pack-year smoking history. He is a retired shipyard worker. On examination, he has oxygen saturations of 95% in air and is afebrile. There is reduced air entry throughout the left lung. Finger clubbing is also noted. A chest X-ray is requested to assess for possible malignancy, pleural effusion, collapse or pneumonia.

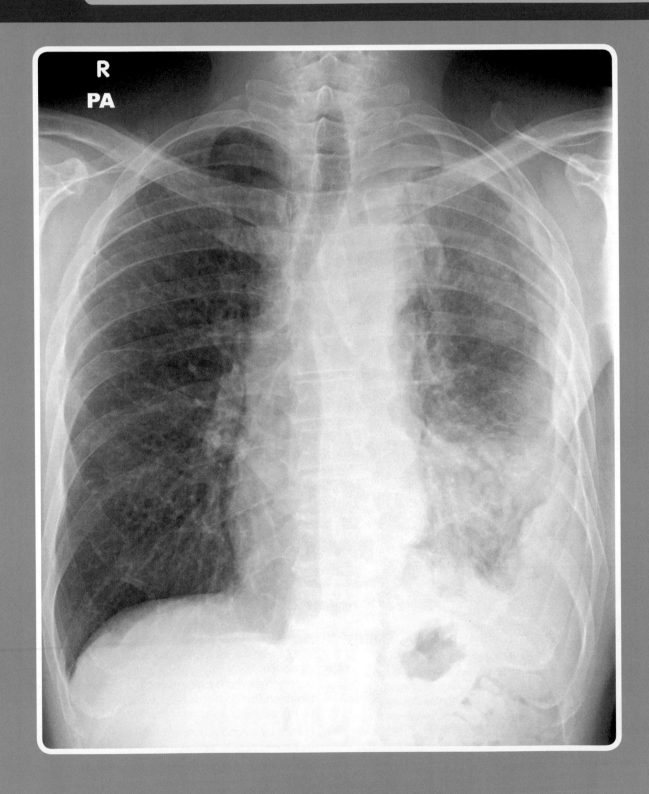

TECHNICAL INFORMATION

Patient ID: Anonymous
Projection: PA
Penetration: Adequate – vertebral bodies just visible behind heart
Inspiration: Adequate – more than seven anterior ribs are visible
Rotation: Not rotated

● AIRWAY

The trachea is displaced to the left of the midline.

● BREATHING

The left hemithorax is diffusely abnormal. There is lobulated opacification within the pleural space, which is concerning for a solid mass. It extends to involve the mediastinal surface. The opacification visible in the left lower zone may represent consolidation or the pleural abnormality seen straight on (en face).

There is coarsening of the lung markings in the right lung in keeping with COPD. The right lung is otherwise clear.

The lungs are not hyperinflated.

Normal pulmonary vascularity.

● CIRCULATION AND MEDIASTINUM

The heart is not enlarged.

The right heart border is clear, and the left is obscured.

The aortic knuckle is obscured.

The mediastinum is central and not widened.

The left hilum is obscured by the pleural abnormality. Normal size, shape and position of the right hilum.

● DIAPHRAGM AND DELICATES

The left hemidiaphragm is obscured by the pleural abnormality. Normal appearance and position of the right hemidiaphragm.

No pneumoperitoneum.

The imaged skeleton is intact with no fractures or destructive bony lesions visible.

The soft tissues are unremarkable.

● EXTRAS AND REVIEW AREAS

No vascular lines, tubes or surgical clips.
Lung apices: Left apical opacification.
Hila: Obscured left hilum, normal right hilum.
Behind heart: Lobulated pleural abnormality in the left retrocardiac location.
Costophrenic angles: Obliterated left costophrenic angle. Normal right costophrenic angle.
Below the diaphragm: Normal.

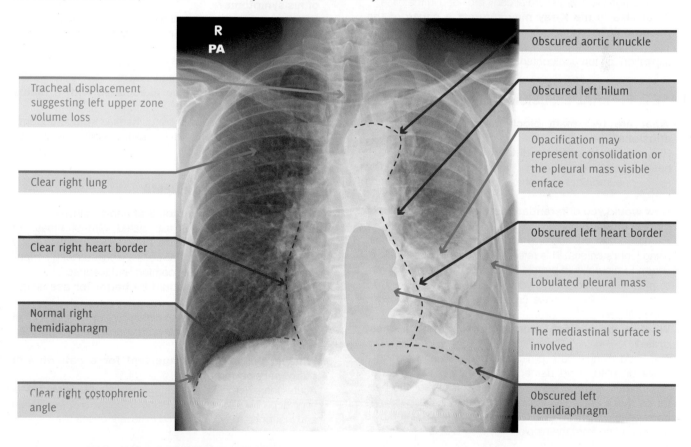

Tracheal displacement suggesting left upper zone volume loss

Clear right lung

Clear right heart border

Normal right hemidiaphragm

Clear right costophrenic angle

Obscured aortic knuckle

Obscured left hilum

Opacification may represent consolidation or the pleural mass visible enface

Obscured left heart border

Lobulated pleural mass

The mediastinal surface is involved

Obscured left hemidiaphragm

SUMMARY, INVESTIGATIONS AND MANAGEMENT

This X-ray demonstrates a diffuse abnormality affecting the left hemithorax which appears to originate in the pleura. The abnormality has lobulated contours. There is volume loss in the left hemithorax as the trachea is displaced to the left. Given the clinical findings, this may represent a malignant process, most likely malignant mesothelioma.

Initial blood tests may include FBC, U&Es, CRP, LFTs and bone profile.

A staging CT chest and abdomen with IV contrast should be performed.

The patient should be referred to respiratory/oncology services for further management, which may include biopsy and MDT discussion. Treatment, which may include surgery, radiotherapy, chemotherapy or palliative treatment, will depend on the outcome of the MDT discussion, investigations and the patient's wishes.

Case Questions and Answers

CASE 1: RIGHT UPPER LOBE CONSOLIDATION

1. **What are common causative organisms of community-acquired pneumonia?**

   In otherwise well patients, the commonest bacterial causes of community-acquired pneumonia are *Streptococcus pneumoniae*, *Chlamydophila pneumoniae* and *Haemophilus influenzae*.

2. **What else would be needed from the clinical review to complete a CURB-65 score?**

   Blood urea nitrogen (>7 mmol/L), respiratory rate (>30 breaths/min) and blood pressure (<90 mm Hg systolic/<60 mm Hg diastolic) need to be evaluated. Confusion status and age (>65 years) are already provided in the case.

3. **What else in the X-ray may suggest a cause of the pneumonia?**

   The hiatus hernia, present on the X-ray, may have led to aspiration of stomach contents.

CASE 2: PLEURAL EFFUSION

1. **What are two main biochemical types of pleural effusions?**

   Pleural effusions can be divided into transudative (e.g. heart failure, kidney failure, liver failure) and exudative (e.g. pneumonia, pulmonary embolism, malignancy) effusions.

2. **How would you differentiate between the two types of pleural effusions?**

   Exudative and transudative effusions can be differentiated using Light's criteria. This refers to a measure of the ratio of serum to pleural fluid protein (>0.5 is exudative) and serum to pleural fluid lactate dehydrogenase (LDH) (>0.6 is exudative). If neither of these criteria are met, the effusion is transudative.

3. **What is the clinical landmark for inserting a chest drain?**

   The 'safe triangle' is a clinical landmark when inserting a chest drain to avoid damage to the chest wall muscles and breast. It is formed by the lateral border of the pectoralis major anteriorly, the lateral border of the latissimus dorsi posteriorly and the fifth intercostal space marked by a horizontal line from the nipple.

CASE 3: LUNG AND HILAR MASSES

1. **What type of tumour is most likely in this individual?**

   This is most likely to be an adenocarcinoma. These tumours are the most common type of lung cancers and are more common in women and less commonly associated with smoking and older age.

2. **What are the common sites of distant metastasis for lung cancer?**

   Lung cancer typically metastasizes to the brain, bone and liver.

3. **What structures pass through the lung hila?**

   The pulmonary arteries, pulmonary veins, the main bronchi, bronchial arteries, bronchial veins, lymphatics and lymph nodes, and the pulmonary nerve plexuses pass through the lung hila.

CASE 4: HIATUS HERNIA

1. **What could be the significance of the patient's gastro-oesophageal reflux disease (GORD) in terms of his symptoms?**

   GORD can be a differential diagnosis for a cough.

2. **What are the risk factors for developing a hiatus hernia?**

   Risk factors for developing a hiatus hernia include age over 50 years old, obesity and pregnancy.

3. **What symptoms could be associated with a hiatus hernia?**

   Symptoms associated with hiatus hernias include abdominal pain, reflux, heartburn, dysphagia, bleeding, weight loss and anaemia.

CASE 5: PULMONARY OEDEMA

1. **What are the other symptoms of heart failure?**

   Left-sided heart failure is associated with shortness of breath, cough, cardiac wheeze, orthopnoea and pink frothy sputum. Right-sided heart failure is associated with peripheral oedema, abdominal discomfort and tiredness.

2. **What X-ray projection would be better for assessing the size of the heart?**

   A PA chest X-ray would more accurately assess the size of the heart as enlargement cannot be adequately assessed when the view is AP.

3. **What is the acute management for a patient with pulmonary oedema?**

   Acute management involves oxygen supplementation (if hypoxic), diuretics and morphine. Noninvasive ventilation and inotropes may be required in severe cases.

CASE 6: RIGHT LOWER LOBE COLLAPSE

1. **What signs might be indicative of lung collapse on a chest X-ray?**

   Signs of lung collapse include a raised hemidiaphragm ipsilaterally, tracheal and mediastinal shift towards the collapsed side, displacement of the hila and narrowing of the space between the ribs compared to the opposite side.

2. **How are pack-years calculated?**

Pack-years are calculated by multiplying the number of years the person has been a smoker with the number of packs smoked per day (one pack is equivalent to 20 cigarettes).

3. **What would be the appearances of a left upper lobe collapse on a chest X-ray?**

Left upper lobe collapse may appear as the veil sign on imaging – the whole lung field would look like it is covered by a veil.

CASE 7: RIGHT UPPER LOBE COLLAPSE

1. **How is a PET-CT used in the assessment of cancer?**

The patient is given radiotracers which accumulate in areas that are more metabolically active, such as cancer cells. Therefore, these areas show up as bright white on the scan.

2. **What would be the indication for a PET-CT in this patient?**

The subtle pulmonary nodule/mass could be further evaluated with PET-CT imaging. The size and morphology of the nodule as well as patient demographic risk factors can be used to determine the risk of malignancy.

3. **What are the two main histological classifications of lung cancer?**

The two main classifications of lung cancer are non–small cell carcinoma – including squamous cell carcinoma, adenocarcinoma and large cell carcinoma – and small cell carcinoma.

CASE 8: LEFT LOWER ZONE CONSOLIDATION

1. **What are the risk factors for developing community-acquired pneumonia?**

Risk factors for community-acquired pneumonias include older age, being immunocompromised, smoking, excess alcohol consumption, living in overcrowded conditions, having regular contact with children, poor dental hygiene and medical comorbidities (e.g. asthma, bronchiectasis, COPD, cystic fibrosis and diabetes mellitus).

2. **How does consolidation differ from pleural effusion in terms of pathology and signs on percussion?**

Consolidation occurs in the alveolar air spaces, whereas pleural effusion occurs between the layers of pleura external to the lungs. Both will be dull to percussion, although an effusion will present with classic stony dullness.

3. **What are the potential complications of pneumonia?**

Complications of pneumonia include sepsis, pleural effusion, acute respiratory distress syndrome, lung abscesses and heart failure.

CASE 9: LEFT UPPER LOBE COLLAPSE

1. **What oxygen saturation level should be aimed for clinically?**

In general, oxygen saturations should be targeted at over 94%. A target level of 88% to 92% is usually used in patients that retain carbon dioxide, such as in COPD patients.

2. **What would constitute a life-threatening asthma exacerbation?**

Markers of a life-threatening exacerbation include peak expiratory flow rate (PEFR) <33% of predicted, oxygen saturations <92%, fatigue, haemodynamic instability, silent chest and confusion.

3. **What are other potential causes of mucus plugging?**

Other than asthma, pneumonia and chronic bronchitis can also cause mucus plugging. Other causes include aspergillosis and hyper-IgE syndromes.

CASE 10: RETROCARDIAC MASS

1. **What are the risk factors for developing lung cancer?**

Risk factors for lung cancer include smoking, occupational exposure to carcinogens (e.g. asbestos), older age and medical comorbidities such as COPD or lung fibrosis.

2. **Which cancers most commonly metastasize to the lungs?**

Breast cancers, colon cancers, prostate cancers, bladder cancers, neuroblastomas and sarcomas commonly metastasize to the lungs.

3. **If this was found to be a metastasis from the patient's testicular cancer, how would it be staged?**

This would be staged using TNM staging with the primary (testicular) tumour rather than the secondary (lung metastasis) tumour. Staging would occur using the appropriate T- and N-values following more detailed imaging. M1 would be assigned due to the metastasis.

CASE 11: LEFT LOWER LOBE CONSOLIDATION

1. **What clinical signs might be noted on examination for a pneumonia?**

Bedside observations may note fever, tachycardia and tachypnoea. On examination of the chest, there may be reduced chest expansion, dullness to percussion, crackles, increased vocal fremitus and bronchial breath sounds.

2. **How important are blood tests in confirming a diagnosis of pneumonia?**

Most chest infections can be diagnosed on clinical history and examination alone, with a chest X-ray to aid diagnosis if there are any doubts. Blood tests are neither essential nor specific for diagnosis but can help if the clinical picture is unclear, if complications are suspected, or to assess response to antibiotics in an initially extremely unwell patient.

3. **What additional bedside imaging modality can be used to assess the pleural effusion?**

Ultrasound is a useful, cost-effective tool to diagnose pleural effusions, measure the volume of the effusion and locate insertion sites for drainage or aspiration.

CASE 12: LINGULA CONSOLIDATION

1. **What is the major anatomical difference between the right and left lungs?**

The left lung has two lobes (upper, lower) while the right lung has three lobes (upper, middle, lower). The upper lobe of the left lung includes the lingula.

2. **What is the lingula?**

The lingula is a tongue-shaped projection found in the left lung and is homologous to the middle lobe of the right lung.

3. **What is the common route of entry of microorganisms causing pneumonia?**

The most common route of infection is through droplet micro-aspiration of airborne pathogens or oropharyngeal secretions.

CASE 13: SWALLOWED FOREIGN BODY

1. **What are common complications of swallowing a foreign body?**

   Complications include dysphagia, vomiting, airway compromise, pleural effusion, oesophageal perforation, intestinal obstruction and peritonitis.

2. **Which metal present in coins can cause sensitivity reactions in some patients?**

   Nickel can lead to systemic signs and symptoms, such as rash or pruritus, if patients have nickel sensitivity.

3. **What further imaging could be used if the foreign body was radiolucent?**

   If ingestion was suspected but there was no evidence of a foreign body on the X-ray, further imaging with ultrasound, CT or MRI can be considered, as these are much more sensitive at detecting radiolucent foreign bodies.

CASE 14: PNEUMOPERITONEUM

1. **What are common causes of pneumoperitoneum in adults?**

   Causes of pneumoperitoneum include perforated peptic ulcer, abdominal trauma, bowel perforation, postoperative free gas and peritoneal dialysis.

2. **How is an erect chest X-ray taken?**

   A patient is asked to sit up for at least 10 minutes, allowing gas (if present) to redistribute into the subdiaphragmatic space. The X-ray is then performed in this position.

3. **Which group of patients are erect chest X-rays difficult to perform on?**

   Paradoxically, very sick patients who may need them most are unable to sit up long enough for air to redistribute. A CT abdomen may be more appropriate in such cases, particularly if the cause of deterioration is unclear.

CASE 15: BILATERAL CONSOLIDATION

1. **Is bilateral pneumonia an indication for intravenous antibiotics?**

   Bilateral pneumonia itself can be treated with oral antibiotics (if tolerated). Intravenous antibiotics may be considered depending on the patient's clinical state and CURB-65 score.

2. **What advice should the mother be given regarding breastfeeding while unwell and on antibiotics?**

   There is little evidence that supports the transmission of many of the causative bacterial agents for pneumonia through breastmilk. Breastfeeding has been shown to be protective against acute respiratory infection. Most antibiotics are safe to give to breastfeeding mothers.

3. **If the left heart border and left hemidiaphragm were obscured, which lobes would be affected by consolidation?**

   Consolidation of the lingula (part of the left upper lobe) can obscure the left heart border. Consolidation of the left lower lobe can lead to obscuration of the left hemidiaphragm

CASE 16: SPONTANEOUS PNEUMOTHORAX

1. **Can a spontaneous pneumothorax develop into a tension pneumothorax?**

   Any type of pneumothorax can lead to tension pneumothorax; hence it is crucial to diagnose pneumothoraces even if they are very small.

2. **What are the radiological features of tension pneumothorax on a chest X-ray?**

   In a tension pneumothorax, there will be general pneumothorax features including darkening of the hemithorax and loss of lung markings due to air in the pleural space. Specific features of tension pneumothorax include mediastinal and tracheal shift away from the pneumothorax with flattening of the hemidiaphragm on the side of the pneumothorax.

3. **What type of cannula should be used for aspiration of a tension pneumothorax?**

   A large-bore cannula should be inserted into the side of the pneumothorax. A 14G-16G cannula is typically used for aspiration.

CASE 17: RIGHT LOWER ZONE CONSOLIDATION

1. **What is the definition of a hospital-acquired pneumonia?**

   A hospital-acquired pneumonia is defined as a pneumonia contracted more than 48 hours after hospital admission that was not incubating at the time of admission.

2. **What are the common causative organisms of hospital-acquired pneumonia?**

   The most common pathogens of hospital-acquired pneumonia are gram-negative bacilli (such as *Pseudomonas Aeruginosa*) and *Staphylococcus aureus*. Antibiotic-resistant organisms remain an important concern.

3. **What measures are taken to reduce the risk of hospital-acquired pneumonia?**

   Important preventative measures include hand hygiene, oral care and bed elevation. It is also important to recognize dysphagia (such as in stroke patients) and reduce the risk of aspiration. Overzealous antibiotic use should be discouraged.

CASE 18: LINES: PERIPHERALLY INSERTED CENTRAL CATHETER (MALPOSITIONED)

1. **What are the common indications for PICC line insertion?**

   PICC lines are commonly used in patients when regular intravenous therapy is needed. These include chemotherapy, parenteral nutrition and long-term antibiotics.

2. **What locations are PICC lines commonly mispositioned?**

   PICC lines can be mispositioned in the internal jugular vein, brachiocephalic vein, subclavian vein as well as within the heart and other vessels within the chest. The risk of malposition of PICC lines is reduced with the use of image guidance.

3. **Where is the tip anatomically located in a correctly positioned PICC line?**

   The tip of the PICC line should ideally be placed in the superior vena cava.

CASE 19: RIGHT MIDDLE AND LOWER LOBE CONSOLIDATION

1. **How much fluid is normally present within the pleural space?**

   Normally, the pleural space contains less than 20 mL of pleural fluid.

2. **How much fluid is needed to detect a pleural effusion on a PA chest X-ray?**

Approximately 200 mL of pleural fluid is needed to start detecting a pleural effusion on a PA chest X-ray.

3. **What is the definition of a simple parapneumonic effusion?**

Simple parapneumonic effusions are sterile exudate pleural effusions in patients with pneumonia.

CASE 20: PNEUMOPERITONEUM

1. **Why is an erect chest X-ray the most sensitive X-ray position for detecting pneumoperitoneum?**

The erect chest X-ray position is most ideal for detecting free air within the peritoneal cavity because air rises to lie beneath the diaphragm. An erect chest X-ray can detect as little as 1 mL of free intraperitoneal air.

2. **What is the commonest cause of pneumoperitoneum?**

The commonest cause of pneumoperitoneum is perforation of a hollow viscus (e.g. perforated peptic ulcer, perforated bowel, perforated diverticula).

3. **How can you differentiate the gas of a pneumoperitoneum from the gas in the normal stomach bubble on a chest X-ray?**

In a pneumoperitoneum, the white line above the gas will be very thin as it consists of the diaphragm only; the white line of the stomach is much thicker. The gas in a stomach bubble is normally well contained within the stomach; hence a greater volume of gas on a chest X-ray is more suggestive of pneumoperitoneum. The presence of gas bilaterally below the diaphragm is also suggestive of a pneumoperitoneum.

CASE 21: PLEURAL EFFUSION

1. **What is granulomatosis with polyangiitis?**

Granulomatosis with polyangiitis is a condition characterized by granulomatous inflammation of small- and medium-sized blood vessels. It commonly affects the respiratory tract and kidneys. Most patients with active disease have antineutrophil cytoplasmic antibodies (ANCA).

2. **What are the clinical manifestations of granulomatosis with polyangiitis?**

The symptoms of granulomatosis with polyangiitis vary depending on the organs and systems affected. A wide range of symptoms may be present from both upper and lower airway involvement, including cough, wheeze and haemoptysis. ENT involvement is extremely common with symptoms such as nasal crusting, hearing loss and sinusitis. Glomerulonephritis is also common and can lead to renal failure.

3. **How is pleurodesis performed to treat recurrent pneumothoraces?**

Pleurodesis can be performed surgically or chemically. Surgical pleurodesis involves the use of video-assisted thoracic surgery (VATS). Chemical pleurodesis involves the use of irritants such as talc and tetracyclines.

CASE 22: LUNG METASTASES

1. **What are the different routes that metastases can spread to the lung?**

Metastases can spread to the lungs through the blood from tumours that have a strong vascular supply, such as breast cancers, kidney cancers and melanomas. Metastases can also spread through lymphatics or through direct invasion of lung tissue.

2. **Which malignancies are associated with causing a 'cannonball' metastasis?**

Breast cancer, renal cell carcinoma, choriocarcinoma and endometrial carcinoma are all strongly associated with causing 'cannonball' metastases.

3. **Other than 'cannonball metastases', how else can pulmonary metastases present on a chest X-ray?**

Pulmonary metastases can also manifest with an ill-defined 'snowstorm' appearance or present as solitary or multiple pulmonary nodules. Cancer cells can invade lymphatics in the lungs and cause a reticular nodular pattern on a chest X-ray; this is known as lymphangitis carcinomatosis. Other potential features include cavitating lesions, pleural effusions and mediastinal lymphadenopathy.

CASE 23: RIGHT UPPER LOBE CONSOLIDATION

1. **What is the major limitation of sputum tests?**

The major difficulty of sputum tests is generating an adequate nonsalivary sample from the patient. The first sputum produced in the morning is preferred as it is usually of the highest quality at this time.

2. **What can be used to induce sputum production in patients who are otherwise unable to provide a sample?**

Nebulized hypertonic saline is sometimes used to induce sputum production in patients who cannot produce a sufficient amount.

3. **What is a potential problem from patients wearing jewellery, such as nipple rings, during a chest X-ray?**

It is common to see jewellery on chest X-rays. A problem with wearing jewellery is that they can create artefacts that can obscure important structures and pathology. Therefore, patients are usually requested to remove all jewellery prior to imaging.

CASE 24: PLEURAL EFFUSION

1. **Why is ultrasound used for pleural procedures, such as chest drain insertion?**

Ultrasound is recommended for all pleural procedures as it can be used to better identify appropriate locations to perform these procedures safely and effectively. Ultrasound can also ensure there are no adjacent structures at risk of damage from the procedure, such as the heart, spleen and liver.

2. **What is the role of PET-CT scans in the assessment of lymphomas?**

PET-CT scans are useful to assess disease spread and hence are used in staging lymphoma. Metabolically active cells, such as malignant cells, can be accurately detected by PET scans. This is also useful to determine if lesions picked up on CT scans are metabolically active or purely benign.

3. **What are the management options for Hodgkin's lymphoma?**

Chemotherapy and radiotherapy are the mainstay of management in patients with Hodgkin's lymphoma. Commonly used chemotherapy agents include doxorubicin, bleomycin, vinblastine and dacarbazine. Steroids can also be used alongside chemotherapy.

CASE 25: LUNG MASS

1. What are the different procedures available to perform a lung tissue biopsy?

Biopsies are commonly performed during bronchoscopy as they allow access to the lower airways. A biopsy can also be performed under radiological guidance using ultrasound or CT imaging. Surgical biopsy using video-assisted thoracoscopic surgery (VATS) can be performed for tumours not accessible by other biopsy procedures.

2. Why is a bone profile blood test performed in suspected lung cancer?

A bone profile is performed to find evidence of bone involvement; increased alkaline phosphatase suggests higher bone turnover, and calcium levels are raised in multiple myeloma and secondary bone cancers.

3. Why is spirometry performed in suspected lung cancer?

Respiratory comorbidities, such as COPD, are frequent in lung cancer patients and may prevent curative treatment. In addition, if surgical resection is being considered, the patient should have adequate lung function demonstrated on spirometry to indicate they can tolerate the loss of lung tissue.

CASE 26: PLEURAL EFFUSION

1. What are the characteristic features of a malignant pleural effusion on pleural fluid analysis?

Malignant pleural effusions are usually exudative effusions with abnormal cytology. Malignant pleural effusions are the most common cause of bloody effusions and half of all malignant pleural effusions appear bloody.

2. Can a pleural effusion cause tracheal deviation?

A pleural effusion, if massive, can cause tracheal deviation away from the affected side.

3. How can you differentiate between a lung collapse and a pleural effusion on a chest X-ray?

The radiological appearance of the trachea is useful to differentiate lung collapse from a pleural effusion. In collapse, the trachea is deviated towards the affected side due to a loss of volume. In a pleural effusion, the trachea is usually central (or if massive, can be pushed towards the opposite side).

CASE 27: NASOGASTRIC TUBE (MALPOSITIONED)

1. What are the indications for NG tube insertion?

An NG tube is most commonly inserted for feeding purposes in malnourished patients who cannot feed orally but have an accessible, functional gastrointestinal tract. For example, it can be used in patients with decreased consciousness or patients who have neurological conditions that cause an unsafe swallow such as in stroke. Other indications for NG tube insertion include assessment of an upper gastrointestinal bleed, aspiration of gastric contents, administration of radiographic contrast, gastric or bowel decompression, and medication delivery.

2. What are the radiological features of a correctly placed NG tube on a chest X-ray?

The NG tube should clearly follow the path of the oesophagus and avoid the contours of the bronchi. It should also bifurcate the carina and cross the diaphragm in the midline. The tip of the NG tube should be seen well below the left hemidiaphragm.

3. Which bronchus is an NG tube more likely to pass through if incorrectly placed in the trachea?

The NG tube is more likely to pass through the right main bronchus and subsequently into the middle and lower lobes of the right lung. This is because the right main bronchus is wider and more vertically orientated compared to the left main bronchus. This also applies to foreign bodies, aspirated materials and endotracheal tubes.

CASE 28: IATROGENIC PNEUMOTHORAX

1. What is the definition of a tension pneumothorax?

A tension pneumothorax is where air enters the pleural space during inspiration but is unable to leave, leading to progressively increasing positive pressure within the chest. It is a medical emergency as the increased pressure can compromise cardiorespiratory function.

2. How is a tension pneumothorax diagnosed?

A tension pneumothorax is a clinical diagnosis and should be treated immediately. Patients with a tension pneumothorax will show signs of respiratory distress and haemodynamic instability (e.g. hypotension, tachycardia).

3. How should a tension pneumothorax be managed?

Once a tension pneumothorax is diagnosed, high-flow oxygen should be administered and patients should undergo needle decompression of the pneumothorax using a large-bore cannula. After immediate decompression of the pneumothorax, a portable chest X-ray is done and a chest drain is inserted to drain the residual pneumothorax.

CASE 29: SPONTANEOUS PNEUMOTHORAX

1. How would you clinically classify this patient's pneumothorax?

This patient has a primary spontaneous pneumothorax. A primary spontaneous pneumothorax develops in the absence of trauma and lung disease and therefore has no apparent cause.

2. How should a large symptomatic primary spontaneous pneumothorax be drained?

Symptomatic patients, or patients who have larger primary spontaneous pneumothoraces (>2 cm), require treatment. First, pleural air is aspirated using a needle and catheter. If aspiration fails to improve the condition, an intercostal chest drain is inserted.

3. How does an intercostal chest drain work to treat a pneumothorax?

The intercostal chest drain is connected to an underwater seal drain that acts as a one-way valve. It allows air to leave the chest but not re-enter. Bubbling of the drain indicates that air is moving out of the pneumothorax into the drain.

CASE 30: IATROGENIC PNEUMOTHORAX

1. What are some common iatrogenic causes of a pneumothorax?

Procedures such as central line insertion, pacemaker insertion and transbronchial biopsy can all cause a pneumothorax. Chest X-rays are routinely performed after these procedures to rule out a pneumothorax.

2. **When is CT thorax imaging performed in pneumothorax patients?**

CT is commonly performed if a pneumothorax cannot be adequately assessed on chest X-ray. CT is considered the gold standard for detecting and accurately estimating the size of a pneumothorax. It can also be used to investigate underlying lung disease in the context of secondary spontaneous pneumothorax. If patients have suffered severe trauma, they may not be able to sit upright for a chest X-ray, so a CT can be performed to ensure a pneumothorax is not missed.

3. **What advice is given on discharge to patients who have had a pneumothorax?**

A follow-up chest X-ray is usually arranged. Patients should be counselled and encouraged to quit smoking. They should also refrain from flying for 1 to 2 weeks and to completely abstain from deep sea diving for life.

CASE 31: LUNG AND HILAR MASSES

1. **What can be used if there is difficulty differentiating pulmonary nodules from the patient's nipples?**

Nipple shadows often mimic nodules as rounded opacities on a chest X-ray. However, they are usually bilateral and appear symmetrical. If there remains uncertainty, taped nipple markers can be used with a repeat X-ray; if the opacities are seen within the nipple markers, then they were likely just nipples.

2. **What are some potential blind spots on a chest X-ray when trying to look for pulmonary nodules?**

Notable blind spots where nodules can be overlooked on a chest X-ray include the lung apices, hilar regions, retrocardiac region and the lung bases.

3. **What are the available treatment options for lung cancer?**

Surgical resection (usually lobectomy or pneumonectomy), chemotherapy and radiotherapy may be used depending on the extent of disease and type of lung cancer. Smoking cessation is also an important aspect of treatment.

CASE 32: RIGHT UPPER LOBE COLLAPSE

1. **What causes lobar collapse?**

Lobar collapse is usually a result of endobronchial obstruction. This obstruction may be due to an intrinsic or extrinsic cause. In adults, the most common causes of intrinsic obstruction are tumours and mucus plugs. Extrinsic compression may be caused by mediastinal masses. In children, inhaled foreign bodies is a common cause of lobar collapse.

2. **What is the significance of a displaced horizontal fissure?**

The horizontal fissure is a useful landmark to determine the type of lobar collapse in the right lung. If it is displaced upwards, it suggests a right upper lobe collapse. Likewise, a downwards displaced horizontal fissure suggests a right lower lobe collapse.

3. **What is the 'Golden S sign' in right upper lobe collapse?**

The Golden S sign refers to the curved 'S' configuration of the horizontal fissure in a right upper lobe collapse. It is highly predictive of a mass obstructing the right main bronchus.

CASE 33: LEFT LOWER LOBE COLLAPSE

1. **What does each hilum consist of?**

Each hilum consists of the pulmonary artery, bronchus, lymph nodes and pulmonary veins.

2. **What is the difference between atelectasis and lobar collapse?**

Lobar collapse and atelectasis are often used synonymously to describe loss of volume within the lung. However, atelectasis more specifically refers to small areas of collapsed alveoli that only affect a part of a lung segment. Lobar collapse is generally used to describe complete loss of volume within an entire lobe or lung.

3. **What is the sail sign of left lower lobe collapse?**

The left lower lobe collapses behind the heart. On a chest X-ray, this appears as a double shadow behind the left heart, creating an apparent double left heart border known as sail sign.

CASE 34: RETROCARDIAC CONSOLIDATION

1. **What is the definition of consolidation?**

Consolidation refers to the filling of alveoli with fluid, pus, cells or other material leading to the lung becoming opacified. Consolidation may be focal, multifocal or diffuse.

2. **What is the definition of air bronchograms?**

Air bronchograms are air-filled bronchi made visible by the consolidation of surrounding alveoli. They appear as dark lines within the opacified lung. Air bronchograms are a specific feature of airspace/alveolar disease.

3. **Why should pneumonia be followed up to resolution?**

If the follow-up chest X-ray at 6 weeks continues to show consolidation, then further investigation is required as a common cause of persistent consolidation is bronchial obstruction, e.g. due to malignancy. A CT scan or bronchoscopy may therefore be needed to exclude an underlying malignancy.

CASE 35: RIGHT MIDDLE LOBE CONSOLIDATION

1. **How can you tell if a chest X-ray is rotated?**

If the spinous process of the vertebrae is equidistant between both clavicle heads, then the image is not rotated. If the distance is less on the left, then the patient is rotated to the right (such as in this case), and vice versa.

2. **Does the presence of consolidation always mean a patient has pneumonia?**

Although consolidation is most commonly seen in pneumonia, consolidation can also occur in many other conditions, such as malignancy, bronchial obstruction and pulmonary oedema.

3. **How does underlying lung disease affect chest X-ray diagnosis of a pneumonia?**

New chest X-ray changes of consolidation may be obscured in patients with underlying chronic lung disease. Pneumonia can also still be suspected based on clinical features, especially in the context of increased inflammatory markers.

CASE 36: PERIPHERALLY INSERTED CENTRAL CATHETER (MALPOSITIONED)

1. **Which veins are commonly used for PICC line insertion?**
   Commonly used veins for PICC line insertion include the brachial, basilic and cephalic veins.
2. **What are some advantages of inserting PICC lines over other types of central lines?**
   PICC lines are safer and easier to insert than central lines and are generally more convenient to manage in the community. The risk of complications from central line insertion, such as pneumothorax and injury to blood vessels in the neck, is lower with PICC lines.
3. **What are some disadvantages of inserting PICC lines over other types of central lines?**
   PICCs are generally associated with a higher rate of catheter-related deep vein thrombosis compared with central lines. The catheter tip of PICC lines can also be difficult to manipulate and there is a higher risk of malposition.

CASE 37: LEFT UPPER LOBE COLLAPSE

1. **Why is the radiological appearance of collapse of the left upper lobe different to the right upper lobe?**
   The majority of the left upper lobe lies anterior to the left lower lobe; it collapses medially and anteriorly, creating the veil-like opacity over the left hemithorax. In contrast, the right upper lobe mostly lies superior to the right middle and lower lobes, so its collapse leads to opacification of the upper medial aspect of the right hemithorax.
2. **What is the 'Luftsichel' sign in a left upper lobe collapse?**
   The Luftsichel sign refers to an area of radiolucency in the left upper zone near the aortic arch that appears in left upper lobe collapse due to a compensatory hyperinflation of the left lower lobe.
3. **What does a complete left lung collapse look like on a chest X-ray?**
   Complete left lung collapse would appear on a chest X-ray as increased opacification of the entire left hemithorax with signs of loss of lung volume, such as tracheal deviation and mediastinal shift. The heart may lie in the left hemithorax. The chest X-ray would resemble that of a left pneumonectomy.

CASE 38: HICKMAN LINE (FRACTURED)

1. **What is a Hickman line?**
   A Hickman line is a type of skin-tunnelled central line. The skin tunnelling aims to reduce the risk of infection by increasing the distance between the skin entry and blood vessel puncture sites. It is usually inserted by an interventional radiologist under local anaesthetic.
2. **What are the common indications for central line insertion?**
   Central lines can be used when peripheral IV access is difficult and/or immediate venous access is required, such as in aggressive fluid resuscitation, drug infusions, transvenous pacing and central venous pressure monitoring. They are also used to administer drugs that are contraindicated peripherally, such as chemotherapy agents and certain vasopressors. Total parenteral nutrition can also be delivered via a central line.

3. **If a pleural effusion develops immediately after central line insertion, what has likely occurred?**
   If a pleural effusion has developed on the same side as central line insertion, then the central line has likely perforated the vein and entered the pleural space. It is also possible that a haemothorax has developed due to vessel injury from the inserted central line.

CASE 39: DEXTROCARDIA

1. **What must be checked on a chest X-ray of a patient with dextrocardia?**
   It is important to check if the orientation of the chest X-ray is correct and to check previous images. This is because the appearances of dextrocardia can often occur due to technical error by radiographers where they mistakenly flip the image. Other organs should also be reviewed, as the condition situs inversus would produce mirroring of other organs in addition to the heart.
2. **What is primary ciliary dyskinesia?**
   Primary ciliary dyskinesia is a genetic disorder that affects the motility of cilia. A common form of this condition is Kartagener syndrome, whereby patients have a triad of situs inversus, recurrent sinusitis and bronchiectasis.
3. **What are the practical aspects of investigating and treating patients with dextrocardia?**
   When the heart is on the right due to dextrocardia, the left lung has three lobes and the right lung has two; hence the location of respiratory pathology must be accurately interpreted. ECG leads, defibrillator pads and pacemakers must also be placed in reverse positions.

CASE 40: BREAST PROSTHESES

1. **Where can prostheses be placed in the breast?**
   Breast prostheses can be placed at the retropectoral position, behind the pectoral muscle. They can also be placed in the retroglandular position, behind the glandular tissue but in front of the pectoral muscle.
2. **In what ways is a chest X-ray useful in patients with suspected pulmonary embolism?**
   Chest X-rays are useful for excluding other differentials such as pneumonia and pneumothorax. A normal chest X-ray in a patient with severe dyspnoea may indicate a pulmonary embolism. There can be subtle radiological features of pulmonary embolism on chest X-ray, including oligaemia and pulmonary artery enlargement.
3. **Which imaging modality is routinely used to diagnose pulmonary embolism?**
   Computed tomography pulmonary angiography (CTPA) is the gold standard for diagnosing pulmonary embolism. It will demonstrate filling defects within the pulmonary arteries.

CASE 41: PNEUMONECTOMY

1. **What conditions are commonly treated by surgical lung resection?**
   Lung cancer is the most common condition treated by lung resection. Resection is also commonly performed for focal infections refractory to medical therapy and to control bleeding in massive haemoptysis.

2. Why does the left lung appear darker than normal?

The left lung has become hyperinflated, so the increased air within the lung leads to increased translucency.

3. What is postpneumonectomy syndrome?

Postpneumonectomy syndrome is a rare condition characterized by severe airway obstruction due to extreme rotation and mediastinal shift after pneumonectomy.

CASE 42: HYDROPNEUMOTHORAX

1. What is the definition of a hydropneumothorax?

A hydropneumothorax is a rare condition where there is fluid and air in the pleural space. There is usually a well-defined air-fluid level.

2. What are the causes of a hydropneumothorax?

Potential causes of hydropneumothorax include thoracentesis, thoracic trauma and bronchopleural fistulas. In this patient, the significant amount of air in the pleural space is concerning for a bronchopleural fistula, whereby air can freely move from the bronchial tree into the pleural space.

3. How should a hydropneumothorax be treated?

An intercostal chest drain can be inserted to drain both the air and fluid.

CASE 43: VAGUS NERVE STIMULATOR

1. When are vagus nerve stimulators used in epilepsy patients?

Vagus nerve stimulators are used as an adjunct to pharmacological therapy in patients who have intractable seizures and are not suitable for surgical procedures.

2. What does vagus nerve stimulation involve?

The vagus nerve stimulator is similar to a pacemaker and it will generate intermittent electrical stimulation of the left vagus nerve. Patients can also use a magnet over the generator to send an extra burst of impulses to help abort an impending seizure.

3. What are the potential side effects of vagus nerve stimulators?

Vagus nerve stimulation can cause adverse events due to irritation of the vagus nerve, such as hoarse voice, cough and throat pain.

CASE 44: EMPHYSEMA

1. What are the radiological features of hyperexpanded lungs on a chest X-ray?

Signs of hyperinflation include a flattened diaphragm, more than 6 anterior ribs or 10 posterior ribs visible above the diaphragm on the midclavicular line.

2. In what ways is a CT thorax useful for assessing patients with COPD?

A CT scan is used to assess for complications of COPD (e.g. bullae) and for lung cancer screening. CT is also better than chest X-ray in evaluating emphysema and can determine if emphysema is centrilobular (seen in smokers) or panlobular (seen in alpha-1-antitrypsin deficiency). CT can also visualize any pulmonary hypertension that may have developed due to COPD.

3. What are the typical spirometry findings in COPD?

Spirometry typically shows an obstructive pattern (reduced FEV_1 and FEV_1/FVC ratio) with air trapping in COPD.

CASE 45: AORTIC DISSECTION

1. What is an aortic dissection?

An aortic dissection is a tear in the intimal layer of the aorta that allows blood to enter the aortic wall. A false lumen is formed that can occlude branching vessels and can rupture.

2. What are potential complications of aortic dissection?

Dissections involving the ascending aorta are associated with a high mortality rate due to the risk of cardiac tamponade, acute aortic regurgitation and acute coronary syndrome. There can also be significant blood loss associated with aortic dissection.

3. Which imaging modality is most commonly performed to diagnose aortic dissection?

CT arteriography is the most common modality used for diagnosing aortic dissection. It has the ability to identify the location of aortic tears, occluded branches and assess for any evidence of pericardial effusion.

CASE 46: ELEVATED RIGHT HEMIDIAPHRAGM

1. Why does the right hemidiaphragm normally lie slightly above the left hemidiaphragm?

The liver is the largest internal organ in the body and pushes superiorly on the right hemidiaphragm.

2. What are the causes of a unilaterally elevated diaphragm?

Phrenic nerve palsy can lead to paralysis of the diaphragm, leading to permanent elevation of the ipsilateral hemidiaphragm. Other causes of unilateral diaphragmatic elevation include liver or subphrenic abscess, and liver metastasis.

3. What are the causes of bilaterally elevated diaphragm?

The entire diaphragm may be elevated due to obesity or hepatosplenomegaly. It can also be caused by an increase in intraabdominal pressure (e.g. pregnancy, ascites).

CASE 47: ANTERIOR MEDIASTINAL MASS

1. What are the boundaries and contents of the anterior mediastinum?

The anterior mediastinal compartment is a space posterior to the sternum and anterior to the pericardium. It extends from the thoracic inlet to the diaphragm. Normally, it only contains the thymus, thyroid gland, lymph nodes, fat and blood vessels.

2. What are the common causes of an anterior mediastinal mass?

The differential diagnosis for an anterior mediastinal mass can be remembered with the five 'T's: thyroid (goitre/neoplasm), teratoma, thymoma, 'terrible' lymph nodes (usually lymphoma) and thoracic aortic aneurysm.

3. What complications can be associated with mediastinal masses?

If large, surrounding structures can be compressed by mediastinal masses. Surrounding structures include airways, nerves, oesophagus and vascular structures (e.g. superior vena cava).

CASE 48: PULMONARY CONTUSIONS PLUS PNEUMOTHORAX

1. What is the definition of a pulmonary contusion?

Pulmonary contusion refers to lung haemorrhage and oedema due to blunt force or penetrating trauma. It can be a life-threatening feature of chest trauma as it can impair oxygenation and lead to complications, such as ARDS and pneumonia.

2. What other conditions can cause acute multifocal consolidation?

Pneumonia, aspiration and lobar collapse can also acutely cause multifocal consolidation.

3. After how long does the consolidation of pulmonary contusions typically appear after chest trauma on a chest X-ray?

The consolidation may not become apparent for 24 to 48 hours after chest trauma.

CASE 49: CLAVICLE FRACTURE

1. What is the most common mechanism of injury in a clavicle fracture?

Clavicle fractures usually occur from a fall on the lateral shoulder, e.g. due to falling from a bicycle.

2. Which part of the clavicle is most vulnerable to injury?

The weakest point of the clavicle is the junction of the middle and outer third. Therefore, the most common site of fracture is the middle third segment of the clavicle.

3. Apart from pain, what are the clinical manifestations of a clavicle fracture?

Patients can develop a sagging shoulder which they have to support with their opposite hand. This occurs because the trapezius muscle cannot support the entire weight of the arm. Significantly displaced fractures can tent the skin over the clavicle as the sternocleidomastoid muscle pulls the inner fragment of the fractured clavicle upwards.

CASE 50: APICAL PNEUMOTHORAX

1. How much air is required to be present in a pneumothorax for it to be visible on a chest X-ray?

On an upright chest X-ray, very small amounts of gas (as little as 50 mL) can be visible at the lung apex, so it is always important to review this area during chest X-ray interpretation.

2. Why is a pneumothorax commonly seen at the apex of the lung?

As free air is less dense than surrounding tissues, it tends to move upwards when sat upright.

3. How is the size of a pneumothorax measured on a chest X-ray?

To measure a pneumothorax, you would measure the horizontal distance from the lung edge to the inside of the chest wall. This should be done at the level of the hilum.

CASE 51: ACUTE RESPIRATORY DISTRESS SYNDROME

1. What is the definition of ARDS?

ARDS is a severe, life-threatening form of microvascular lung injury. This lung injury can be triggered by a number of intrathoracic or extrathoracic conditions, e.g. pneumonia, sepsis, acute pancreatitis.

2. What are the radiological features of ARDS on a chest X-ray?

A chest X-ray typically shows widespread bilateral alveolar infiltrates that can mimic cardiogenic pulmonary oedema.

3. What are the potential complications of tracheostomy tube placement?

Surrounding structures such as the recurrent laryngeal nerve and vocal cords can be damaged during tracheostomy tube placement. There is also a risk of bleeding, pneumothorax and tracheomalacia.

CASE 52: AORTIC DISSECTION

1. What is the Stanford system of classifying aortic dissection?

In Stanford type A, the ascending aorta is affected with or without involvement of the descending aorta. In Stanford type B, the descending aorta is affected with no involvement of the ascending aorta.

2. How are dissections that involve the ascending aorta managed differently from those that involve the descending aorta only?

Dissections involving the ascending aorta are surgical emergencies, whereas descending aortic dissections are usually treated medically.

3. What is the role of echocardiography in the diagnosis of aortic dissection?

A transoesophageal echocardiogram is a useful diagnostic test for aortic dissection. It is generally not as readily available as CT, although it does have a high sensitivity for both ascending and descending aortic dissections. It also has an advantage of helping identify complications, such as cardiac tamponade and aortic regurgitation.

CASE 53: TRAUMATIC PNEUMOTHORACES

1. What is the commonest cause of rib fractures in adults?

In adults, rib fractures are most commonly due to blunt force trauma to the chest wall, such as a major fall as seen in this patient.

2. Why are the upper and lower two ribs less commonly fractured?

The upper two ribs are protected by the clavicle. The lower two ribs are not attached to the anterior chest wall and swing freely.

3. Why are rib fractures rare in children?

The chest wall is highly elastic in children, so rib fractures in children are rare as it requires a lot of force to break a rib.

CASE 54: LUNG MASS

1. What is the role of PET scans in the assessment of lung cancer?

PET scans are used before curative surgery or radiotherapy to ensure that there are no occult metastases.

2. What are radioisotope bone scans used for in the assessment of lung cancer?

Radioisotope bone scans (also known as bone scintigraphy) can identify bone metastases in lung cancer patients. It is considered in patients with bone pain and blood tests demonstrating hypercalcaemia or high alkaline phosphatase.

3. **What paraneoplastic syndrome should be suspected if the patient complained of weakness that improves after exercise?**

Lambert-Eaton myasthenic syndrome is associated with lung cancer. It often presents with hyporeflexia and weakness that improves after exercise. Other features include gait difficulty and autonomic dysfunction.

CASE 55: VENTRICULOATRIAL SHUNT

1. **What are the causes of hydrocephalous?**

The most common causes of hydrocephalous include congenital malformations, tumours and inflammation (e.g. haemorrhage, meningitis).

2. **What are the management options for hydrocephalous?**

The underlying cause of hydrocephalous should be treated. Many types of hydrocephalous require a ventricular shunt for definitive treatment. Shunts most commonly connect the right lateral ventricle to the peritoneal cavity (known as a ventriculoperitoneal shunt). Rarely, a shunt can be placed to the right atrium (known as a ventriculoatrial shunt), as has been done in this patient.

3. **What are the complications of ventricular shunts?**

Shunts are at risk of infection, which may require them to be removed and replaced. Shunts can also malfunction because of a mechanical obstruction or because of a fracture in the tubing. Shunt malfunction can be dangerous as it can lead to a sudden increase in intracranial pressure.

CASE 56: PULMONARY OEDEMA

1. **What are the causes of dilated cardiomyopathy?**

There are many causes of dilated cardiomyopathy, including genetic defects, autoimmune diseases (e.g. SLE), infections (e.g. coxsackievirus), toxins (e.g. alcohol), pregnancy and metabolic conditions (e.g. wet beriberi). Many cases of dilated cardiomyopathy are idiopathic.

2. **What are Kerley B lines on a chest X-ray?**

Kerley B lines are caused by engorgement of the interlobular septa. On a normal chest X-ray, interlobular septa are invisible. They become visible when thickened by fluid, such as in pulmonary oedema. Kerley B lines are very fine, are seen peripherally and lie directly perpendicular to the pleura.

3. **On imaging, how can you differentiate between cardiogenic pulmonary oedema and pulmonary oedema due to ARDS?**

The presence of Kerley B lines and cardiomegaly is more suggestive of cardiogenic pulmonary oedema. Ground-glass opacities with air bronchograms can also be visible in ARDS unlike in cardiogenic pulmonary oedema where this is unlikely. Most patients with ARDS will be intubated; hence the absence of an endotracheal tube on a chest X-ray is more suggestive of cardiogenic pulmonary oedema.

CASE 57: SURGICAL EMPHYSEMA

1. **What is surgical emphysema?**

Surgical emphysema refers to the presence of free gas within soft tissues.

2. **What are the causes of surgical emphysema?**

Free gas can be introduced into the soft tissues from the internal or external environment. Air can be introduced internally from various sources, such as a pneumothorax, ruptured oesophagus or visceral perforation. It can be iatrogenically introduced from the external environment through insertion of chest drains or central lines.

3. **What is the prognosis of surgical emphysema?**

The majority of surgical emphysema has low morbidity and is self-limiting. Rarely, patients can have a massive surgical emphysema that can lead to complications such as compartment syndrome, reduced chest expansion and tracheal compression.

CASE 58: MILIARY NODULES

1. **What are the stages of TB infection?**

Primary TB refers to the initial lesion, which is usually solitary and asymptomatic. Latent TB is a noninfectious state where the TB infection remains dormant. Patients with latent TB can develop reactivation at a later time which is known as post-primary TB. Miliary TB occurs when TB is acutely disseminated by the blood throughout the body.

2. **What are the radiological features of lung TB on a chest X-ray?**

A chest X-ray may demonstrate consolidation, cavitation (typically in the upper lobe) and evidence of pleural effusions. Mediastinal lymphadenopathy may also be present. Miliary TB is characterized by the appearance of multiple dot-like opacities ('millet seeds') throughout the lung fields.

3. **What is the management of TB?**

In the majority of patients, treatment involves the use of a prolonged course of combination antimicrobial therapy. One example of this is rifampicin, isoniazid, pyrazinamide and ethambutol (RIPE).

CASE 59: NASOGASTRIC TUBE (MALPOSITIONED)

1. **Other than using a chest X-ray, how can the position of an NG tube be checked to see if it is appropriately placed?**

The position of the NG tube should be checked by assessing the pH of gastric aspirate. If the pH is below 5.5, it confirms the NG tube is positioned adequately within the stomach.

2. **What are the potential complications of an incorrectly placed NG tube?**

If the NG tube is incorrectly placed in the lung, there is a high risk of patients developing severe aspiration pneumonia when the feeding solution is infused. The NG tube can cause trauma to the tissue it passes, leading to epistaxis, haemorrhage and perforation. Rarely, NG tubes may pass through a base of skull fracture into the brain which can be fatal.

3. **What should you do if there are concerns regarding the position of the NG tube?**

If there are any concerns regarding the positioning of the NG tube, then feeding must not commence. The chest X-ray should be reviewed with a senior and the findings should be documented in patient notes. If the NG tube is incorrectly placed, then it must be removed and reinserted. A repeat chest X-ray can be performed following reinsertion to confirm its position if necessary.

CASE 60: PACEMAKER LEAD (MALPOSITIONED)

1. What is a pacemaker?

A pacemaker is an electronic device that is inserted under the skin, usually in the upper left chest wall. It can monitor cardiac rhythm and deliver electrical impulses to maintain an adequate heart rate (e.g. in severe bradycardia) or synchronize ventricular contraction (e.g. in atrioventricular block). The pacemaker box is attached to wires, which are inserted into the heart using the central veins.

2. What are the different types of pacemakers?

There are three main types of pacemakers. A single-chamber pacemaker consists of one lead implanted into the right atrium or ventricle. A dual-chamber pacemaker consists of two leads – one lead in the right atrium and the other lead in the right ventricle. A biventricular pacemaker, also known as cardiac resynchronization therapy, consists of leads in the right atrium, right ventricle and left ventricle.

3. How can you differentiate a pacemaker from an implantable cardioverter defibrillator (ICD) on a chest X-ray?

Unlike pacemakers, ICDs have a thick segment in the distal part of the ventricular lead as it generates a shock in response to an arrhythmia. This thick segment can be easily seen on a chest X-ray.

CASE 61: ENDOTRACHEAL TUBE, INTERNAL JUGULAR LINE AND NASOGASTRIC TUBE

1. If a central venous catheter is correctly placed, what anatomical landmark should the catheter tip be superior to on a chest X-ray?

The carina is the anatomical landmark used when determining the tip position of central venous catheters. The carina is a cartilaginous ridge found at the bifurcation of the trachea, which usually sits at the level of the sternal angle. The tip of the central venous catheter should lie just above the level of the carina.

2. What are the complications of a misplaced ET tube?

ET tubes positioned too low can selectively intubate the right or left bronchus, which can overinflate the ipsilateral lung while collapsing the contralateral lung. An ET tube positioned too high can cause vocal cord trauma.

3. What do ring shadows suggest on a chest X-ray?

Ring shadows are indicative of cystic bronchiectasis but also can be seen if a bronchus is imaged end-on.

CASE 62: LUNG ABSCESS

1. What are the causes of an air-fluid level on a chest X-ray?

The most common cause for an air-fluid level on a chest X-ray is an abscess; other rare causes include malignancy and tuberculosis.

2. What are some risk factors for developing lung abscesses?

Alcoholism, infective endocarditis, sepsis, intravenous drug use, bronchiectasis and cystic fibrosis all increase the risk of developing a lung abscess.

3. How might this patient's oral intake be assessed and managed to prevent future lung abscess development?

As part of this patient's management plan, they should receive a swallow assessment by the speech and language team (SALT). Nasogastric feeding and feeding modification, such as thickened fluids, could be considered to reduce the risk of aspiration and subsequent abscesses.

CASE 63: TRAUMATIC PNEUMOTHORAX

1. What is the most suitable next imaging modality for the patient?

Following this chest X-ray, the patient should receive a chest CT with contrast to gain a more accurate assessment of the described injuries. CT head, cervical spine, abdomen and pelvis may also be appropriate given the history of trauma, but these should be guided by the clinical picture of the patient.

2. What is considered a small pneumothorax on a chest X-ray?

A pneumothorax is considered small if there is <2 cm visible rim of air between the chest wall and the lung rim on a chest X-ray at the level of the hilum.

3. What nerves may be damaged in a fracture of the humerus?

There are three important nerves that run closely with the humerus – the axillary, radial and ulnar; they may be damaged, respectively, in fractures of the humeral neck, midshaft and distal end.

CASE 64: CHILAIDITI'S SIGN

1. What would be the next appropriate investigation if there was suspicion of abdominal visceral perforation but the X-ray was unclear?

The next appropriate investigation would be CT abdominal imaging. This has higher sensitivity for picking up perforation. It can clearly demonstrate the presence of loops of bowel between the diaphragm and liver (Chilaiditi's sign) or free intraperitoneal air in visceral perforation.

2. How can you differentiate between Chilaiditi's sign and pneumoperitoneum on an erect chest X-ray?

In Chilaiditi's sign, there will be haustral markings of bowel that indicate the gas is within bowel and is not free.

3. Which parts of the patient's history indicate that this patient should be treated as being at least intermediate risk, by CURB-65 criteria?

This patient is confused, which is the most worrying feature of their presentation and would give them a point on the CURB-65 score. In combination with his age (over 65 years old), his CURB-65 score is at least 2, placing him at least at intermediate risk. It may be higher depending on their renal function, respiratory rate and blood pressure.

CASE 65: TRAUMATIC PNEUMOTHORAX

1. What is a pneumothorax?

A pneumothorax describes the presence of air within the potential space between the visceral and parietal pleura in the thorax. This increase in pressure can result in lung collapse. Pneumothoraces can be categorized into simple, tension and open, and further categorized into traumatic and atraumatic.

2. What pathologies can cause tracheal deviation away from the side of the lesion?

A large pleural effusion and a tension pneumothorax can both cause the trachea to deviate away from the pathology. This is due to volume expansion, due to either air or fluid, within the pleural cavity. Other causes include retrosternal goitre and mediastinal masses.

3. What are the examples of iatrogenic causes of a pneumothorax?

Pulmonary needle biopsy, positive pressure ventilation and central line insertion can all result in a pneumothorax.

CASE 66: HUMERUS FRACTURE

1. What is the difference between the anatomical and the surgical neck of the humerus?

The anatomical neck of the humerus describes the narrowing distal to the head of the humerus and acts as a division between the head of the humerus and the tubercles. This is the attachment point for the joint capsule of the shoulder. The surgical neck of the humerus describes the narrowing of the humerus located inferior to the greater and lesser tubercles. The surgical neck is a common site for fractures to the humerus; fractures of the anatomical neck of the humerus are very rare.

2. What scoring tool could be used to calculate this patient's risk of having another fracture in the next 10 years?

The FRAX tool is a fracture risk calculator used to calculate a patient's risk of having a major osteoporotic fracture in the next 10 years. It uses risk factors alongside DEXA scan measurements to assess risk.

3. What medications may be used to reduce this patient's risk of osteoporotic fractures in the future?

To reduce the risk of osteoporosis and osteoporotic fractures, calcium and vitamin D supplementation alongside bisphosphonates can be used.

CASE 67: HIATUS HERNIA

1. What drugs can be used for managing hiatus hernias?

Medical management is indicated in symptomatic cases of hiatus hernias with GORD. Potential drugs that can be used include proton pump inhibitors, histamine 2 receptor antagonists and antacids.

2. If the right heart border could not be seen, where in the lungs would the pneumonia most likely be?

A right middle lobe pneumonia would result in a silhouette sign, causing loss of clarity of the right heart border. A sharp horizontal fissure may also be seen.

3. What are the long-term complications of hiatus hernias?

Hiatus hernias can increase the risk of GORD and consequently increase the risk of oesophageal ulcers, strictures and bleeding. There is also an associated increased risk of oesophageal adenocarcinoma due to Barrett's oesophagus with long-term reflux. In rare cases, the hernia can also become incarcerated.

CASE 68: RIGHT MIDDLE LOBE CONSOLIDATION

1. What is the initial imaging modality of choice for hydatid cysts?

Ultrasound is the imaging modality of choice for diagnosing hydatid cysts. This can then be complemented by CT or MRI imaging.

2. What is the most likely causative organism for a hydatid cyst?

Hydatid cysts are most commonly caused by tapeworms, *Echinococcus granulosus*, in their larval stage.

3. What are the surgical treatment options for a hydatid cyst?

The management of hydatid cysts is generally surgical with either radical or percutaneous drainage.

CASE 69: CALCIFIED PLEURAL PLAQUES

1. What lung pathologies are associated with asbestos inhalation?

Apart from pleural plaques, asbestos inhalation increases the risk of developing lung fibrosis, atelectasis, adenocarcinoma and mesothelioma.

2. What is the prognosis of pleural plaques?

Pleural plaques are seen as benign thickenings of the parietal pleura with a good prognosis. They do not impair respiratory function and are not associated with malignant change. While exposure to asbestos increases the risk of developing mesothelioma, having a pleural plaque does not increase this risk.

3. Which area of the lungs is typically affected in asbestosis?

Asbestosis is diffuse interstitial lung fibrosis that typically affects the lower lobes of the lungs bilaterally.

CASE 70: SUPINE PLEURAL EFFUSION

1. What chest X-ray appearances may be seen in a haemothorax?

The chest X-ray of a haemothorax would not look different to that of a pleural effusion. It may show blunting of the costophrenic angle, fluid in the lung fissures and a meniscus. If it is a large haemothorax, there may be an element of tracheal or mediastinal deviation.

2. What is the initial management of a haemothorax?

The patient should have an A to E assessment and be resuscitated according to the ATLS algorithm. This may include the insertion of large-bore cannulas, cardiac monitoring and oxygen monitoring. The next step in the management of a haemothorax is intercostal drainage via a chest drain. This drainage has two main objectives: drain the pleural space to allow for expansion of the lung, and allow assessment of the rate of blood loss.

3. What are the key complications associated with the insertion of a chest drain?

Early complications include damage to nearby solid organs and structures, and recurrent pneumothoraces. Air leaks and surgical emphysema can also occur after chest drain insertion. As with any invasive procedure, there is an infection risk.

CASE 71: SARCOIDOSIS

1. **What electrolyte abnormality is most commonly associated with sarcoidosis?**

   Hypercalcaemia is the electrolyte abnormality most commonly associated with sarcoidosis. Despite it being the most common abnormality, less than 10% of cases have hypercalcaemia.

2. **What pulmonary manifestations of sarcoidosis would show up on imaging of the chest?**

   Sarcoidosis can be visualized on chest X-ray and CT chest. Signs such as bilateral hilar lymphadenopathy, pulmonary infiltrates, pulmonary fibrosis and pulmonary nodules are suggestive of sarcoidosis.

3. **What test can be used to support a histological diagnosis of sarcoidosis?**

   The diagnosis of sarcoidosis can be made clinically and supported histologically using a bronchoscopy with ultrasound-guided biopsy of mediastinal lymph nodes. The biopsy would show noncaseating granulomas with epithelioid cells.

CASE 72: DOUBLE LUNG TRANSPLANT

1. **What are the most common features of late-stage cystic fibrosis on a chest X-ray?**

   Most patients with late-stage cystic fibrosis will have features of chronic bronchiectasis on their chest X-ray. They can also have hyperinflation, lung collapse and pulmonary arterial enlargement.

2. **What type of incisions are used for lung transplants?**

   For a unilateral lung transplant, a lateral thoracotomy incision is used. For a bilateral lung transplant, the classic incision is a clamshell incision, although bilateral sternal sparing anterior thoracotomies can also be used if the bilateral transplant is given as a bilateral single lung transplant.

3. **What are the complications associated with immunosuppression after organ transplantation?**

   There are many complications associated with lifelong immunosuppression. There are side effects specific to the long-term use of steroids, including diabetes, osteoporosis and Cushing's syndrome. The risk of the development of other cancers, particularly squamous cell carcinoma of the skin, increases with immunosuppression. There is also an increased risk of developing life-threatening or atypical infections.

CASE 73: HILAR LYMPHADENOPATHY

1. **What is the difference between the contents of the right and left hilum?**

   The left hilum has one bronchus referred to as the principal bronchus, whereas the right hilum has two bronchi.

2. **What conditions can cause symmetrical bilateral hilar enlargement?**

   Sarcoidosis is the most common cause of bilateral symmetrical hilar lymphadenopathy. Other causes include viral infections (such as adenovirus or mononucleosis), lymphoma, fungal infections and mycobacterial infections.

3. **What pathologies can cause an abnormal hilar position?**

   Pathologies that cause an increase in lung volume or pressure would push the hila away from the affected side; these include a pneumothorax or a large pleural effusion.

Pathologies that cause reduced volume in one haemothorax will pull the hila to the affected side, such as lobar collapse and pulmonary fibrosis.

CASE 74: PULMONARY OEDEMA

1. **What is the physiological difference between cardiogenic pulmonary oedema and noncardiogenic pulmonary oedema?**

   Cardiogenic pulmonary oedema is when decompensated left ventricular failure increases the pulmonary venous pressure. This increased pressure increases the capillary hydrostatic pressure, which then results in the accumulation of fluid in the alveoli and parenchyma. Noncardiogenic pulmonary oedema is the accumulation of fluid secondary to an increase in capillary permeability.

2. **What are the most common causes of cardiogenic pulmonary oedema?**

   The causes of cardiogenic pulmonary oedema can be split into acute and chronic. The most common causes of acute cardiogenic pulmonary oedema are acute coronary syndrome, cardiac arrhythmias, valvular heart disease and cardiac tamponade. The most common chronic conditions include left ventricular failure, congestive heart failure, cardiomyopathy and valvular heart disease.

3. **What features seen on a chest X-ray would suggest pulmonary oedema?**

   The following features on a chest X-ray are associated with pulmonary oedema: bat wing shadowing, Kerley B lines, enlarged upper lobe vessels, interstitial oedema, peribronchial cuffing, pleural effusion and associated cardiomegaly.

CASE 75: ANTERIOR SHOULDER DISLOCATION

1. **What fossa of the shoulder socket articulates with the head of the humerus?**

   The glenoid fossa articulates with the head of the humerus.

2. **What nerve is commonly damaged during an anterior shoulder dislocation and which muscles are consequently weakened?**

   The axillary nerve is the most commonly damaged nerve after an anterior shoulder dislocation. This results in muscle weakness in the deltoid and teres minor.

3. **What is the eponymous name for a compression fracture of the posterolateral head of the humerus caused by anterior dislocation of the shoulder?**

   Hill-Sachs defects are compression fractures of the posterolateral head of the humerus that can occur following anterior glenohumeral dislocation.

CASE 76: PECTUS EXCAVATUM

1. **What is pectus excavatum?**

   Pectus excavatum is a congenital condition where the sternum is curved inwards and connects to the ribs. This chest wall deformity causes a 'funnel chest' appearance that becomes more noticeable during puberty.

2. **What connective tissue disorders are commonly associated with pectus excavatum?**

   Marfan syndrome, Ehlers-Danlos syndrome and Noonan syndrome are all commonly associated with pectus excavatum.

3. **Based on the obscure right heart border and midzone opacification on this chest X-ray, what are the possible differential diagnoses?**
In addition to pectus excavatum, other differential diagnoses to consider are right-sided consolidation, atelectasis and tissue masses.

CASE 77: UPPER ZONE FIBROSIS WITH MYCETOMAS

1. **What are the most common causes of mycetoma?**
Mycetoma can be categorized as eumycetoma or actinomycetoma, caused by fungi and bacteria, respectively. Eumycetoma is often caused is *Madurella mycetomatis*, while actinomycetoma are often caused by *Nocardia brasiliensis* and *Streptomyces somaliensis*.
2. **What are some risk factors for developing a mycetoma?**
Occupational exposure and lack of protective clothing can increase the risk of developing a mycetoma due to the increased contact with colonized soil and water. It most commonly affects males between 20 and 40 years old and those with low socioeconomic status. The disease is highly prevalent in tropical and subtropical regions.
3. **What are the clinical features of mycetoma?**
Patients with mycetoma often present with localized painless soft tissue swelling. These progressively develop draining sinuses with a purulent discharge of contagious grains (aggregates of the causative organism). Patients are often afebrile but can develop scarring from healed sinuses.

CASE 78: LIVER ABSCESS

1. **What features may make you suspect a liver abscess on a chest X-ray?**
Clues of a liver abscess on chest X-rays include the presence of basilar atelectasis, elevation of the right hemidiaphragm and right-sided pleural effusion.
2. **What key clinical manifestations of a liver abscess would be found on physical examination?**
The classic triad includes right upper quadrant tenderness, fever and hepatomegaly.
3. **When would surgical drainage of a liver abscess be preferred over percutaneous drainage?**
Surgical drainage would be preferred if there were multiloculated abscesses over 5 cm in diameter. This would also apply if the abscess has ruptured or if the patient is not responding to first-line treatment.

CASE 79: PNEUMOMEDIASTINUM

1. **How may asthma cause pneumomediastinum?**
Pneumomediastinum may develop in cases of severe asthma attacks due to the sudden increase in airway pressure and overexpansion. This causes alveolar rupture and air leakage into the mediastinum.
2. **Why would a younger patient be more prone to developing pneumomediastinum?**
Pneumomediastinum mainly affects young adults. The mediastinum becomes progressively more fibrous as one ages, making it harder for air to penetrate.

3. **What finding on auscultation would suggest pneumomediastinum?**
Hamman's sign can be heard over the praecordium in pneumomediastinum. This is defined as a crunching or clicking noise synchronous with the heartbeat that is louder on inspiration.

CASE 80: ANTERIOR MEDIASTINAL MASS

1. **What clinical signs would you see if the mass has compressed the superior vena cava?**
Superior vena cava obstruction (SVCO) would present with facial and upper limb oedema, bilateral swelling of the upper body, Pemberton's sign and headache. This is an oncological emergency that needs to be treated immediately, usually with an SVC stent.
2. **What type of cells found on a lymph node biopsy would indicate Hodgkin's lymphoma?**
A hallmark of Hodgkin's lymphoma is large, abnormal lymphocytes called Reed-Sternberg cells. They are often multinucleated or are known as Hodgkin's cells if they are mononucleated.
3. **What differences may be seen in the clinical presentation of Hodgkin's and non-Hodgkin's lymphoma?**
Hodgkin's lymphoma can present with lymphadenopathy that can become painful after consuming alcohol; otherwise, lymphadenopathy is painless in both Hodgkin's and non-Hodgkin's lymphoma. Rapid weight loss and fever in early stages can also suggest Hodgkin's lymphoma as these usually occur in later stages of non-Hodgkin's lymphoma.

CASE 81: GROUND-GLASS OPACIFICATION

1. **What is the difference between ground-glass opacification and consolidation on a chest X-ray?**
Both ground-glass opacification and consolidation describe increased opacity in the lung field; however, ground-glass opacification is less opaque and does not obscure the margins of the pulmonary vessels and bronchi.
2. **What is the management for acute eosinophilic pneumonia?**
In addition to antibiotics, supplemental oxygen and glucocorticoids should be given in acute cases of eosinophilic pneumonia. Dosage of the glucocorticoids is adjusted based on the severity of the condition and is crucial in preventing respiratory failure.
3. **What is the difference in the immunological aetiology between eosinophilic pneumonia and hypersensitivity pneumonitis?**
Eosinophilic pneumonia is Th2-mediated, whereas hypersensitivity pneumonitis is Th1-mediated.

CASE 82: LEFT LOWER LOBE CONSOLIDATION AND PSEUDOTUMOUR

1. **What condition is commonly associated with developing pseudotumours?**
Preexisting congestive cardiac failure increases the risk of developing pleural effusions and, subsequently, pseudotumours.

2. **How may pneumonia cause a pleural effusion?**
If left untreated, the infection from pneumonia can cause a local inflammatory reaction leading to increased permeability in the pulmonary microvascular structures. This allows the invasion of fluids into the pleural space, resulting in a parapneumonic pleural effusion.

3. **What are the most common organisms that cause atypical pneumonia?**
The most common bacteria that cause atypical pneumonia include *Mycoplasma pneumoniae*, *Legionella pneumophila* and *Chlamydia pneumoniae*.

CASE 83: LUNG NODULES

1. **Are lung nodules likely to be malignant or benign?**
Most pulmonary nodules are benign, particularly if they are calcified.

2. **What model might be used to estimate the risk of malignancy in pulmonary nodules?**
The Brock model is used to estimate lung cancer risk. This multivariable model uses the various information from a thoracic CT scan, older age, female sex and family history of lung cancer. If the risk is equal or greater than 10%, further assessment should be conducted with PET-CT scan with subsequent risk prediction using the Herder model.

3. **How are lung nodules managed?**
Most lung nodules do not require treatment as they are small and nonmalignant. However, if the nodule is malignant or obstructs the airway, surgical procedures may be undertaken to remove the nodule using VATS or thoracotomy.

CASE 84: AZYGOS LOBE

1. **How does the vascular supply and bronchi of an azygos lobe differ from other lobes of the lung?**
An azygos lobe embryologically stems from the right upper lobe. Therefore, it does not have its own bronchial or vascular supply as it is not a separate lobe.

2. **What are some differential diagnoses of an azygos lobe on a chest X-ray?**
Paratracheal abnormalities, such as abscesses and bullae, can mimic an azygos lobe. Scars, bullae and displaced fissures can also be mistaken as an azygos fissure.

3. **How might an azygos lobe impede clinical procedures?**
Although this is a normal variant, an azygos lobe can potentially increase the risk of bleeding and neurovascular damage during thoracotomy.

CASE 85: LUNG MASS PLUS RIB DESTRUCTION

1. **What is the most appropriate next investigation for chest X-ray appearances suggestive of lung cancer?**
CT chest with contrast is important to accurately determine the location and nature of the lesion. It is also important to include the neck, abdomen and pelvis for staging and assessment of metastases. After this, more specialist investigations, such as bronchoscopy, may be considered following discussion at the MDT.

2. **What is the most common type of lung cancer?**
Adenocarcinomas are the most common type of lung cancer and these tumours are more common in women and nonsmokers.

3. **What paraneoplastic endocrine syndromes are associated with small cell lung cancer?**
Small cell lung cancers can secrete both antidiuretic hormone (ADH) and adrenocorticotropic (ACTH). ADH secretion causes syndrome of inappropriate antidiuretic hormone (SIADH). ACTH secretion can cause ectopic Cushing's syndrome as it causes excess cortisol release.

CASE 86: DESTRUCTIVE SCAPULAR LESION

1. **What are the clinical features of the bone pain caused by bone tumours?**
The bony pain associated with bone tumours can be progressive, localized to the site of the lesions and painful with palpation. It may also worsen at night and on mobilization.

2. **What are the risk factors for developing primary bone cancer?**
Li-Fraumeni syndrome and familial retinoblastoma increase the risk of osteosarcomas. Tuberous sclerosis increases the risk of chordoma development in childhood. Bone diseases, such as Paget's disease, increase the risk of osteosarcoma. Environmental factors, such as radiation exposure, also increase the risk of developing a primary bone tumour.

3. **What is the pathological difference between osteolytic and osteoblastic bone metastases?**
Osteolytic lesions are caused by the destruction of normal bone due to increased activity of the osteoclasts. Osteoblastic lesions are caused by the deposition of new bone. There can also be mixed bone metastases, whereby there are simultaneously osteolytic and osteoblastic lesions.

CASE 87: RETAINED SURGICAL SWAB

1. **How might you prevent retained surgical foreign bodies (RSB)?**
Swab and instrument counting measures can be used to avoid RSB. There are several points at which counting surgical materials are recommended. Counts should occur before the procedure begins (this is known as the initial count), whenever a new additional item is used during the operation, before the surgeon closes the body cavity, when the surgeon begins to close the wound and when the surgeon closes the skin (this is known as the final count).

2. **What postoperative complications can occur from retained swabs in the abdominal cavity?**
RSB inside the abdominal cavity can lead to intraabdominal abscesses, obstructive ileus, intraabdominal bleeding, intestinal perforation and fistula formation. It can also cause long-term pain for the patient. In addition, it may be misdiagnosed as suspicious for tumour development if detected on radiological imaging.

3. **What are the signs of postoperative pneumoperitoneum on a chest X-ray?**
Pneumoperitoneum is a normal postoperative finding following a hemicolectomy. This appears as subdiaphragmatic free gas on a chest X-ray. Cupola sign can also be present, which describes an area of radiolucency overlying the lower thoracic vertebral bodies due to air underneath the central tendon of the diaphragm.

CASE 88: NIPPLE SHADOWS

1. What features may be seen on the chest X-ray of patients with COPD?

Flattened hemidiaphragms and lung hyperexpansion (which can cause the lungs to appear hyperlucent) can be seen in COPD due to overinflation. There can also be evidence of bullae and increased bronchovascular markings.

2. What is the pathophysiology behind bullae?

Bullae describe large abnormal air spaces in the lungs caused by emphysema. In emphysema, there is damage to the alveoli and destruction of the adjoining walls of the alveoli. This causes fusion of adjacent alveoli, producing large pockets of air in the lungs.

3. What is the function of nipple markers on a chest X-ray?

On chest X-rays, it is common to see nipple shadows on women. Nipple markers can be used to determine whether the radiodensity seen is in fact a nipple shadow or pathological. These radio-opaque markers are stuck to the chest, either with the nipple inside or stuck directly onto the nipple, and a repeat scan is taken. If the nodule in question is found inside the marker, then it confirms it was a nipple shadow.

CASE 89: PLEURAL MASS

1. What two types of pleura are in the thorax?

Pleura describes a serous membrane formed of squamous cells and connective tissue. In the chest, there is both parietal and visceral pleura. The parietal pleura covers the internal surface of the thoracic cavity. The visceral pleura covers the surface of the lungs.

2. If the projection was not documented on the image, what feature on a chest X-ray would help you determine if it was a PA or AP projection?

For a PA X-ray, the scapulae are retracted laterally; therefore, minimal scapulae are visible over the lung fields and allow for better visualization of the lungs. For an AP X-ray, the scapulae are not retracted laterally, so they are visible within the lung fields.

3. Which condition in this patient's medical history would make the lesion more likely to be an invasive thymoma?

A history of myasthenia gravis (MG) would increase the risk of this being a thymoma because MG is strongly associated with thymic hyperplasia and thymomas. Other conditions associated with an increased risk of developing thymomas include red cell aplasia, hypogammaglobulinemia, SLE and rheumatoid arthritis.

CASE 90: RIB METASTASES

1. How is breast cancer screened and how often is screening done for the general population?

Breast cancer is often screened in the general population using a mammogram. Different countries have different age groups screened and varying screening intervals; in the United Kingdom, mammograms are offered every 3 years for women between the ages of 50 and 70.

2. What are the treatment options available for breast cancer?

Management is dependent on the stage and grade of the cancer as well as the patient's baseline health. Most breast cancer patients are offered surgery, including mastectomy or wide local excision depending on the spread and size of the tumour. Radiotherapy is often offered post-surgery to lower the chance of recurrence. Chemotherapy may be offered to downstage the tumour prior to surgery. Finally, hormonal or biological therapies are considered in patients for patients with positive hormone receptors.

3. What genetic mutations are the most common cause of hereditary breast cancer?

Mutations in the *BRCA1* or *BRCA2* genes are the most common cause of hereditary breast cancer.

CASE 91: LUNG MASS AND MEDIASTINAL LYMPHADENOPATHY

1. How does the lung mass in this case cause Horner's syndrome?

The location of the ipsilateral left apical mass is in keeping with a Pancoast tumour, which can compress the paravertebral sympathetic chain to produce Horner's syndrome.

2. What are the classic signs of Horner's syndrome?

Horner's syndrome consists of ptosis, miosis and anhidrosis.

3. What are the common causes of lymphangitis carcinomatosis?

Lymphangitis carcinomatosis is most commonly caused by breast, lung and stomach cancer. Other causes include cancer of the cervix, colon, prostate, pancreas, thyroid and larynx.

CASE 92: RIGHT MIDDLE LOBE COLLAPSE

1. Which fissures separate the right middle lobe from the right upper and lower lobes?

The right middle lobe is separated from the right upper and lower lobe by the right horizontal and right oblique fissures, respectively.

2. How might preexisting COPD increase the risk of lung collapse?

Chronic inflammation from COPD can cause tissue destruction and allow air to leak and build in the pleural cavity, resulting in secondary spontaneous pneumothorax.

3. Why might a primary malignancy in the right middle lobe have worse prognosis than malignancy in the other lung lobes?

Primary lung cancer originating in the right middle lobe can have a worse prognosis compared to other lobe tumours due to its proximity to the mediastinal lymph nodes and consequent propensity to metastasize.

CASE 93: APICAL LUNG MASS

1. Which histological classification of lung cancer would this lung mass likely fall under?

Lung masses in the apex are usually non–small cell lung cancers (NSCLCs). Within this classification, the most common types of apical lung mass include squamous cell carcinomas and bronchial adenocarcinoma.

2. What are the signs of Pancoast syndrome?

Pancoast syndrome classically consists of a triad of ipsilateral effects, including shoulder and arm pain, weakness and atrophy of the hand muscles, and Horner's syndrome.

3. **What part of the brachial plexus, if invaded, will deem a Pancoast tumour inoperable?**

The tumour is deemed inoperable if it extends beyond the lower trunk of the brachial plexus or the C8 nerve root.

CASE 94: LOCULATED PLEURAL COLLECTION

1. **What is the pathological difference between an empyema and a lung abscess?**

A build-up of purulent fluid occurs in the pleural space in empyema, compared to purulent fluid accumulation in the lung parenchyma in lung abscesses.

2. **How might an empyema differ from a lung abscess on CT imaging?**

Findings that suggest an empyema instead of a lung abscess include thickening and separation of the adjacent pleura, thinner and smoother walls, and distortion instead of abruptly cutting off adjacent bronchovascular structures.

3. **Why is it important to differentiate between an empyema and a lung abscess?**

Distinguishing between the two is crucial as their management strategies are different. An empyema is managed with drainage using a chest drain and antibiotics. Lung abscesses are treated with intravenous antibiotics and chest physiotherapy; if needed, drainage through postural manoeuvres or surgical intervention may be considered.

CASE 95: LEFT ATRIAL ENLARGEMENT

1. **What are the common causes of left atrial enlargement?**

Left atrial enlargement is caused by an increase in atrial pressure or volume. This commonly occurs as a result of hypertension, atrial fibrillation, mitral valve dysfunction (stenosis or regurgitation) and left ventricular failure.

2. **What ECG changes may be seen in left atrial enlargement?**

Left atrial enlargement can produce a broad, bifid P wave in lead II, and/or a broad, deepened downward deflection of the P wave in lead V_1.

3. **What anatomical structures produce the double right heart border?**

The double right heart border occurs due to the extension of the enlarged left atrium behind the right atrial border.

CASE 96: SCLEROTIC BONE METASTASES

1. **Which primary malignancies commonly metastasize to bone?**

In addition to prostate cancer (such as in this case), bony metastases can arise from malignancies of the breast, kidney, thyroid or lungs. The mnemonic 'lead kettle' or PB-KTL can be useful to help remember these malignancies.

2. **What is an unfolded thoracic aorta and what is its clinical significance?**

An unfolded aorta refers to the widening of the mediastinum due to disproportionate growth of the ascending aorta with age. Calcification is often associated with this finding, indicating atherosclerosis.

3. **What are the differences in the radiological features of lytic and sclerotic bone metastases on a chest X-ray?**

This case demonstrated sclerotic (osteoblastic) metastases characterized by bone formation. The increased bone density can be seen in the whiter areas on the X-ray. Lytic (osteolytic) metastases are characterized by bone destruction and appear radiolucent (dark) on the X-ray. Some patients may present with a mixed pattern of sclerotic and lytic bone lesions.

CASE 97: SICKLE CELL ANAEMIA

1. **How do you calculate the cardiothoracic ratio?**

The cardiothoracic ratio is the ratio between the maximal width of the cardiac borders and the maximal width of the thoracic cavity at its widest point (inner rib to inner rib). It should be assessed on a PA chest X-ray as the cardiac size can be exaggerated on an AP view. A normal ratio is equal or less than 50% in adults.

2. **What is acute chest syndrome in the context of sickle cell disease?**

This is defined as a new pulmonary infiltrate on X-ray in a patient with known sickle cell disease, accompanied by respiratory symptoms and/or fever.

3. **What are the aetiological mechanisms of sickle cell acute chest syndrome in adults?**

Infection is the most common cause of acute chest syndrome in sickle cell disease. Other causes include fat emboli and pulmonary infarction.

CASE 98: CALCIFIED LEFT VENTRICULAR ANEURYSM

1. **What classification system is commonly used to classify the symptoms of heart failure?**

The New York Heart Association (NYHA) Functional Classification is commonly used to classify heart failure patients according to their symptoms. Stages I to IV range from no limitation to physical activity through to being unable to carry out any physical activity without discomfort.

2. **What clinical features are suggestive of right-sided heart failure?**

Peripheral pitting oedema, jugular venous distension, ascites and hepatosplenomegaly are clinical features consistent with right-sided heart failure.

3. **What are the potential complications of ventricular aneurysms?**

Complications of ventricular aneurysms include heart failure, thromboembolism, ventricular rupture and ventricular arrhythmias.

CASE 99: HIATUS HERNIA

1. **What are the different types of hiatus hernias?**

Sliding hernias, whereby the gastro-oesophageal junction is displaced above the diaphragm, account for most cases of hiatus hernias. In rolling (para-oesophageal) hernias, the gastro-oesophageal junction remains in place but a portion of the stomach is herniated through the oesophageal hiatus.

2. **What type of hiatus hernia is more likely to cause acid reflux?**

Compared to rolling hernias, sliding hernias are more likely to cause acid reflux because the lower oesophageal sphincter often becomes incompetent.

3. **How are hiatus hernias managed?**

Hiatus hernias are mainly managed conservatively with changes in diet to smaller, more frequent meals and smoking cessation. Patients should be advised to lose weight. Drug therapies, such as proton pump inhibitors, are indicated for patients with symptoms of GORD. If this fails, or if there are complications from GORD, then surgical repair can be performed; Nissen fundoplication is the most commonly performed surgery for hiatus hernias.

CASE 100: MESOTHELIOMA

1. **What occupational hazard is strongly associated with malignant mesothelioma?**

The strongest risk factor for malignant mesothelioma is asbestos exposure. This patient was likely exposed to the substance from his past occupation as a shipyard worker and remained asymptomatic for decades.

2. **Apart from pleural masses, what other X-ray findings might be found in mesothelioma?**

Other X-ray findings in a patient with mesothelioma may include pleural effusion or pleural thickening.

3. **Apart from imaging, what investigations are used to make a definitive diagnosis of mesothelioma?**

A diagnosis of mesothelioma should be established using pleural fluid cytology. If results are inconclusive, biopsy by VATS or thoracotomy is used. At least two positive mesothelial and two negative adenocarcinoma immunohistochemical markers should be used to rule out adenocarcinoma.

Case Index

Index